Paleo Diet Recipes for Beginners

500 Easy and Most Delicious Recipes to Help You Lose Weight, Improve Your Health, and Live a Healthy Lifestyle

By

Olivia Sanders

Copyright © 2019 by Olivia Sanders- All rights reserved.

The follow eBook is reproduced below with the goal of providing information that is as accurate and reliable as possible. Regardless, purchasing this eBook can be seen as consent to the fact that both the publisher and the author of this book are in no way experts on the topics discussed within and that any recommendations or suggestions that are made herein are for entertainment purposes only. Professionals should be consulted as needed prior to undertaking any of the action endorsed herein.

This declaration is deemed fair and valid by both the American Bar Association and the Committee of Publishers Association and is legally binding throughout the United States.

Furthermore, the transmission, duplication or reproduction of any of the following work including specific information will be considered an illegal act irrespective of if it is done electronically or in print. This extends to creating a secondary or tertiary copy of the work or a recorded copy and is only allowed with express written consent from the Publisher. All additional right reserved.

The information in the following pages is broadly considered to be a truthful and accurate account of facts and as such any inattention, use or misuse of the information in question by the reader will render any resulting actions solely under their purview. There are no scenarios in which the publisher or the original author of this work can be in any fashion deemed liable for any hardship or damages that may befall them after undertaking information described herein.

Additionally, the information in the following pages is intended only for informational purposes and should thus be thought of as universal. As befitting its nature, it is presented without assurance regarding its prolonged validity or interim quality. Trademarks that are mentioned are done without written consent and can in no way be considered an endorsement from the trademark holder.

TABLE OF CONTENTS

Introduction 1
The Benefits of Paleo Diet 2
How Paleo Helps to Lose Weight? 4
What Can We Eat on a Paleo Diet? 5
What Not to Eat When Going Paleo 6
Types of Paleo Diets 7
Getting Started 8
Breakfast Recipes 9

    Breakfast Granola 9
    Green Smoothie 9
    Muffins Breakfast 9
    Special Burrito 10
    Coconut and Almonds Granola 10
    Red Breakfast Smoothie 10
    Tomato and Eggs Breakfast 11
    Plantain Pancakes 11
    Strawberry and Kiwi Breakfast Smoothie ... 11
    Turkey Breakfast Sandwich 11
    Sweet Potato Breakfast 12
    Pork Skillet 12
    Squash Blossom Frittata 12
    Maple Nut Porridge 13
    Breakfast Waffles 13
    Nuts Porridge 13
    Eggplant French Toast 14
    Blueberry Smoothie 14
    Spinach Frittata 14
    Eggs and Ham 15
    Italian Style Eggs 15
    Orange and Dates Granola 15
    Bacon Muffins 16
    Parsley and Pear Smoothie 16

Peach and Coconut Smoothie 16
Bacon and Egg Breakfast Sandwich 17
Sausage Balls 17
Portobello Sandwich 17
Paleo Kale Frittata 17
Spicy Eggs 18
Eggs and Artichokes 18
Breakfast Pancakes 19
Avocado Muffins 19
Spinach Omelet 20
Pumpkin Muffins 20
Zucchini and Chocolate Muffins 20
Special Breakfast Dish 21
Breakfast Burrito 21
Wrapped Eggs 22
Cereal Bowl 22
Apple Omelet 22
Banana Pancakes 23
Sweet Potato Waffles 23
Breakfast Burger 23
Sausage Frittata 24
Breakfast Sandwich 24
Orange and Vanilla Breakfast Delight 24
Burger 25
Blueberry Muffins 25
Chicken Waffles 25
Beef and Squash Skillet 26
Ham and Mushroom Breakfast 26
Porridge 27
Chorizo Breakfast Skillet 27
Apple Pancakes 27
Steak and Veggie Breakfast 28

Breakfast Sliders 28
Bacon Waffles 28
Coconut Pancakes 29
Veggie Omelet Cupcakes 29

Side Dish Recipes 30
Ginger Cauliflower Rice 30
Side Salad 30
Roasted Cabbage Side Dish 30
French Fries 31
Asparagus and Mushrooms Side Dish 31
Asparagus Side Dish 31
Roasted Okra 32
Mashed Cauliflower Dish 32
Braised Cabbage Side Dish 32
Roasted Beets 33
Kale Dish 33
Roasted Bell Peppers 33
Roasted Cherry Tomatoes 34
Sweet Potatoes Dish 34
Pumpkin Salad 34
Roasted Beets 35
Fennel Side Dish 35
Zucchini and Leeks Side Dish 35
Veggie Mix 36
Sautéed Spinach Dish 36
Butternut Squash 36
Kale and Beets 37
Grilled Artichokes 37
Slow Cooked Mushrooms 37
Pumpkin Fries 38
Roasted Cauliflower 38
Mushrooms and Thyme Side Dish 38
Mashed Sweet Potatoes 38
Roasted Carrots 39

Butternut Squash Mix 39
Pumpkin and Bok Choy 39
Side Dish 40
Butternut Squash Side Dish 40
Roasted Green Beans 40
Poached Kohlrabi Dish 41
Stir Fried Side Dish 41
Mushrooms and Red Chard Side Dish 41
Mashed Carrots 42
Spaghetti Squash 42
Squash and Cranberries 42
Mint Zucchini 43
Spicy Sweet Potatoes 43
Chard Side Dish 43
Basil Zucchini Spaghetti 43
Turnips and Sauce 44
Eggplant and Mushrooms 44
Cauliflower and Leeks 44
Taro Dish 44
Roasted Brussels Sprouts 45
Roasted Broccoli 45
Stuffed Artichokes 45
Paleo Tapioca Root Fries 46
Plantain Fries 46
Plantain Mash 46
Creamy Mashed Pumpkin 47
Brussels Sprouts Side Dish 47
Broccoli and Tasty Hazelnuts 47
Dill Carrots 47
Kale Dish 48

Soups & Stews Recipes 49
Veggie and Chorizo Stew 49
Coconut and Zucchini Soup 49
Healthy Veggie Stew 50

Veggie Soup	50
Cauliflower Cream	50
Beef and Plantain Stew	51
Lemon and Garlic Soup	51
Chicken Stew	52
Brussels Sprouts Soup	52
Tasty Turkey Soup	52
Chicken Soup	53
Delicious Paleo Soup	53
Clam Soup	54
Tomato and Basil Soup	54
Beef Soup	54
Cauliflower Soup	55
Sweet Potato Soup	55
Seafood Soup	55
Easy Paleo Soup	56
Oxtail Stew	56
Beef Stew	57
Asparagus Soup	57
Mushroom Cream	58
Gazpacho	58
French Chicken Stew	58
Beef Stew	59
Broccoli Soup	59
Root Soup	60
Pork Stew	60
Chicken Soup	61
Chicken Soup	61
Zucchini Soup	62
Nettles Soup	62
Roasted Veggie Stew	62
Oxtail Stew	63
Paleo Stew	63
Beef Stew	64
Kale and Sausage Soup	64
Squash Soup	64
Onion Soup	65
Chorizo Stew	65
Eggplant Stew	65
Shrimp and Chicken Soup	66
Celery Soup	66
Slow Cooker Stew	66
Eggplant Stew	67
Chicken Stew	67
African Style Stew	67
Veggie Soup	68
Lamb and Coconut Stew	68
Mexican Paleo Stew	69
Cucumber Soup	69
Green Soup	69
Vietnamese Stew	70
Beef and Sweet Potatoes Stew	70
Lamb Stew	71
Slow Cooked Paleo Stew	71
French Chicken Stew	72
Hearty Meat Stew	72
Beef Stew	72

Seafood & Fish Recipes ... 73

Grilled Calamari	73
Shrimp and Cauliflower Rice	73
Lobster with Sauce	74
Shrimp Dish	74
Steamed Clams	74
Paleo Scallops	75
Glazed Salmon	75
Roasted Cod	76
Glazed Salmon	76
Salmon and Chives	76

Shrimp and Zucchini Noodles	77
Scallops with Delicious Puree	77
Smoked salmon and veggies	77
Salmon Dish	78
Salmon Pie	78
Tuna and Chimichurri Sauce	79
Paleo Salmon	79
Fish Dish	79
Thai Shrimp Delight	80
Salmon Skewers	80
Shrimp Dish	81
Salmon Tartar Delight	81
Salmon and Chili Sauce	81
Salmon with Avocado Sauce	82
Roasted Trout	82
Fish Tacos	83
Lobster and Sauce	83
Tuna Dish	84
Salmon and Lemon Relish	84
Salmon and Spicy Slaw	84
Grilled Salmon with Peaches	85
Stuffed Salmon Fillets	85
Shrimp Burgers	86
Salmon Delight	86
Scallops Tartar	87
Shrimp Skewers	87
Infused Clams	87
Halibut and Tasty Salsa	88
Shrimp with Mango and Avocado Mix	88
Grilled Oysters	88
Stuffed Calamari	89
Shrimp Cocktail	89
Grilled Calamari	90
Grilled Salmon and Avocado Sauce	90
Crusted Salmon	90
Salmon Tartar	91
Tuna and Salsa	91
Crab Cakes and Red Pepper Sauce	91
Tilapia Surprise	92
Shrimp and Zucchini Noodles	92
Squid and Guacamole	92
Swordfish	93
Spicy Shrimp	93
Scallops Tartar	93
Salmon and Tomato Pesto	94
Crusted Snapper	94
Cod and Herb Sauce	94
Mussels Mix	95
Mahi Mahi Dish	95
Roasted Cod	96

Meat Recipes 97

Beef Dish	97
Turkey Casserole	97
Beef Lasagna	98
Beef and Bok Choy	98
Grilled Steaks	98
Pulled Pork	99
Beef Casserole	99
Grilled Lamb Chops	99
Pork Dish with Delicious Blueberry Sauce	100
Stuffed Quail	100
Beef in Tomato Marinade	101
Lamb Chops and Mint Sauce	101
Lamb Casserole	101
Paleo Steak	102
Lamb Chops with Mint Sauce	102
Beef Kabobs	103
Pork Chops	103

Chicken Thighs with Tasty Squash 103
Sausage Casserole 104
Mexican Steaks 104
Beef Tenderloin with Special Sauce..................... 104
Roasted Duck Dish 105
Steaks and Scallops.. 105
Beef Stir Fry 106
Pork with Pear Salsa 106
Pork Tenderloin with Carrot Puree 106
Pork with Strawberry Sauce 107
Beef and Veggies 107
Chicken Meatballs 108
Chicken and Veggies Stir Fry 108
Beef and Brussels Sprouts 109
Steaks and Apricots 109
Beef and Wonderful Gravy 109
Sheppard's Pie 110
Barbeque Ribs.. 110
Souvlaki 111
Turkey Casserole 111
Moroccan Lamb 112
Carne Asada 112
Steak and Blueberry Sauce 113
Filet Mignon and Special Sauce 113
Veal Rolls 113
Roasted Lamb 114
Beef Curry 114
Beef Teriyaki 115
Beef Skillet 115
Thai Curry 115
Hamburger Salad 116
Lamb Chops 116
Beef and Cabbage Delight 117
Slow Cooked Lamb Shanks 117

Rosemary Lamb Chops 117
Slow-Cooked Beef 118
Lamb and Eggplant Puree 118
Beef and Spinach 119
Lavender Lamb Chops 119
Beef Patties 119
Thai Lamb Chops 120
Greek Beef Bowls.. 120
Beef and Basil 121

Salad Recipes 122
Pear Salad with Tasty Dressing.......................... 122
Carrot and Cucumber Salad 122
Broccoli Salad 122
Cabbage and Salmon Slaw 123
Beef Salad 123
Lobster Salad... 123
Summer Salad 124
Special Salad 124
Summer Salad 124
Shrimp Salad 125
Egg Salad 125
Chicken Salad 125
Chicken Salad 126
Winter Salad 126
Shrimp and Radish Salad 127
Scallops Salad.. 127
Potato Salad 127
Taco Salad... 128
Chorizo Salad 128
Paleo Salad 129
Brussels Sprouts Salad 129
Kale and Carrots Salad 130
Chicken Salad 130
Radish Salad 130

Salmon Salad 131

Summer Salad 131

Sashimi Salad 131

Steak Salad 131

Pomegranate Salad 132

Green Apple and Shrimp Salad 132

Quick Paleo Salad 133

Eggplant and Tomato Salad 133

Salmon and Strawberry Salad 134

Cucumber Salad 134

Sweet Potato Salad 134

Swiss Chard Salad 135

Dinner Salad 135

Steak Salad 135

Fresh Salad 136

Awesome Pork Salad 136

Broccoli and Carrots Salad 136

Seafood Salad 137

Red Cabbage Salad 137

Cuban Radish Salad 137

Shrimp Cobb Salad 138

Avocado Salad 138

Watermelon Salad 138

Rich Salad 139

Hearty Chicken Salad 139

Autumn Salad 139

Russian Salad 140

Tomato Salad 140

Tomato and Chicken Salad 140

Radish and Eggs Salad 141

Beetroot Salad 141

Cucumber and Tomato Salad 142

Kale and Avocado Salad 142

Grilled Shrimp Salad 142

Chicken Salad and Raspberry Dressing 143

Figs and Cabbage Salad 143

Vegetable Recipes 144

Tomato and Mushroom Skewers 144

Potato Bites 144

Stuffed Zucchinis 145

Veggie Mix and Scallops 145

Broccoli and Cauliflower Fritters 145

Stuffed Mushrooms 146

Baked Yuka with Tomato Sauce 146

Onion Rings 146

Stuffed Eggplant 147

Eggplant Jam 147

Veggies and Fish Mix 147

Roasted Tomatoes 148

Cucumber Salsa 148

Veggies Dish with Tasty Sauce 149

Surprise Dinner Dish 149

Watercress Soup 150

Kohlrabi Dish 150

Avocado Spread 151

Celery Casserole 151

Bell Peppers Stuffed with Tuna 151

Falafel 152

Eggplant Dish 152

Endive Bites 152

Zucchini Noodles and Capers Sauce 153

Grilled Cherry Tomatoes 153

Rutabaga Noodles and Cherry Tomatoes 154

Stuffed Baby Peppers 154

Garlic Sauce 154

Paleo Pancakes 155

Sweet Potatoes and Cabbage Bake 155

Mexican Stuffed Peppers 155

Artichokes and Tomatoes Dip	156
Artichokes with Horseradish Sauce	156
Zucchini Noodles with Tomatoes and Spinach	156
Eggplant Hash	157
Stuffed Peppers	157
Spinach and Mushroom Dish	158
Cherry Mix	158
Stuffed Poblanos	158
Tomato Quiche	159
Liver Stuffed Peppers	159
Stuffed Portobello Mushrooms	159
Zucchini Noodles and Pesto	160
Spaghetti Squash and Tomatoes	160
Daikon Rolls	161
Glazed Carrots	161
Cauliflower Pizza	161
Cucumber Wraps	162
Garlic Tomatoes	162
Grilled Artichokes	162
Pork Stuffed Bell Peppers	163
Carrots and Lime	163
Eggplant Casserole	163
Warm Watercress Mix	164
Artichokes Dish	164
Cucumber Noodles and Shrimp	164
Baked Eggplant	165
Purple Carrots	165
Stuffed with Beef	166
Carrot Hash	166

Snacks & Appetizers Recipes 167

Stuffed Mushrooms	167
Avocado Boats	167
Pepperoni Bites	167
Egg Cups	168
Roasted Eggplant Spread	168
Cauliflower Popcorn	168
Cabbage Chips	168
Appetizer Salad	169
Sun Dried Tomatoes Spread	169
Hummus	169
Mixed Snack	170
Baked Zucchini Chips	170
Stuffed Eggs	170
Coconut Bars	171
Paleo Hummus	171
Party Meatballs	171
Chicken Appetizer	172
Delicious Crackers	172
Beef Jerky	172
Watermelon Wraps	173
Chicken Skewers	173
Chicken Strips	173
Zucchini Rolls	173
Guacamole	174
Butternut Squash Bites	174
Mushroom and Broccoli Appetizer	174
Mushroom Boats	175
Nuts Snack	175
Carrot Balls	175
Cucumber Rolls	176
Cauliflower Mini Hot Dogs	176
Fried Peppers	176
Apricot Bites	177
Chicken Bites	177
Wrapped Olives	177
Kale Chips And Yummy Dip	178
Rosemary Crackers	178
Scallops Bites	179

Oyster Spread 179

Dessert Recipes 180

Cherry Sorbet 180

Pumpkin Custard 180

Pumpkin Pudding 180

Chocolate Parfait 181

Avocado Pudding 181

Raspberry Popsicles 181

Poached Rhubarb 181

Passion Fruit Pudding 182

Pomegranate Fudge 182

Summer Carrot Cake 182

Green Apple Smoothie 183

Cupcakes 183

Hazelnut Balls 183

Strawberry Cobbler 184

Caramel Ice Cream 184

Fruit Jelly 184

Stuffed Apples 185

Carrot Cupcakes 185

Intense Cheesecake 185

Hazelnut Pancakes 186

Tomato Cake 186

Dessert Smoothie Bowl 187

Pumpkin Cookies 187

Summer Sorbet 187

Summer Energy Bars 188

Coconut Macaroons 188

Cherry Jam 188

Chia Seeds Pudding 189

Muffins 189

Spring Cheesecake 189

Mango Granita 190

Fruits Mix and Vinaigrette 190

Fruit Cream 190

Almond and Fig Dessert 191

Chocolate Butter Cups 191

Berry and Cashew Cake 191

Almond Bars 192

Summer Lemon Fudge 192

Grapefruit Granita 192

Spring Ice Cream 193

Introduction

The Paleo diet also called as caveman diet. This Diet is based mainly on foods presumed to have been available to Stone-Age man. The Paleo diet is about consuming food which existing since Paleolithic period.

The Paleolithic period was pre-agricultural period. In Paleo diet the technique of consuming food goes back to fundamental way of eating. Paleolithic diets are about consuming food the way our predecessors did

Our prehistoric ancestors ate and lived very differently. The result was that they lived longer and their lives were healthier. So if we can return to a lifestyle more in line with how they lived, our lives will improve as well. We'll have more energy, live more honestly, be sick less often, reduce our weight and bring ourselves in line with how we're supposed to live. Our lives will return to something as close to natural as is possible in this modern-day world.

Unlike most fad diets, the Paleo diet is a sustainable, long-term diet. It regulates hormonal balance and positive gene expression. This leads to better health and well-being, enhanced athletic performance and body composition. The Paleo diet is a one of the most widely supported diets in the world. Celebrities, clinical experts and dietitians recommend it as the best way to restore balance, fight medical conditions and reduce the waistline.

Also known as the caveman diet, the stone-age diet or hunter-gatherer diet, the Paleo Diet is low in carbohydrates, while being high in protein and fat. It focuses on the consumption of fruits, vegetables and nuts and rejects processed and man-made foods. The diet's central premise is that humanity has not changed much since our hunter-gatherer past. Thus we should shift away from modern culinary inventions. Instead we should focus on eating the way we did back then in order for us to live longer and healthier lives.

It was originally conceived by Walter L. Voegtlin, a famous gastroenterologist, in the 1970s. His version was meat-based and contained few carbohydrates. The diet gained mainstream attention in the 1980s through the work of Melvin Konner and S. Boyd Eaton. They modified it so that it included some foods not available to hunter-gatherers, like whole-grain bread.

Whatever the name or the specific guidelines, you can't deny the diet's benefits. Millions swear by it, convinced it has changed their lives for the better. It's not just them. Every year, new studies supporting their claims that it has physical and psychological health benefit are published.

So what are you waiting for? Don't live a junk life, don't choose for junk food. Instead, opt for a healthier way of life, choose less stress, choose reduced depression, and choose less medicine. Choose Paleo.

The Benefits of Paleo Diet

1. Weight Loss
The Paleo diet is a low carbohydrate diet getting rid of junk and refined food will radically cut carbohydrate which results in weight loss. By restricting carbohydrates intake, Paleo helps to eliminate unnecessary weight gain. Paleo plays a major part in reducing waist lines and stubborn fat by burning excess fat.

2. Better Digestion and Absorption
Eating of food that has adapted over thousands of years ago. This means that food was consumed in its simplest form and therefore was easy on digestion. If digestive problems are recurring, trying Paleo diet for at least a month will make you feel healthier for sure.

3. Provide Vitamins & Minerals
The Paleo diet advocates consuming the "rainbow", the diverse colors of vegetables. Vegetables are a great component of the Vitamins. Eating vegetables and fruits is the best way to stock up on the essential nutrients. The diverse colors of vegetables indicate the presence of a variety of nutrients.

4. Enhance Brain Function
The supplies of protein and fat recommended by the Paleo diet emerges from wild salmon. Salmon is full of omega 3 fatty acids which is deficient in the standard diet. Since omega 3 fatty acids have DHA, acknowledged to be excellent for eyes, heart, and improvement brain and multi-tasking

5. Fewer Allergies
The Paleo diet eliminate allergic foods. Food which are unable to digest like seeds, grains, and dairy which is the reason for which the Paleo diet advocates the elimination of these food products, when most diets do not skip these food, and the people affected are considerably in control of their allergies after the Paleo regime.

6. Improve Health
Sugar, salt, artificial fats, and other refined edibles cause inflammation inside the intestinal tract. Sadly, when unnecessary amount of processed foods met with a lot of anxiety, the result the intestinal walls are infringed and things that do not generally leave the passage end up seeping out

Clearly a person wants to keep the fare in the digestive tract until it is all set to be brought to your cells, so that energy can be produced.

Eating Paleo can help indefinitely with the problem, because processed food and sugars are eliminated, leaving little to no chance of a mishap occurring

7. Healthy Cells
Each cell in the body is made with a combination of saturated and unsaturated fat. The Paleo diet offers an ideal equilibrium of fats, since both saturated and unsaturated fats exist in adequate quantities in the Paleo diet, while other diets lack one or the other fat

8. Reduce Inflammation
Studies show that inflammation is the primary issue behind cardiovascular disease. The Paleo diet focuses solely on food items that are anti-inflammatory, thereby reducing the risk of heart disease significantly. The presence of omega 3 fatty acids is one of the reasons for which the Paleo diet is anti-inflammatory.

9. New Energy
Breakfast cereals and any food that are advertised to give energy really drain you of it. When following the Paleo diet, there has been reported significant increase in energy due to the high protein content.

10 Increased Insulin Sensitivity

When a person regularly supplies their body with sugary and junk food, in time the body numbs itself to the food as it does not desire or require them. This is where the surplus sugar and carbohydrates store up, because they do not have a specific use for their energy, the cells reject them. This leads to insulin sensitivity where the body will be inept in identifying when the cells are filled or not.

How Paleo Helps to Lose Weight?

The paleo diet converts the body from a principally carbohydrate-burning machine into a fat-burning machine. This is the reason why many find that Paleo diet to be a successful way for losing weight. This is because the human body almost derives its ideal source of energy from fats

Fat takes a lot of time to be burned and it is more resourceful for the body. But as soon as we acquire extra carbohydrates more than what is required for our energy use, the body store the rest as fat for later, in case starvation is on the horizon. Fortunately, a large amount of people will in no way be in risk of starvation

Hence, a person has no means of using the stored fat meant for emergencies for energy; so instead of burning the fat that has already been stored up in the body, people just keep piling more over again

This is the key reason for majority of western countries have an obesity epidemic. The Paleo diet revolutionizes this problem with one simple strategy: eliminate plain carbohydrates from everyday meals.

Mainly, it simply means that by cutting down the quantity of carbohydrate intake, the Paleo diet permits the body to initiate the route of burning fat, hence leading to prominent weight loss

What Can We Eat on a Paleo Diet?

The Paleo diet is more of a lifestyle change. Sometimes it helps to educate yourself about just how unhealthy processed foods can be for you. It can also help to start growing your own garden so you have access to nutritious fruits and vegetables that you helped to cultivate yourself. Not only is it easy on the wallet, but it's empowering

The foods you are allowed to eat on a Paleo diet can be broken down to these basic essentials:

1. Vegetables
An unfortunate aspect of the SAD diet is how it treats fruits and vegetables. Only a few vegetables are commonly eaten: potatoes, corn, and, every once in a while, broccoli. And usually these are lathered with butter and cheese.

The Paleo diet demands great utilization of vegetables, preferably as raw as possible to guarantee the ability to detoxify the body of toxins, including the BPA all too often consumed from canned vegetables and fruit.

2. Fruits
Fruits should be organic whenever possible to prevent consumption of pesticides into the body that can lead to disruptions in hormonal functions and other complications. Fruits are a good substitute for artificially sweetened snacks and desserts that are typically found in the SAD diet

3. Nuts
It is rare to stumble upon a person who eats enough nuts and seeds in their diet. Nuts can be a bit pricey, possibly because there is such a low demand for them, and many people suffer from nut allergies

However, they are full of proteins, healthy fats, and oils that were used by our ancestors to stay alert. They contribute to positive muscle growth and make a great snack when you're on the go.

4. Meat
Meat may be most people's favorite part of the Paleo diet. Meat is full of proteins that help build our muscles and maintain athleticism, and our ancestors often depended upon meat from a hunt for survival

Stay away from factory farmed foods; the animals are treated cruelly and are served a cocktail of antibiotics and growth hormones that find their way into our bodies. As you can imagine, these are toxins that ultimately worsen our health and impede weight-loss and other positive results of the Paleo diet.

5. Seeds
Seeds offer great nutritional benefits, but because they are high in fat, it's possible for them to become rancid, so be careful not to buy more than you can eat in a reasonable amount of time and store them in dark, cool places with low humidity

If the seeds have already been removed from their hulls they will expire faster. Seeds are full of great things like iron (sometimes having even more than meat!), calcium, niacin, fiber, and folic-acid.

What Not to Eat When Going Paleo

Every diet ends up with restrictions. In the case of the Paleo diet, there are a few things you'll want to stay away from.

- Processed/boxed foods
- Canned fruits and vegetables
- Most dairy products (They are full of growth hormones)
- Anything with artificial ingredients. (nitrates, MSG, calcium sorbate, aspartame, artificial colors, saccharin, sorbic acid, potassium bromate, any and all GMOs, and all artificial sweeteners)
- Oils full of trans fats or partly hydrogenated oils
- Fast food
- High Fructose Corn Syrup. (in most junk foods)
- Legumes (phytic acid)
- Grains and pseudograins. (phytic acid)
- Potatoes
- Soda.

Our ancestors survived just fine without most of these things. Although many were present during the time of the caveman and used for survival, in order to maintain a Paleo diet that not only provides us with great health but also helps us to lose weight and maintain lean muscle, we will need to make a few sacrifices

Types of Paleo Diets

One of the greatest features of the Paleo diet is that it can be tailored to your exact health requirements or conditions, such as food allergy, religious practices, or moral restraints.

There are many types of paleo but here we focus on three widely followed types of paleo diet.

1. The Basic Paleo
This is the standard Paleo diet rejects grains, dairy, soy, refined and processed foods. It also omits bogus fats, in addition to vegetable oils that are excessively processed

2. The Ketogenic Paleo
The most vital in low-carbohydrate, the ketogenic diet makes the body into a state of ketosis where fat is the main fuel as an alternative of glucose. Ketogenic consumption can be prepared inside the restrictions of a Paleo regimen.

Ketogenic Paleo is mainly consumed by those who have a great amount of weight to lose, diabetics, or body builders. It can, moreover, be made use of to keep up a wellness arrangement for epilepsy

3. The 80/ 20 Paleo
When Paleo was originally growing to be accepted, some supporters advised being Paleo 80% of the time, while saving the remaining 20% for non-Paleo foods.

This can be taken up by people who are in the Paleo lifestyle as they are a family unit, or persons who have by now accomplished their physical condition targets

Getting Started

Paleo diet is not like other classical diets. You need to open your mind and widen your understanding of what Paleolithic diet really means and how you will advance in it.

Paleo diet is not about calculating calories, carbohydrates, or fat. The diet works not because of calorie counting but for the body is getting rid of stored up fat, along with a lot of harmful things that would eventually be a threat

There are two types of Paleolithic followers:

1. Classic Followers:

These type of Paleo followers go accurately. They will not permit grains of any category, refined sugar, everything dairy, will look for pasture-fed meats and natural fruits and vegetables, consume freshly caught game, and aspire to pursue the set of rules word for word

2. Modern Followers:

These type of Paleo followers take a laidback approach, and understand that in the current world it is not realistic to eat precisely like a caveman, and they include some contemporary comfort into their Paleo style

They may add little dairy every so often, or be happy with pseudo-grains, or even include a non-Paleo meal per month. Regardless of which way one chooses the Paleo diet will work, as you simply follow its basic principles. One does consume much better food, cutting oneself off from the fast food that surrounds us each day

1. In Early Weeks:

In early weeks of Paleo can be little tough, mainly for those who don't try any kind of diet earlier

Purging sugar from the system can be tough for individuals who have consumed a diet loaded with sugary substances. Eliminating bread and other grain-based food can also be rough. The early various person to person but it is typically 4 to 8 weeks.

2. After Early Weeks:

After early weeks, your path will not be rocky anymore. The diet starts working; you begin to drop weight until you attain a physically healthy weight. You have more energy than in the past. This is wonderful comes alive.

Breakfast Recipes

Breakfast Granola

(**Prep + Cook Time**: 55 minutes | **Servings**: 6)

Ingredients:
- 2 tsp. cinnamon powder
- 1½ cups almond flour
- 2 tsp. nutmeg; ground
- 1/2 cup coconut flakes
- 2 tsp. vanilla extract
- 1/2 cup walnuts; chopped
- 1/3 cup coconut oil
- 1/4 cup hemp hearts

Instructions:
1. In a bowl; combine almond flour with coconut flakes, walnuts, cinnamon, nutmeg, vanilla, hemp and walnuts, stir well and spread on a baking sheet.
2. Bake in the oven at 275 °F and bake for 50 minutes, stirring every 10 minutes. Transfer to plates when the granola is cold and serve for breakfast.

Nutrition Facts Per Serving: Calories: 250; Fat: 23g; Fiber: 4g; Carbs: 5g; Protein: 6g

Green Smoothie

(**Prep + Cook Time**: 5 minutes | **Servings**: 3)

Ingredients:
- 1 small cucumber; peeled and chopped
- 1 green apple; chopped
- Juice of 1/2 lemon
- Juice of 1/2 lime
- 1 tbsp. ginger; finely grated
- 1 tbsp. gelatin powder
- 1 cup kale; chopped
- 1 cup coconut water

Instructions:
1. In your kitchen blender, mix the apple with cucumber, ginger and kale and pulse a few times.
2. Add lime and lemon juice, coconut water and gelatin powder and blend a few more times. Transfer to glasses and serve right away.

Nutrition Facts Per Serving: Calories: 180; Fat: 1g; Carbs: 42g; Fiber: 7g; Sugar: 0g, protein: 7g

Muffins Breakfast

(**Prep + Cook Time**: 40 minutes | **Servings**: 4)

Ingredients:
- 1 cup kale; chopped
- Some coconut oil for greasing the muffin cups
- 1/4 cup chives; finely chopped
- 1/2 cup almond milk
- 6 eggs
- Black pepper to the taste

Instructions:
1. In a bowl; mix eggs with chives and kale and whisk very well.
2. Add black pepper to the taste and almond milk and stir well.
3. Divide this into 8 muffin cups after you've greased it with some coconut oil.
4. Introduce this in preheated oven at 350 °F and bake for 30 minutes. Take muffins out of the oven, leave them to cool down, transfer them to plates and serve warm.

Nutrition Facts Per Serving: Calories: 100; Fat: 5g; Protein: 14; Sugar: 0

Special Burrito

(Prep + Cook Time: 25 minutes | **Servings**: 2)

Ingredients:
- 1/4 cup canned green chilies; chopped
- 1 small yellow onion; chopped
- 4 eggs; egg yolks and whites divided
- 1/4 cup cilantro; chopped
- 1 red bell pepper; finely cut in strips
- 2 tomatoes; chopped
- 1/2 cup beef; ground and browned for 10 minutes
- 1 avocado; peeled, pitted and chopped
- Some hot sauce for serving
- A drizzle of olive oil

Instructions:
1. Heat up a pan with a drizzle of olive oil over medium high heat, add half of the egg whites after you've whisked them in a bowl; spread evenly and cook for 1 minute.
2. Flip them cook for 1 minute more, transfer to a plate and repeat the action with the rest of the egg whites.
3. Heat up the same pan over medium high heat, add onions, stir and cook for 1 minute.
4. Add chilies, bell pepper, tomato, meat and cilantro, stir and cook for 5 minutes. Add egg yolks, stir well and cook until they are done.
5. Arrange egg whites tortillas on 2 plates, divide eggs and meat mix between them, add some chopped avocado and hot sauce, roll and serve them for breakfast.

Nutrition Facts Per Serving: Calories: 255; Fat: 23g; Fiber: 3g; Carbs: 7g; Protein: 12g

Coconut and Almonds Granola

(Prep + Cook Time: 45 minutes | **Servings**: 4)

Ingredients:
- 3 cups coconut flakes
- 1½ cups almonds; chopped
- 1/2 cup sesame seeds
- 1/2 cup sunflower seeds
- 1/2 tsp. cinnamon; ground
- 2 tbsp. chia seeds
- 1/2 cup maple syrup
- A pinch of cardamom
- 1 tsp. vanilla extract
- 2 tbsp. olive oil

Instructions:
1. In a bowl; mix almonds with sunflower seeds, sesame seeds, coconut, chia seeds, cardamom and cinnamon and stir.
2. Meanwhile; heat up a small pot over medium heat, add oil, vanilla and maple syrup, stir well and cook for about 1 minute.
3. Pour this over almonds mix, stir everything, spread on a baking sheet, bake in the oven at 300 °F for 25 minutes, stirring the mixture after 15 minutes. Leave your special granola to cool down before dividing it between plates and serving it.

Nutrition Facts Per Serving: Calories: 270; Fat: 13g; Fiber: 5g; Carbs: 7g; Protein: 8g

Red Breakfast Smoothie

(Prep + Cook Time: 5 minutes | **Servings**: 2)

Ingredients:
- 1 small red bell pepper; seeded and roughly chopped
- 5 strawberries; cut in halves
- 1 tomato; cut into 4 wedges
- 1 cup red cabbage; chopped
- 1/2 cup raspberries
- 8 oz. water
- 2 ice cubes for serving

Instructions:
1. In your food processor, mix cabbage with bell pepper, tomato, strawberries and raspberries and pulse well until you obtain cream.
2. Add water and pulse well a few more times. Transfer to glasses and serve with ice cubes.

Nutrition Facts Per Serving: Calories: 189; Fat: 2g; Carbs: 40g; Fiber: 7; Sugar: 1g; Protein: 5g

Tomato and Eggs Breakfast

(Prep + Cook Time: 40 minutes | **Servings**: 2)

Ingredients:
- 2 tomatoes
- 2 eggs
- A pinch of black pepper
- 1 tsp. parsley; finely chopped

Instructions:
1. Cut tomatoes tops, scoop flesh and arrange them on a lined baking sheet.
2. Crack an egg in each tomato.
3. Season with salt and pepper. Introduce them in the oven at 350 °F and bake for 30 minutes.
4. Take tomatoes out of the oven, divide between plates, season with pepper, sprinkle parsley at the end and serve.

Nutrition Facts Per Serving: Calories: 186g; Protein: 14; Fat: 10; Sugar: 6

Plantain Pancakes

(Prep + Cook Time: 20 minutes | **Servings**: 1)

Ingredients:
- 1/2 plantain; peeled and chopped
- 1 tbsp. shaved coconut; toasted for serving
- 1 tbsp. coconut milk for serving
- 3 eggs
- 1/4 cup coconut flour
- 1/4 cup coconut water
- 1 tsp. coconut oil
- 1/4 tsp. cream of tartar
- 1/4 tsp. baking soda
- 1/4 tsp. chai spice

Instructions:
1. In your food processor, mix eggs with coconut water and flour, plantain, cream of tartar, baking soda and chai spice and blend well.
2. Heat up a pan with the coconut oil over medium heat, add 1/4 cup pancake batter, spread evenly, cook until it becomes golden, flip pancake and cook for 1 more minute and transfer to a plate.
3. Repeat this with the rest of the batter. Serve pancakes with shaved coconut and coconut milk.

Nutrition Facts Per Serving: Calories: 372; Fat: 17g; Carbs: 55g; Fiber: 12; Sugar: 21g; Protein: 23g

Strawberry and Kiwi Breakfast Smoothie

(Prep + Cook Time: 10 minutes | **Servings**: 2)

Ingredients:
- 1½ cups kiwi; chopped
- 1½ cups frozen strawberries; chopped
- 8 mint leaves
- 2 cups crushed ice
- 2 oz. water

Instructions:
1. In your blender, mix kiwi with strawberries and mint and pulse well.
2. Add water and crushed ice and pulse again.

Transfer to glasses and serve right away.

Nutrition Facts Per Serving: Calories: 133; Fat: 1g; Carbs: 34g; Fiber: 4; Sugar: 9g; Protein: 1.3

Turkey Breakfast Sandwich

(Prep + Cook Time: 5 minutes | **Servings**: 1)

Ingredients:
- 2 oz. turkey meat; roasted and thinly sliced
- 2 tbsp. pecans; toasted and chopped
- 2 slices paleo coconut bread
- 2 tbsp. cranberry chutney
- 1/4 cup arugula

Instructions:
1. In a bowl; mix pecans with chutney and stir well.

2. Spread this on bread slice, add turkey slices and arugula and top with the other bread slice. Serve right away.

Nutrition Facts Per Serving: Calories: 540; Fat: 11g; Carbs: 52g; Fiber: 4; Sugar: 13g; Protein: 32

Sweet Potato Breakfast

(Prep + Cook Time: 25 minutes | **Servings:** 4)

Ingredients:
- 2 Italian sausages; casings removed
- 4 tbsp. coconut oil
- 1 small green bell pepper; chopped
- 1/2 cup onion; chopped
- 2 garlic cloves; minced
- 2 cups sweet potato; chopped
- 1 avocado; peeled, pitted, cut into halves and thinly sliced
- 3 eggs
- 2 cups spinach

Instructions:
1. Heat up a pan with the oil over medium high heat, add onion, stir and cook for 3 minutes.
2. Add garlic and bell pepper, stir and cook for 1 minute.
3. Add sausage meat, stir and brown for 4 minutes more.
4. Add sweet potato, stir and cook for 4 minutes.
5. Add spinach, stir and cook for 2 minutes.
6. Make 3 holes in this mix, crack an egg in each, introduce pan in preheated broiler and cook for 3 minutes. Divide this tasty mix on plates, add avocado pieces on the side and serve.

Nutrition Facts Per Serving: Calories: 200; Fat: 4g; Fiber: 2g; Carbs: 6g; Protein: 9g

Pork Skillet

(Prep + Cook Time: 30 minutes | **Servings:** 4)

Ingredients:
- 8 oz. mushrooms; chopped
- 1 lb. pork; ground
- 1 tbsp. olive oil
- Black pepper to the taste
- 2 zucchinis; cut in halves and then in half moons
- 1/2 tsp. garlic powder
- 1/2 tsp. basil; dried
- A pinch of sea salt
- 2 tbsp. Dijon mustard

Instructions:
1. Heat up a pan with the oil over medium high heat, add mushrooms, stir and cook for 4 minutes.
2. Add zucchinis, a pinch of salt and black pepper, stir and cook for 4 minutes more.
3. Add pork, garlic powder and basil, stir and cook until meat is done. Add mustard, stir well, cook for a couple more minutes, divide between plates and serve.

Nutrition Facts Per Serving: Calories: 200; Fat: 4g; Fiber: 2g; Carbs: 5g; Protein: 12g

Squash Blossom Frittata

(Prep + Cook Time: 50 minutes | **Servings:** 4)

Ingredients:
- 10 eggs; whisked
- Black pepper to the taste
- 1/4 cup coconut cream
- 1 yellow onion; finely chopped
- 1 leek; thinly sliced
- 2 scallions; thinly sliced
- 2 zucchinis; chopped
- 8 squash blossoms
- 2 tbsp. avocado oil

Instructions:
1. In a bowl; mix eggs with coconut cream and black pepper to the taste and stir well.
2. Heat up a pan with the oil over medium high heat, add leek and onions, stir and cook for 5 minutes.
3. Add zucchini, stir and cook for 10 more minutes.

4. Add eggs, spread, reduce heat to low, cook for 5 minutes.
5. Sprinkle scallions and arrange squash blossoms on frittata, press blossoms into eggs, introduce everything in the oven at 350 °F and bake for 20 minutes. Take frittata out of the oven, leave it to cool down, cut, arrange on plates and serve it.

Nutrition Facts Per Serving: Calories: 123; Fat: 8g; Protein: 7g; Carbs: 2; Sugar: 0

Maple Nut Porridge

(Prep + Cook Time: 10 minutes | **Servings**: 2)

Ingredients:
- 2 tbsp. coconut butter
- 1/2 cup pecans; soaked
- 3/4 cup hot water
- 1 banana; peeled and chopped
- 1/2 tsp. cinnamon
- 2 tsp. maple syrup

Instructions:
1. In your food processor, mix pecans with water, coconut butter, banana, cinnamon and maple syrup and blend well.
2. Transfer this to a pan, heat up over medium heat until it thickens, pour into bowls and serve.

Nutrition Facts Per Serving: Calories: 170; Fat: 9g; Carbs: 20g; Fiber: 6g; Protein: 6g

Breakfast Waffles

(Prep + Cook Time: 20 minutes | **Servings**: 4)

Ingredients:
- 2 eggs
- 1/2 cup almond milk
- 2 tbsp. coconut oil; melted
- 1/2 tsp. cinnamon; ground
- 1 tbsp. baking powder
- 1 tbsp. coconut flour
- 2 tbsp. honey
- 1½ cups almond flour
- 1/4 cup tapioca flour
- 1½ tsp. vanilla extract
- Pure maple syrup for serving

Instructions:
1. In your mixer bowl; combine coconut flour with almond flour, tapioca flour, baking powder and cinnamon and stir.
2. Add egg yolks, almond milk, coconut oil, honey and vanilla extract and blend very well.
3. In another bowl; whisk egg whites with your mixer.
4. Add them to waffles mix and stir everything very well.
5. Pour this into your waffle iron and make 8 waffles. Divide them on plates, top with maple syrup and serve.

Nutrition Facts Per Serving: Calories: 160; Fat: 11g; Fiber: 2g; Carbs: 7g; Protein: 6g

Nuts Porridge

(Prep + Cook Time: 15 minutes | **Servings**: 2)

Ingredients:
- 1/2 cup pecans; soaked overnight and drained
- 1/2 banana; mashed
- 3/4 cup hot water
- 2 tbsp. coconut butter
- 1/2 tsp. cinnamon
- 2 tsp. maple syrup

Instructions:
1. In a blender, mix pecans, with water, banana, coconut butter, cinnamon and maple syrup, pulse really well and transfer to a small pot.
2. Heat everything up over medium heat, cook until it's creamy, transfer to serving bowls and serve.

Nutrition Facts Per Serving: Calories: 150; Fat: 2g; Fiber: 2g; Carbs: 4g; Protein: 6g

Eggplant French Toast

(Prep + Cook Time: 10 minutes | **Servings**: 2)

Ingredients:
- 1 eggplant; peeled and sliced
- 1 tsp. vanilla extract
- 2 eggs
- Stevia to the taste
- 1 tsp. coconut oil
- A pinch of cinnamon

Instructions:
1. In a bowl; mix eggs with vanilla, stevia and cinnamon and whisk well.
2. Heat up a pan with the coconut oil over medium-high heat.
3. Dip eggplant slices in eggs mix, add to heated pan and cook until they become golden on each side. Arrange them on plates and serve.

Nutrition Facts Per Serving: Calories: 125; Fat: 5g; Protein: 7.8g; Carbs: 13g; Fiber: 7.8

Blueberry Smoothie

(Prep + Cook Time: 5 minutes | **Servings**: 2)

Ingredients:
- 2 cups blueberries
- 1 tsp. lemon zest
- 1/2 cup coconut milk
- A pinch of cinnamon
- Water as needed

Instructions:
1. In your kitchen blender, mix coconut milk with blueberries, lemon zest and a pinch of cinnamon and pulse a few times.
2. Add water as needed to thin your smoothie and pulse a few more times. Transfer to a tall glass and serve.

Nutrition Facts Per Serving: Calories: 177; Fat: 3g; Carbs: 45g; Fiber: 7; Sugar: 12g; Protein: 3g

Spinach Frittata

(Prep + Cook Time: 50 minutes | **Servings**: 4)

Ingredients:
- 1/2 lb. sausage; ground
- 2 tbsp. ghee
- 1 cup mushrooms; thinly sliced
- 1 cup spinach leaves; chopped
- 10 eggs; whisked
- 1 small yellow onion; finely chopped
- Black pepper to the taste

Instructions:
1. Heat up a pan with the ghee over medium-high heat, add onion and some black pepper, stir and cook until it browns.
2. Add sausage, stir and also cook until it browns. Add spinach and mushrooms and cook for 4 minutes, stirring from time to time.
3. Take the pan off the heat, add eggs, spread evenly, introduce frittata in the oven at 350 °F and bake for 20 minutes.
4. Take frittata out of the oven, leave it aside for a few minutes to cool down, cut, arrange on plates and serve.

Nutrition Facts Per Serving: Calories: 233; Fat: 13g; Carbs: 4g; Fiber: 1.2; Sugar: 1g; Protein: 21g

Eggs and Ham

(Prep + Cook Time: 25 minutes | **Servings**: 4)

Ingredients:
- 4 eggs
- 10 ham slices
- 4 tbsp. scallions
- A pinch of black pepper
- A pinch of sweet paprika
- 1 tbsp. melted ghee

Instructions:
1. Grease a muffin pan with melted ghee.
2. Divide ham slices in each muffin mold to form your cups. In a bowl; mix eggs with scallions, pepper and paprika and whisk well.
3. Divide this mix on top of ham, introduce your ham cups in the oven at 400 °F and bake for 15 minutes. Leave cups to cool down before dividing on plates and serving.

Nutrition Facts Per Serving: Calories: 250; Fat: 10g; Fiber: 3g; Carbs: 6g; Protein: 12g

Italian Style Eggs

(Prep + Cook Time: 25 minutes | **Servings**: 1)

Ingredients:
- 2 eggs
- 1/4 tsp. rosemary; dried
- 1/2 cup cherry tomatoes halved
- 1½ cups kale; chopped
- 1/2 tsp. coconut oil
- 3 tbsp. water
- 1 tsp. balsamic vinegar
- 1/4 avocado; peeled and chopped

Instructions:
1. Heat up a pan with the oil over medium high heat, add water, kale, rosemary and tomatoes, stir; cover and cook for 4 minutes.
2. Uncover pan, stir again and add eggs.
3. Stir and scramble eggs for 3 minutes.
4. Add vinegar, stir everything and transfer to a serving plate. Top with chopped avocado and serve.

Nutrition Facts Per Serving: Calories: 185; Fat: 10g; Fiber: 1g; Carbs: 6g; Protein: 7g

Orange and Dates Granola

(Prep + Cook Time: 25 minutes | **Servings**: 6)

Ingredients:
- 5 oz. dates; soaked in hot water
- 1/2 cup pumpkin seeds
- Juice from 1 orange
- Grated rind of 1/2 orange
- 1 cup desiccated coconut
- 1/2 cup silvered almonds
- 1/2 cup linseeds
- 1/2 cup sesame seeds
- Almond milk for serving

Instructions:
1. In a bowl; mix almonds with orange rind, orange juice, linseeds, coconut, pumpkin and sesame seeds and stir well.
2. Drain dates, add them to your food processor and blend well. Add this paste to almonds mix and stir well again.
3. Spread this on a lined baking sheet, introduce in the oven at 350 °F and bake for 15 minutes, stirring every 4 minutes.
4. Take granola out of the oven, leave aside to cool down a bit and then serve with almond milk.

Nutrition Facts Per Serving: Calories: 208g; Protein: 6g; Fiber: 5; Fat: 9; Sugar: 0

Bacon Muffins

(Prep + Cook Time: 40 minutes | **Servings**: 4)

Ingredients:
- 4 oz. bacon slices
- 3 garlic cloves; minced
- 1 small yellow onion; chopped
- 1 zucchini; thinly sliced
- A handful spinach; torn
- 6 canned and pickled artichoke hearts; chopped
- 8 eggs
- 1/4 tsp. paprika
- A pinch of black pepper
- A pinch of cayenne pepper
- 1/4 cup coconut cream

Instructions:
1. Heat up a pan over medium high heat, add bacon, stir; cook until it's crispy, transfer to paper towels, drain grease and leave aside for now.
2. Heat up the same pan over medium heat again, add garlic and onion, stir and cook for 4 minutes.
3. In a bowl; mix eggs with coconut cream, onions, garlic, paprika, black pepper and cayenne and whisk well.
4. Add spinach, zucchini and artichoke pieces and stir everything.
5. Divide crispy bacon slices in a muffin pan, add eggs mixture on top, introduce your muffins in the oven and bake at 400 °F for 20 minutes. Leave them to cool down before serving them for breakfast.

Nutrition Facts Per Serving: Calories: 270; Fat: 12g; Fiber: 4g; Carbs: 6g; Protein: 12g

Parsley and Pear Smoothie

(Prep + Cook Time: 5 minutes | **Servings**: 6)

Ingredients:
- 1 apple pear; chopped
- 1 bunch parsley; roughly chopped
- 1 small avocado; stoned and peeled
- 1 pear; peeled and chopped
- 1 green apple; chopped
- 1 Granny Smith apple; chopped
- 6 bananas; peeled and roughly chopped
- 2 plums; stoned
- 1 cup ice
- 1 cup water

Instructions:
1. In your kitchen blender, mix parsley with avocado, apple pear, pear, green apple, Granny Smith apple, plums and bananas and blend very well.
2. Add ice and water and blend again very well. Transfer to tall glasses and serve right away.

Nutrition Facts Per Serving: Calories: 208g; Carbs: 48g; Fiber: 13; Fat: 3g; Protein: 3; Sugar: 28

Peach and Coconut Smoothie

(Prep + Cook Time: 5 minutes | **Servings**: 2)

Ingredients:
- 1 cup ice
- 2 peaches; peeled and chopped
- Lemon zest to the taste
- 1 cup cold coconut milk
- 1 drop lemon essential oil

Instructions:
1. In your kitchen blender, mix coconut milk with ice and peaches and pulse a few times.
2. Add lemon zest to the taste and 1 drop lemon essential oil and pulse a few more time. Pour into glasses and serve right away.

Nutrition Facts Per Serving: Calories: 200; Fat: 5g; Fiber: 4g; Carbs: 6g; Protein: 8g

Bacon and Egg Breakfast Sandwich

(Prep + Cook Time: 20 minutes | **Servings**: 2)

Ingredients:
- 2 cups bell peppers; chopped
- 1/2 tbsp. avocado oil
- 3 eggs
- 4 bacon slices

Instructions:
1. Heat up a pan with the oil over medium high heat, add bell peppers, stir and cook until they are soft.
2. Heat up another pan over medium heat, add bacon, stir and cook until it's crispy.
3. In a bowl; whisk eggs really well and add them to bell peppers.
4. Cook until eggs are done for about 8 minutes. Divide half of the bacon slices between plates, add eggs, top with bacon slices and serve.

Nutrition Facts Per Serving: Calories: 200; Fat: 4g; Fiber: 3g; Carbs: 6g; Protein: 10g

Sausage Balls

(Prep + Cook Time: 30 minutes | **Servings**: 8)

Ingredients:
- 2 eggs
- 1 tsp. baking soda
- 1 lb. sausage; chopped
- 1/4 cup coconut flour
- Black pepper to the taste
- 1 tsp. smoked paprika

Instructions:
1. In your food processor, mix sausage with eggs, baking soda, flour, pepper and paprika and pulse really well.
2. Shape medium balls from this mix, arrange them on a lined baking sheet and bake them in the oven at 350 °F for 20 minutes. Divide them between plates and serve in the morning.

Nutrition Facts Per Serving: Calories: 150; Fat: 7g; Fiber: 3g; Carbs: 4g; Protein: 6g

Portobello Sandwich

(Prep + Cook Time: 15 minutes | **Servings**: 1)

Ingredients:
- 2 Portobello mushroom caps
- Some lettuce leaves
- 2 avocado slices
- 1/2 lb. bacon; chopped

Instructions:
1. Heat up a pan over medium high heat, add bacon, cook until it's crispy, transfer to paper towels and drain grease.
2. Heat up the pan with the bacon fat over medium high heat, add mushroom caps, cook for 2 minutes on each side and take off heat.
3. Put 1 mushroom cap on a plate, add bacon, avocado slices and lettuce leaves, top with the other mushroom cap and serve.

Nutrition Facts Per Serving: Calories: 200; Fat: 4g; Fiber: 2g; Carbs: 4g; Protein: 6g

Paleo Kale Frittata

(Prep + Cook Time: 40 minutes | **Servings**: 4)

Ingredients:
- 3 bacon slices; cooked and crumbled
- 1/3 cup yellow onion; chopped
- 1 tbsp. coconut oil
- 1/2 cup red bell pepper; chopped
- 2 cups kale; torn
- 1/2 cup almond milk
- 8 eggs
- A pinch of black pepper

Instructions:
1. In a bowl; whisk eggs with some black pepper and almond milk.
2. Heat up a pan with the oil over medium high heat, add bell pepper and onion, stir and cook for 3 minutes.
3. Add kale, stir; cover pan and cook for 5 minutes more.
4. Uncover your pan, add bacon and eggs, spread evenly around the pan and cook for 4 minutes.
5. Introduce your pan in the oven at 350 °F and bake for 15 minutes. Take frittata out of the oven, leave it to cool down a bit before cutting and serving it for breakfast.

Nutrition Facts Per Serving: Calories: 240; Fat: 13g; Fiber: 2g; Carbs: 5g; Protein: 15g

Spicy Eggs

(Prep + Cook Time: 35 minutes | **Servings**: 4)

Ingredients:
- 4 bacon slices; cooked and crumbled
- 12 cherry tomatoes; halved
- 1/2 tsp. turmeric
- 1/2 onion; chopped
- 5 eggs
- 2 Serrano peppers; chopped
- 1 green bell pepper; chopped
- Black pepper to the taste
- A pinch of sea salt

Instructions:
1. In a bowl; whisk eggs with a pinch of salt, black pepper, Serrano peppers, green pepper and turmeric.
2. Heat up a pan over medium heat, add bacon, stir and cook for 3 minutes.
3. Add onion, stir and cook for 2 minutes more.
4. Add eggs and tomatoes, stir; cook for 6 minutes and then bake in the oven at 350 °F for 15 minutes. Leave your eggs to cool down before slicing and serving it.

Nutrition Facts Per Serving: Calories: 240; Fat: 8g; Fiber: 3g; Carbs: 6g; Protein: 8g

Eggs and Artichokes

(Prep + Cook Time: 50 minutes | **Servings**: 2)

Ingredients:
- 1 egg white
- 4 whole eggs
- 3/4 cup balsamic vinegar
- 4 oz. bacon; chopped
- 4 artichoke hearts
- A pinch of sea salt
- Black pepper to the taste

For the sauce:
- 1 tbsp. lemon juice
- 3/4 cup ghee
- 4 egg yolks
- A pinch of paprika

Instructions:
1. Put artichoke hearts in a bowl; add vinegar, toss a bit and leave aside for 20 minutes.
2. Put the ghee in a pan and melt it over medium high heat.
3. In a bowl; mix 4 egg yolks with paprika and lemon juice and stir well. Put some water into a pot and bring to a simmer over medium heat.
4. Put the bowl with the egg yolks on top of simmering water and stir constantly.
5. Add melted ghee gradually, stir until sauce thickens and take off heat.
6. Drain artichokes, place them on a lined baking sheet, brush tops with 1 egg white, add bacon on top and season with black pepper and a pinch of sea salt.
7. Introduce them in the oven at 375 °F and bake for 20 minutes.
8. Meanwhile; heat up a pot with water and bring to a simmer over medium high heat.
9. Crack 4 eggs into simmering water but make sure you only crack one at a time.
10. Poach eggs for 1 minute and transfer them to plates. Add artichokes and bacon on the side, drizzle the sauce you've made earlier on top and served.

Nutrition Facts Per Serving: Calories: 270; Fat: 24g; Fiber: 0g; Carbs: 5g; Protein: 16g

Breakfast Pancakes

(Prep + Cook Time: 40 minutes | **Servings**: 4)

Ingredients:
- 12 bacon slices; chopped
- 8 eggs
- Black pepper to the taste
- 1½ tbsp. coconut oil
- 10 grain-free pancakes

For the pancakes:
- 1 cup arrowroot
- 1/2 cup almond flour
- 1/2 cup coconut flour
- 1/2 tsp. baking soda
- 1 tsp. cinnamon
- 1 cup almond milk
- 2 eggs
- 1 tsp. vanilla extract
- 3 tbsp. maple syrup
- 2 tbsp. coconut oil

Instructions:
1. In a bowl; mix arrowroot with almond flour, coconut flour, baking soda and cinnamon and stir.
2. Add almond milk, 2 eggs, vanilla extract and maple syrup and stir well until you obtain a smooth batter.
3. Heat up a pan with 2 tbsp. coconut oil over medium high heat, pour some of the batter, spread in the pan, cook for 1 minute, flip, cook for 2 minutes more and transfer pancake to a plate.
4. Repeat with the rest of the batter.
5. You will obtain 10 pancakes.
6. Heat up a pan with 1/2 tbsp. coconut oil over medium high heat, add bacon, cook until it's crispy, transfer to paper towels, drain grease and leave it aside in a bowl for now.
7. In another bowl; whisk 8 eggs with some black pepper.
8. Heat up a pan with 1 tbsp. oil over medium high heat, add whisked eggs, cook until they are done and then mix them with cooked bacon.
9. Stir everything well and take off heat. Divide this on your pancakes, roll them and serve for breakfast.

Nutrition Facts Per Serving: Calories: 260; Fat: 7g; Fiber: 4g; Carbs: 5g; Protein: 10g

Avocado Muffins

(Prep + Cook Time: 40 minutes | **Servings**: 12)

Ingredients:
- 6 thin bacon slices; chopped
- 1 yellow onion; chopped
- 4 avocados; pitted, peeled and chopped
- 4 eggs
- 1/2 cup coconut flour
- 1 cup coconut milk
- 1/2 tsp. baking soda
- A pinch of sea salt
- Black pepper to the taste

Instructions:
1. Heat up a pan over medium high heat, add bacon and onion, stir well and cook until they brown.
2. Meanwhile; put avocado in a bowl and mash with a fork.
3. Add eggs, a pinch of salt, black pepper, milk, baking soda and coconut flour and stir everything well.
4. Add almost all of the bacon and onions, stir well again and divide into muffin pans.
5. Sprinkle the rest of the bacon and onions on top, place in the oven at 350 °F and bake for 20 minutes. Leave your avocado muffins to cool down before dividing them on plates and serving.

Nutrition Facts Per Serving: Calories: 240; Fat: 4g; Fiber: 4g; Carbs: 7g; Protein: 3g

Spinach Omelet

(Prep + Cook Time: 25 minutes | **Servings**: 4)

Ingredients:
- 2 eggs; whisked
- 1 tbsp. ghee; melted
- A pinch of black pepper
- 1 handful baby spinach; torn
- 1 onion; chopped
- 4 thyme springs; chopped
- 3 garlic cloves; minced
- 1 red bell pepper; chopped
- 1 green bell pepper; chopped
- 3 tbsp. olive oil
- 1 cup cherry tomatoes; halved
- 1 red chili pepper; chopped

Instructions:
1. Heat up a pan with the ghee over medium high heat, add eggs, black pepper, stir a bit, cook until eggs are done, add spinach, stir gently, cook for a few minutes and divide between plates.
2. Heat up another pan with the oil over medium high heat, add onion, stir and cook for 3 minutes.
3. Add garlic, stir and cook for 1 minute more. Add thyme, tomatoes, red, yellow pepper and chili pepper, stir; cook for 5 minutes more and divide on top of the omelet. Serve hot.

Nutrition Facts Per Serving: Calories: 200; Fat: 5g; Fiber: 3g; Carbs: 4g; Protein: 4g

Pumpkin Muffins

(Prep + Cook Time: 35 minutes | **Servings**: 10)

Ingredients:
- 1¼ cup almond meal
- 2 tbsp. flax meal
- 1 tbsp. flax seeds
- 3/4 cup coconut flour
- 1 tsp. baking soda
- 2 tsp. pumpkin pie spice
- 1/2 tsp. nutmeg; ground
- 1/2 tsp. ginger powder
- 5 eggs
- 1/4 cup coconut oil
- 1/4 cup agave
- 1 cup pumpkin puree
- 1 cup blueberries
- 1 cup walnuts; chopped

Instructions:
1. In a bowl; mix almond meal with flax meal, flax seeds, coconut flour, baking soda, nutmeg, ginger and pumpkin spice and stir.
2. In another bowl; mix eggs with oil, agave, pumpkin puree, walnuts and blueberries and whisk well.
3. Combine the 2 mixtures and stir using your mixer.
4. Divide this into a lined muffin tray, place in the oven at 350 °F and bake for 25 minutes. Leave your muffins to cool down, divide them between plates and serve.

Nutrition Facts Per Serving: Calories: 240; Fat: 3g; Fiber: 2g; Carbs: 4g; Protein: 6g

Zucchini and Chocolate Muffins

(Prep + Cook Time: 40 minutes | **Servings**: 8)

Ingredients:
- 4 eggs
- 1/4 cup honey
- 1/4 cup melted ghee
- 1/4 cup coconut milk
- 1/4 cup coconut flour
- 1/2 cup almond flour
- 1 tsp. baking soda
- 1/4 cup cocoa powder
- 1 zucchini; grated
- 4 oz. dark chocolate; chopped
- 1 tsp. vanilla extract

Instructions:
1. In a bowl; mix eggs with ghee and whisk using a mixer.
2. Add coconut milk, honey and vanilla and whisk well again.
3. In another bowl; mix coconut flour with baking soda, almond flour and cocoa powder and stir well.
4. Combine the 2 mixtures and stir again.

5. Add chocolate pieces and zucchini, stir gently, divide into a lined muffin tray and bake in the oven at 350 °F for 30 minutes. Serve your muffins cold.

Nutrition Facts Per Serving: Calories: 230; Fat: 4g; Fiber: 2g; Carbs: 4g; Protein: 6g

Special Breakfast Dish

(Prep + Cook Time: 45 minutes | **Servings**: 8)

Ingredients:
- 1 lb. pork meat; ground
- 1 lb. chorizo; ground
- A pinch of sea salt
- Black pepper to the taste
- 8 eggs
- 3 tbsp. ghee
- 1 avocado; pitted, peeled and chopped
- 1 tomato; chopped
- 1/2 cup red onion; chopped
- 2 tbsp. Paleo enchilada sauce

Instructions:
1. In a bowl; mix pork with chorizo, a pinch of salt and black pepper and stir well.
2. Spread this on a lined baking sheet, shape a circle out of it and spread enchilada sauce all over.
3. Place in the oven and be at 350 °F for 25 minutes.
4. Heat up a pan with the ghee over medium heat, add eggs, stir and scramble them.
5. Spread them over pork mix and then add onion, tomato and avocado. Divide between plates and serve.

Nutrition Facts Per Serving: Calories: 345; Fat: 23g; Fiber: 3g; Carbs: 6g; Protein: 23g

Breakfast Burrito

(Prep + Cook Time: 17 minutes | **Servings**: 4)

Ingredients:
- 1 small yellow onion; finely chopped
- 4 eggs; egg yolks and whites separated
- 1/4 cup canned green chilies; chopped
- 2 tomatoes; chopped
- 1 red bell pepper; cut into thin strips
- 1/4 cup cilantro; finely chopped
- 1/2 cup chicken meat; already cooked and shredded
- Black pepper to the taste
- A drizzle of extra virgin olive oil
- 1 avocado; pitted, peeled and chopped
- Hot sauce for serving

Instructions:
1. Put egg whites in a bowl; add some black pepper, whisk them well and leave them aside for now.
2. Heat up a pan with a drizzle of oil over medium-high heat, add half of the egg whites, spread evenly, cook for 30 seconds, cover pan, cook for 1 minute and then slide on a plate.
3. Repeat this with the rest of the egg whites and leave the two "tortillas" aside.
4. Heat up the same pan with another drizzle of oil over medium-high heat, add onions, stir and cook for 1 minute.
5. Add red bell pepper, green chilies, tomato, meat and cilantro and stir.
6. Add egg yolks to the pan and scramble the whole mix.
7. Add avocado, stir; take off heat and spread evenly on the two egg whites "tortillas". Roll them, arrange on plates and serve with some hot sauce.

Nutrition Facts Per Serving: Calories: 170; Fat: 5g; Carbs: 1; Sugar: 0.6g; Fiber: 0g; Protein: 6g

Wrapped Eggs

(**Prep + Cook Time**: 25 minutes | **Servings**: 2)

Ingredients:
- 4 bacon slices
- 2 bacon slices; chopped
- 4 eggs
- 1/2 yellow onion; chopped
- 1 sweet potato; peeled and chopped
- 1 tbsp. olive oil
- A pinch of sea salt
- Black pepper to the taste

Instructions:
1. Heat up a pan over medium high heat, add 4 bacon slices, cook until it's crispy, transfer to paper towels, drain grease and line 4 muffin molds with it.
2. Crack an egg into each bacon cup, season with salt and pepper, place in the oven at 375 °F and bake for 15 minutes.
3. Meanwhile; heat up a pan with the oil over medium high heat, add onion and sweet potato, stir and cook for a few minutes.
4. Add the rest of the bacon, stir and cook for a few more minutes. Divide wrapped eggs on plates, add sweet potato mix on the side and serve.

Nutrition Facts Per Serving: Calories: 200; Fat: 5g; Fiber: 3g; Carbs: 6g; Protein: 5g

Cereal Bowl

(**Prep + Cook Time**: 10 minutes | **Servings**: 2)

Ingredients:
- 2 tbsp. pumpkin seeds
- 2 tbsp. almonds; chopped
- 1 tbsp. chia seeds
- A handful blueberries
- 1/3 cup water
- 1/3 cup almond milk

Instructions:
1. Put half of the pumpkin seeds in your food processor and blend them.
2. In 2 bowls, divide water, milk, the rest of the pumpkin seeds, chia seeds and almonds and stir.
3. Add blended pumpkin seeds and stir gently everything. Serve with blueberries on top.

Nutrition Facts Per Serving: Calories: 150; Fat: 3g; Fiber: 4g; Carbs: 5g; Protein: 6g

Apple Omelet

(**Prep + Cook Time**: 25 minutes | **Servings**: 1)

Ingredients:
- 1 apple; peeled, cored and sliced
- 2 tsp. ghee
- 3 tsp. maple syrup
- 1/2 tsp. cinnamon powder
- 2 eggs; whites and yolks separated
- 2 tbsp. almond milk
- A pinch of sea salt
- Black pepper to the taste
- 2 tbsp. walnuts; toasted and chopped

Instructions:
1. Heat up a pan with half of the ghee over medium high heat, add apple slices and cook them for about 5 minutes.
2. Sprinkle them with cinnamon, drizzle maple syrup, stir gently, cook for 1 minute, transfer them to a plate and leave aside for now.
3. In a bowl; whisk egg yolks with milk, a pinch of salt and black pepper and leave aside for now.
4. In another bowl; whisk egg whites well using your mixer.
5. Combine egg yolks with egg whites.
6. Heat up a pan with the rest of the ghee over medium heat, add eggs mix, stir and cook for 3 minutes.
7. Add apple slices, cover pan, cook eggs for 6 minutes more and transfer everything to a plate. Top with walnuts and serve.

Nutrition Facts Per Serving: Calories: 150; Fat: 1g; Fiber: 3g; Carbs: 4g; Protein: 12g

Banana Pancakes

(Prep + Cook Time: 20 minutes | **Servings**: 2)

Ingredients:
- 2 bananas; peeled and chopped
- 1/4 tsp. baking powder
- 4 eggs
- Cooking spray

Instructions:
1. In a bowl; mix eggs with chopped bananas and baking powder and whisk well.
2. Transfer this to your food processor and blend very well. Heat up a pan over medium high heat after you've sprayed it with some cooking oil.
3. Add some of the pancakes batter, spread in the pan, cook for 1 minute, flip and cook for 30 seconds and transfer to a plate.
4. Repeat this with the rest of the batter, arrange pancakes on plates and serve.

Nutrition Facts Per Serving: 120; Fat: 2g; Carbs: 2; Sugar: 1g; Protein: 4g

Sweet Potato Waffles

(Prep + Cook Time: 20 minutes | **Servings**: 4)

Ingredients:
- 2 sweet potatoes; peeled and finely grated
- 1/2 tsp. nutmeg; ground
- 2 tbsp. melted coconut oil
- 3 eggs
- 1 tsp. cinnamon powder
- Some apple sauce for serving

Instructions:
1. In a bowl; mix eggs with sweet potatoes, coconut oil, cinnamon and nutmeg and whisk very well.
2. Cook waffles in your waffle iron, arrange them on plates and serve with apple sauce drizzled on top.

Nutrition Facts Per Serving: Calories: 227; Fat: 6g; Carbs: 37g; Fiber: 2; Sugar: 9g; Protein: 6g

Breakfast Burger

(Prep + Cook Time: 30 minutes | **Servings**: 4)

Ingredients:
- 5 eggs
- 1 lb. ground beef meat
- 1/2 cup sausages; ground
- 8 slices bacon
- 3 sun-dried tomatoes; chopped
- 2 tbsp. almond meal
- 2 tsp. basil leaves; chopped
- 1 tsp. garlic; finely minced
- A drizzle of avocado oil
- Black pepper to the taste

Instructions:
1. In a bowl; mix beef meat with 1 egg, almond meal, tomatoes, basil, pepper and garlic, stir well and form 4 burgers.
2. Heat up a pan over medium high heat, add burgers, cook them 5 minutes on each side, transfer them to plates and leave aside for now.
3. Heat up the same pan over medium-high heat, add sausages, stir; cook for 5 minutes and transfer them to a plate.
4. Heat up the pan again, add bacon, cook for 4 minutes, drain excess grease and also leave aside on a plate.
5. Fry the 4 eggs in a pan with a drizzle of oil over medium-high heat and place them on top of burgers. ,Add sausage and bacon and serve.

Nutrition Facts Per Serving: Calories: 264; Fat: 12g; Carbs: 5g; Fiber: 0.3; Sugar: 0.7g; Protein: 32

Sausage Frittata

(Prep + Cook Time: 40 minutes | **Servings**: 4)

Ingredients:
- 10 eggs
- 2 tbsp. melted ghee
- 1 cup spinach; chopped
- 1/2 lb. sausage; chopped
- 1 cup mushrooms; chopped
- 1 small yellow onion; chopped
- A pinch of sea salt
- Black pepper to the taste

Instructions:
1. Heat up a pan with the ghee over medium high heat, add sausage pieces, stir and brown for a couple of minutes.
2. Add onion, mushroom, spinach, a pinch of salt and black pepper to the taste, stir and cook for a few more minutes.
3. Add whisked eggs, spread evenly and stir gently.
4. Place in the oven at 350 °F and bake for 20 minutes. Leave your Paleo breakfast to cool down before slicing and serving it.

Nutrition Facts Per Serving: Calories: 260; Fat: 8g; Fiber: 2g; Carbs: 4g; Protein: 9g

Breakfast Sandwich

(Prep + Cook Time: 20 minutes | **Servings**: 2)

Ingredients:
- 3.5 oz. pumpkin flesh; peeled
- 4 slices paleo coconut bread
- 1 small avocado; pitted and peeled
- 1 carrot; finely grated
- 1 lettuce leaf; torn into 4 pieces

Instructions:
1. Put pumpkin in a tray, introduce in the oven at 350 °F and bake for 10 minutes.
2. Take pumpkin out of the oven, leave aside for 2-3 minutes, transfer to a bowl and mash it a bit. Put avocado in another bowl and also mash it with a fork.
3. Spread avocado on 2 bread slices, add grated carrot, mashed pumpkin and 2 lettuce pieces on each and top them with the rest of the bread slices.

Nutrition Facts Per Serving: Calories: 340; Fat: 7g; Protein: 4g; Carbs: 13g; Fiber: 8; Sugar: 4

Orange and Vanilla Breakfast Delight

(Prep + Cook Time: 10 minutes | **Servings**: 2)

Ingredients:
- 2 cups coconut milk
- 1/2 cup chia seeds
- Juice from 1/4 lemon
- Zest from 1 orange
- 1 tbsp. vanilla extract
- 1 tbsp. maple syrup

Instructions:
1. Divide coconut milk, lemon juice, chia, orange zest, vanilla extract and maple syrup into 2 breakfast bowls.
2. Stir well and keep in the fridge until you serve them.

Nutrition Facts Per Serving: Calories: 200; Fat: 3g; Fiber: 2g; Carbs: 5g; Protein: 4g

Burger

(Prep + Cook Time: 30 minutes | **Servings:** 4)

Ingredients:
- 8 bacon slices; chopped and cooked
- 5 eggs
- 1 lb. beef; ground
- 1/2 cup sausage; ground
- 3 sun-dried tomatoes; chopped
- 2 tbsp. almond meal
- 2 tsp. basil
- 2 tbsp. coconut oil
- 1 tsp. garlic; minced

Instructions:
1. In a bowl; mix beef with garlic, basil, tomatoes, almond meal and 1 egg, stir well and shape 4 burgers.
2. Heat up a grill over medium high heat, add burgers, cook them for 5 minutes on each side, transfer to plates and leave them aside.
3. Heat up a pan over medium high heat, add sausage, cook until it's done and divide into burgers. Add cooked bacon on top of sausages and leave aside for now.
4. Heat up a pan with the coconut oil over medium high heat, crack one egg at a time, fry them well and divide them on burgers.

Nutrition Facts Per Serving: Calories: 340; Fat: 20g; Fiber: 3g; Carbs: 7g; Protein: 20g

Blueberry Muffins

(Prep + Cook Time: 35 minutes | **Servings:** 10)

Ingredients:
- 1/2 tsp. baking soda
- 2½ cups almond flour
- 1 tbsp. vanilla extract
- 1/4 cup coconut oil
- 1/4 cup coconut milk
- 2 eggs
- 1/4 cup maple syrup
- 1 tbsp. coconut flour
- 3 tbsp. cinnamon powder
- 1 cup blueberries

Instructions:
1. In a bowl; mix almond flour with baking soda and coconut flour and stir.
2. Add eggs, oil, coconut milk, cinnamon, maple syrup, vanilla and blueberries and stir everything using your mixer.
3. Divide this into muffin cups, place in the oven at 350 °F and bake for 25 minutes. Leave your muffins to cool down a bit, divide between plates and serve them for breakfast.

Nutrition Facts Per Serving: Calories: 240; Fat: 3g; Fiber: 1g; Carbs: 3g; Protein: 1g

Chicken Waffles

(Prep + Cook Time: 20 minutes | **Servings:** 4)

Ingredients:
- 1½ cups chicken; cooked and shredded
- 1/2 cup hot sauce
- 1 cup almond flour
- 2 green onions; chopped
- 1/2 cup tapioca flour
- 2 eggs
- 6 tbsp. coconut flour
- A pinch of cayenne pepper
- 3/4 tsp. baking soda
- 1 tsp. garlic powder
- 1 cup coconut milk
- 1/4 cup ghee+ some more for the waffle iron
- A pinch of sea salt

Instructions:
1. In a bowl; mix almond flour with tapioca flour, coconut one, baking soda, garlic powder and a pinch of salt and stir well.
2. Add chicken, hot sauce, green onions, eggs, milk and 1/4 cup ghee and blend using your mixer.
3. Pour some of the batter into your greased waffle iron, close the lid and make your waffle. Repeat with the rest of the batter, divide waffles between plates and serve them in the morning.

Nutrition Facts Per Serving: Calories: 200; Fat: 11g; Fiber: 1g; Carbs: 7g; Protein: 8g

Beef and Squash Skillet

(**Prep + Cook Time**: 30 minutes | **Servings**: 3)

Ingredients:
- 15 oz. beef; ground
- 2 tbsp. ghee
- 3 garlic cloves; minced
- 2 celery stalks; chopped
- 1 yellow onion; chopped
- A pinch of sea salt
- White pepper to the taste
- 1/2 tsp. coriander; ground
- 1 tsp. cumin; ground
- 1 tsp. garam masala
- 1/2 butternut squash; chopped and already cooked
- 3 eggs
- 1 small avocado; peeled, pitted and chopped
- 15 oz. spinach

Instructions:
1. Put spinach in a heatproof bowl; place in your microwave and cook for 1 minute.
2. Squeeze spinach and leave it aside.
3. Heat up a pan with the ghee over medium heat, add onion, garlic, celery, a pinch of salt and white pepper, stir and cook for 3 minutes.
4. Add beef, cumin, garam masala and coriander, stir and cook for a few minutes more.
5. Add squash flesh and spinach, stir and make 3 holes in this mix.
6. Crack an egg into each, cover pan, place in the oven at 375 °F and bake for 15 minutes. Divide this mix on plates and serve with avocado on top.

Nutrition Facts Per Serving: Calories: 400; Fat: 23g; Fiber: 7g; Carbs: 8g; Protein: 24g

Ham and Mushroom Breakfast

(**Prep + Cook Time**: 20 minutes | **Servings**: 1)

Ingredients:
- 2 tbsp. ghee
- 1/4 cup coconut milk
- 3 eggs
- 3.5 oz. smoked ham; chopped
- 3 oz. mushrooms; sliced
- 1 cup arugula; torn
- A pinch of black pepper

Instructions:
1. Heat up a pan with half of the ghee over medium heat, add mushrooms, stir and cook for 3 minutes.
2. Add ham, stir; cook for 2-3 minutes more and transfer everything to a plate.
3. In a bowl; mix eggs with coconut milk and black pepper and whisk well.
4. Heat up the pan with the rest of the ghee over medium heat, add eggs, spread into the pan, cook for a couple of minutes, start stirring and cook until eggs are completely done.
5. Transfer this to a serving bowl; add mushrooms mix on top and arugula. Toss everything to coat well and serve right away.

Nutrition Facts Per Serving: Calories: 356; Fat: 23g; Fiber: 2g; Carbs: 6g; Protein: 25g

Porridge

(Prep + Cook Time: 16 minutes | **Servings**: 3)

Ingredients:
- 1 big plantain; peeled and mashed
- 1/4 cup flax meal
- 2 cups coconut milk
- 3/4 cup almond meal
- 1 tsp. cinnamon; powder
- A pinch of cloves; ground
- 1/2 tsp. ginger powder
- A pinch of nutmeg; ground
- Maple syrup for serving
- Some unsweetened coconut flakes for serving

Instructions:
1. In a small pan, mix plantain with flax meal, almond meal, coconut milk, cinnamon, cloves, ginger and nutmeg, stir well, bring to a simmer over medium heat and cook for about 6 minutes.
2. Divide your porridge into bowls, top with coconut flakes and maple syrup and serve.

Nutrition Facts Per Serving: Calories: 140; Fat: 3g; Fiber: 2g; Carbs: 5g; Protein: 6g

Chorizo Breakfast Skillet

(Prep + Cook Time: 40 minutes | **Servings**: 2)

Ingredients:
- 1 small avocado; peeled, pitted and chopped
- 1/2 cup beef stock
- 1 lb. chorizo; chopped
- 2 poblano peppers; chopped
- 1 cup kale; chopped
- 8 mushrooms; chopped
- 1/2 yellow onion; chopped
- 3 garlic cloves; minced
- 1/2 cup cilantro; chopped
- 4 bacon slices; chopped
- 4 eggs

Instructions:
1. Heat up a pan over medium heat, add chorizo and bacon, stir and cook until they are browned.
2. Add garlic, peppers and onions, stir and cook for 6 minutes more.
3. Add stock, mushrooms and kale, stir and cook for 4 minutes more.
4. Make holes in this mix, crack an egg in each, place in the oven at 350 °F and bake for 12 minutes. Divide this mix on plates, sprinkle cilantro and avocado on top and serve.

Nutrition Facts Per Serving: Calories: 200; Fat: 6g; Fiber: 3g; Carbs: 6g; Protein: 10g

Apple Pancakes

(Prep + Cook Time: 30 minutes | **Servings**: 18)

Ingredients:
- 2 cups apples; peeled, cored and chopped
- 1 tbsp. coconut oil
- 4 eggs
- 2 tsp. cinnamon powder
- 2 tbsp. honey
- 1 cup almond milk+ 3 tablespoons
- 1 tsp. vanilla extract
- 1/2 cup coconut flour
- A pinch of nutmeg
- 1/2 tsp. baking soda
- 3 tbsp. ghee
- 2 tbsp. maple syrup

Instructions:
1. Heat up a pan with 1 tbsp. oil over medium heat, add apples and cinnamon, stir and cook for 5 minutes.
2. In a bowl; whisk eggs with vanilla, 1 cup milk, honey, baking soda, coconut flour and nutmeg and whisk. Add apples and the rest of the almond milk and stir again well.
3. Heat up a pan with the ghee over medium high heat, pour some of the pancake batter, spread, cook until it's done on one side, flip, cook on the other side as well and transfer to a plate.
4. Repeat with the rest of the batter and serve your pancakes with maple syrup on top.

Nutrition Facts Per Serving: Calories: 340; Fat: 14g; Fiber: 4g; Carbs: 7g; Protein: 12g

Steak and Veggie Breakfast

(**Prep + Cook Time**: 35 minutes | **Servings**: 4)

Ingredients:
- 2 sweet potatoes; chopped
- 3/4 lb. sirloin steak; cut into small pieces
- 1 yellow onion; chopped
- 1 green bell pepper; chopped
- 1 red bell pepper; chopped
- 2 tbsp. bacon fat
- Black pepper to the taste
- A pinch of sea salt
- 1 tomato; sliced
- 4 eggs

Instructions:
1. Heat up a pan with half of the fat over medium high heat, add steak, cook for a few minutes until it browns and takes off heat.
2. Heat up the same pan with the rest of the fat over medium high heat, add green and red peppers and onions, stir and cook for 5 minutes. Add sweet potatoes, stir and cook for 10 minutes more.
3. Add steak pieces, stir well, make 4 holes, crack an egg in each, arrange tomato slices, sprinkle black pepper and a pinch of salt, place in the oven at 350 °F and bake for 12 minutes. Serve warm.

Nutrition Facts Per Serving: Calories: 180; Fat: 4g; Fiber: 3g; Carbs: 6g; Protein: 8g

Breakfast Sliders

(**Prep + Cook Time**: 25 minutes | **Servings**: 3)

Ingredients:
- 3 Portobello mushroom caps
- 4 bacon slices
- 3 eggs
- 4 oz. smoked salmon

Instructions:
1. Heat up a pan over medium high heat, add bacon, cook until it's crispy, transfer to paper towels and drain grease.
2. Heat up the pan with the bacon grease over medium heat and place egg rings in it.
3. Crack and egg in each, cook them for 6 minutes and transfer them to a plate.
4. Heat up the pan again over medium high heat, add mushroom caps, cook the for 5 minutes and transfer them to a platter. Top each mushroom cap with bacon, salmon and eggs. Serve hot.

Nutrition Facts Per Serving: Calories: 180; Fat: 3g; Fiber: 5g; Carbs: 7g; Protein: 8g

Bacon Waffles

(**Prep + Cook Time**: 40 minutes | **Servings**: 4)

Ingredients:
- 2 eggs
- 6 bacon slices
- 1/2 cup coconut milk
- 1 tsp. vanilla extract
- 2 tbsp. maple syrup
- 1/2 tsp. baking soda
- 1¾ cups almond flour
- 2 tbsp. ghee
- Maple syrup for serving

Instructions:
1. Place bacon slices on a lined baking sheet, place in the oven at 400 °F and bake for 20 minutes.
2. Transfer bacon to paper towels, drain grease, crumble them and leave them aside.
3. In a bowl; mix almond flour with baking soda.
4. In another bowl; whisk eggs with vanilla extract, ghee, 2 tbsp. maple syrup and coconut milk.
5. Combine the wet and dry mixtures and stir well.
6. Add crumbled bacon, stir again and pour some of the batter in your waffle iron.
7. Close the lid, cook your waffle for 5 minutes and transfer it to a plate. Repeat with the rest of the batter, divide waffles between plates and serve them with maple syrup on top.

Nutrition Facts Per Serving: Calories: 200; Fat: 12g; Fiber: 4g; Carbs: 7g; Protein: 10g

Coconut Pancakes

(Prep + Cook Time: 20 minutes | **Servings**: 8)

Ingredients:
- 1/4 cup coconut milk
- 1/4 cup coconut flour
- 1/8 tsp. baking soda
- 3 eggs
- 2 tbsp. coconut oil
- 1/2 tsp. vanilla extract
- 2 tbsp. honey
- Maple syrup for serving
- 2 tbsp. melted ghee

Instructions:
1. In a bowl; whisk eggs with honey and coconut oil. Add vanilla, coconut milk, baking soda and coconut flour and stir very well.
2. Heat up a pan with the ghee over medium heat, add some of the batter, spread into the pan, cook until it's golden, flip and cook on the other side as well.
3. Repeat with the rest of the batter, divide your pancakes between plates and serve with maple syrup on top.

Nutrition Facts Per Serving: Calories: 300; Fat: 5g; Fiber: 2g; Carbs: 4g; Protein: 10g

Veggie Omelet Cupcakes

(Prep + Cook Time: 30 minutes | **Servings**: 4)

Ingredients:
- 4 bacon slices; chopped
- A handful spinach; chopped
- 1 white onion; chopped
- 1 red bell pepper; chopped
- 1 green bell pepper; chopped
- 1 yellow bell pepper; chopped
- 1 tomato; chopped
- 8 eggs
- A pinch of sea salt
- Black pepper to the taste

Instructions:
1. Heat up a pan over medium high heat, add bacon, stir; cook until it's crispy, transfer to paper towels, drain grease and leave aside for now.
2. Heat up the same pan with the bacon fat over medium high heat, add onion, stir and cook for 3 minutes.
3. Add tomato, all bell peppers, a pinch of salt and black pepper, stir; cook for a couple more minutes and take off heat.
4. In a bowl; whisk eggs with a pinch of salt and black pepper and mix with veggies and bacon.
5. Stir, divide this into a lined muffin tray, place in the oven at 350 °F and bake for 17 minutes. Leave you special muffins to cool down, divide between plates and serve.

Nutrition Facts Per Serving: Calories: 200; Fat: 4g; Fiber: 2g; Carbs: 5g; Protein: 7g

Side Dish Recipes

Ginger Cauliflower Rice

(Prep + Cook Time: 20 minutes | **Servings**: 4)

Ingredients:
- 5 cups cauliflower florets
- 3 tbsp. coconut oil
- 4 ginger slices; grated
- 1 tbsp. coconut vinegar
- 3 garlic cloves; minced
- 1 tbsp. chives; minced
- A pinch of sea salt
- Black pepper to the taste

Instructions:
1. Put cauliflower florets in a food processor and pulse well.
2. Heat up a pan with the oil over medium high heat, add ginger, stir and cook for 3 minutes.
3. Add cauliflower and garlic, stir and cook for 7 minutes. Add a pinch of salt, black pepper, vinegar and chives, stir; cook for a few seconds more, divide between plates and serve.

Nutrition Facts Per Serving: Calories: 100; Fat: 2g; Fiber: 5g; Carbs: 6g; Protein: 8g

Side Salad

(Prep + Cook Time: 10 minutes | **Servings**: 2)

Ingredients:
- 2 cups arugula
- 1 tbsp. olive oil
- 1 tbsp. balsamic vinegar
- 2 cups kale; torn
- 3 tbsp. red onion; chopped
- 4 kumquats; sliced
- 1 small avocado; pitted, peeled and cubed
- 3 figs; chopped
- 1/2 cup walnuts; chopped

Instructions:
1. In a bowl; mix vinegar with the oil, whisk well and leave aside for now.
2. In a salad bowl; mix arugula with kale, onion, kumquats, avocado, figs and walnuts and stir. Add salad dressing, toss to coat and serve.

Nutrition Facts Per Serving: Calories: 100; Fat: 1g; Fiber: 0g; Carbs: 0g; Protein: 4g

Roasted Cabbage Side Dish

(Prep + Cook Time: 40 minutes | **Servings**: 4)

Ingredients:
- 1 green cabbage head; cut into medium wedges
- A pinch of sea salt
- Black pepper to the taste
- A pinch of red chili flakes
- A pinch of garlic powder
- 2 tbsp. extra virgin olive oil
- Juice from 2 lemons

Instructions:
1. Brush cabbage wedges with olive oil, season with a pinch of sea salt and pepper to the taste, sprinkle garlic powder and pepper flakes and arrange them on a lined baking sheet.
2. Introduce in preheated oven at 450 °F and bake for 15 minutes.
3. Flip cabbage wedges, bake for 15 more minutes, take out of the oven and divide them between plates. Serve as a side dish with lemon juice squeezed on top.

Nutrition Facts Per Serving: Calories: 67; Fat: 6g; Carbs: 1g; Fiber: 2g; Protein: 0; Sugar: 0

French Fries

(Prep + Cook Time: 40 minutes | **Servings**: 3)

Ingredients:
- 2 lbs. sweet potatoes; cut into wedges
- A pinch of sea salt
- Black pepper to the taste
- 1/4 cup ghee
- 3 tsp. thyme and rosemary; dried

Instructions:
1. In a bowl; mix potato wedges with ghee, a pinch of salt and pepper to the taste and dried herbs and toss to coat.
2. Spread potatoes on a lined baking sheet and bake in the oven at 425 °F for 25 minutes. Take potatoes out of the oven, leave them aside for 5 minutes, divide between plates and serve as a side dish.

Nutrition Facts Per Serving: Calories: 120g; Carbs: 12g; Fiber: 4; Sugar: 1g; Protein: 12g

Asparagus and Mushrooms Side Dish

(Prep + Cook Time: 20 minutes | **Servings**: 4)

Ingredients:
- 1 lb. asparagus; trimmed
- A pinch of sea salt
- Black pepper to the taste
- 8 green onions; thinly sliced
- 2 tbsp. coconut oil
- 2 tbsp. red wine vinegar
- 2 tbsp. hazelnuts; toasted and chopped
- 1 lb. mushrooms; chopped

Instructions:
1. In a bowl; mix vinegar with a pinch of sea salt, pepper to the taste and half of the oil and whisk well.
2. Put some water in a pot, bring to a boil over medium heat, add asparagus, cook for 3 minutes, drain and transfer to a bowl filled with cold water.
3. Heat up a pan with the rest of the oil over medium-high heat, add mushrooms and cook them for 4-5 minutes stirring from time to time.
4. Add onions, stir and cook for 1 minute.
5. Add drained asparagus, stir; cook 3 more minutes and take off heat.
6. Add vinegar mix, stir and transfer to plates. Sprinkle hazelnuts at the end and serve as a side dish!

Nutrition Facts Per Serving: Calories: 70; Fat: 2.5g; Carbs: 7g; Fiber: 3.2; Sugar: 2g; Protein: 5g

Asparagus Side Dish

(Prep + Cook Time: 20 minutes | **Servings**: 4)

Ingredients:
- 1/4 cup caramelized pecans; chopped
- 4 bacon slices; already cooked and crumbled
- 1½ lbs. asparagus
- A pinch of sea salt
- Black pepper to the taste
- 2 garlic cloves; minced
- 1 shallot; finely chopped
- 1/2 tsp. red chili flakes
- 2 tsp. mustard
- 1 tsp. maple syrup
- 2 tbsp. ghee
- 2 tsp. balsamic vinegar

Instructions:
1. In a bowl; mix vinegar with mustard, maple syrup, sea salt and pepper to the taste and stir well.
2. Heat up a pan with the ghee over medium high heat, add garlic, shallots and pepper flakes, stir and cook for 2 minutes.
3. Add asparagus, stir and cook for 5 minutes.
4. Add vinegar mix and more pepper, toss to coat and cook for 3 minutes more. Transfer to plates, top with bacon and pecans and serve as a side dish.

Nutrition Facts Per Serving: Calories: 80; Fat: 4g; Carbs: 4g; Fiber: 2; Sugar: 0g; Protein: 2g

Roasted Okra

(Prep + Cook Time: 35 minutes | **Servings**: 3)

Ingredients:
- 18 okra pods; sliced
- A pinch of sea salt
- Black pepper to the taste
- Sweet paprika to the taste
- 1 tbsp. extra virgin olive oil

Instructions:
1. Put okra in a baking dish, season with, paprika, a pinch of salt and pepper to the taste and drizzle olive oil.
2. Introduce in preheated oven at 425 °F and bake for 15 minutes. Take okra out of the oven, leave them to cool down, divide between plates and serve as a side dish.

Nutrition Facts Per Serving: Calories: 76; Fat: 0.8g; Carbs: 16g; Fiber: 7.3; Sugar: 2.7g; Protein: 4.6

Mashed Cauliflower Dish

(Prep + Cook Time: 35 minutes | **Servings**: 4)

Ingredients:
- 4 bacon slices; already cooked and crumbled
- 2 garlic cloves; finely chopped
- 6 cups cauliflower florets
- 2 green onions; thinly sliced
- A pinch of sea salt
- Black pepper to the taste
- 3 tbsp. ghee

Instructions:
1. Put water in a pot, place on stove over medium-high heat and bring to a boil.
2. Add cauliflower, cook for 20 minutes, drain water and leave cauliflower in the pot.
3. Add a pinch of salt, pepper to the taste and the ghee and mash everything using a hand mixer. Transfer to plates, sprinkle crumbled bacon and chopped green onions on top and serve as a side dish.

Nutrition Facts Per Serving: Calories: 70; Fat: 15g; Carbs: 9; Sugar: 2g; Fiber: 3g; Protein: 7g

Braised Cabbage Side Dish

(Prep + Cook Time: 30 minutes | **Servings**: 4)

Ingredients:
- 1 small cabbage head; shredded
- 2 tbsp. water
- 6 oz. bacon; chopped
- A pinch of black pepper
- A pinch of sweet paprika
- 1 tbsp. dill; chopped

Instructions:
1. Put bacon in a pan and heat up over medium high heat.
2. Stir and cook for 8 minutes.
3. Add cabbage and 1 tbsp. water, stir and cook for 5 minutes.
4. Add the rest of the water, black pepper, paprika and dill, stir and cook for 5 minutes more. Divide between plates and serve as a side dish!

Nutrition Facts Per Serving: Calories: 90; Fat: 2g; Fiber: 2g; Carbs: 8g; Protein: 6g

Roasted Beets

(Prep + Cook Time: 1 hour 10 minutes | **Servings**: 4)

Ingredients:
- 2 tbsp. extra virgin olive oil
- 6 beets; cut into quarters and then thinly sliced
- A pinch of sea salt
- Black pepper to the taste
- 1/2 cup balsamic vinegar
- 1 tsp. orange zest
- 2 tsp. maple syrup

Instructions:
1. Arrange beets on a lined baking sheet, add a pinch of salt and pepper and the olive oil, toss to coat well, introduce in preheated oven at 325 °F and roast for 45 minutes.
2. Heat up a pan over medium heat, add vinegar and maple syrup, stir well, cook until vinegar is reduced and take off heat.
3. Take beets out of the oven, leave them to cool down a bit, transfer to plates, drizzle the glaze on top, sprinkle orange zest and serve right away as a side dish.

Nutrition Facts Per Serving: Calories: 80; Fat: 1g; Carbs: 8g; Fiber: 2; Sugar: 7g; Protein: 2g

Kale Dish

(Prep + Cook Time: 18 minutes | **Servings**: 4)

Ingredients:
- 3 oz. bacon; chopped
- 1 bunch kale; roughly chopped
- 1/2 cup veggie stock
- 1 tbsp. lemon juice
- 1 garlic clove; minced
- Black pepper to the taste

Instructions:
1. Put bacon in a pan and heat it up over medium high heat.
2. Cook for 3 minutes, stirring all the time.
3. Add kale, stock and black pepper to the taste, stir and cook for 4 minutes. Add lemon juice and garlic, stir; cook for 1 minute more, divide between plates and serve as a side dish.

Nutrition Facts Per Serving: Calories: 150; Fat: 5g; Fiber: 2g; Carbs: 4g; Protein: 3g

Roasted Bell Peppers

(Prep + Cook Time: 1 hour 10 minutes | **Servings**: 4)

Ingredients:
- 6 bell peppers (green; yellow and red)
- 1 garlic clove; finely minced
- 2 tbsp. capers
- 2 tbsp. extra virgin olive oil
- 1/4 cup red wine vinegar
- A pinch of sea salt
- Black pepper to the taste
- 2 tbsp. parsley; finely chopped

Instructions:
1. Arrange bell peppers on a lined baking sheet, introduce them in the oven at 400 °F and bake for 40 minutes.
2. Transfer bell peppers to a bowl; cover and leave them aside for 15 minutes.
3. Peel bell peppers, discard seeds, cut into strips and transfer them to a bowl.
4. Add a pinch of sea salt and pepper to the taste, vinegar, oil, garlic, capers and parsley and toss to coat. Divide between plates and serve as a side dish.

Nutrition Facts Per Serving: Calories: 98; Fat: 1g; Carbs: 10g; Fiber: 3; Sugar: 2g; Protein: 2g

Roasted Cherry Tomatoes

(Prep + Cook Time: 25 minutes | **Servings**: 4)

Ingredients:
- 2 tbsp. extra virgin olive oil
- 20 oz. colored cherry tomatoes; cut in halves
- 6 garlic cloves; finely minced
- A pinch of sea salt
- Black pepper to the taste
- 1 tbsp. basil leaves; finely chopped

Instructions:
1. In a large bowl; mix tomatoes with a pinch of sea salt, pepper to the taste, olive oil, garlic and basil and toss to coat.
2. Spread these on a lined baking dish, introduce in the oven at 375 °F and bake for 20 minutes.
3. Take tomatoes out of the oven, leave them to cool down, divide to plates and serve as a side dish for a frittata for example.

Nutrition Facts Per Serving: Calories: 35; Fat: 2.4g; Carbs: 2g; Fiber: 0.4; Sugar: 0g; Protein: 0.4

Sweet Potatoes Dish

(Prep + Cook Time: 55 minutes | **Servings**: 4)

Ingredients:
- 3 sweet potatoes; pricked with a fork and ends cut off
- A pinch of sea salt
- 1/2 cup coconut milk
- 1/4 cup coconut; toasted and shredded
- 2 tbsp. cilantro; chopped
- Seeds from 1 pomegranate
- 1 lime; cut into wedges

Instructions:
1. Arrange potatoes on a lined baking sheet, introduce in the oven at 400 °F and bake for 45 minutes.
2. Take sweet potatoes out of the oven, leave them to cool down, peel and mash them with a fork and put in a bowl.
3. Add a pinch of sea salt, shredded coconut, coconut milk and pomegranate seeds and stir well. Transfer to plates and serve as a side dish.

Nutrition Facts Per Serving: Calories: 160; Fat: 1g; Carbs: 20g; Fiber: 4; Sugar: 2g; Protein: 5g

Pumpkin Salad

(Prep + Cook Time: 40 minutes | **Servings**: 6)

Ingredients:
- 1 tbsp. honey + 2 tsp. honey
- 2 tbsp. olive oil + 2 tsp. olive oil
- 21 oz. pumpkin; peeled, seeded and cut into medium pieces
- 2 tsp. sesame seeds
- 1 tbsp. lemon juice
- 2 tsp. mustard
- 4 oz. baby spinach
- 2 tbsp. pine nuts; toasted
- A pinch of sea salt
- Black pepper to the taste

Instructions:
1. In a bowl; mix pumpkin with a pinch of salt, black pepper, 2 tsp. oil and 2 tsp. honey, toss to coat well, spread on a lined baking sheet, place in the oven at 400 °F and bake for 25 minutes.
2. Leave pumpkin pieces to cool down a bit, add sesame seeds, toss to coat, place in the oven again and bake for 5 minutes more.
3. In a bowl; mix lemon juice with 1 tbsp. honey, 2 tbsp. oil and mustard and stir well.
4. Leave pumpkin to completely cool down and transfer it to a salad bowl.
5. Add baby spinach and pine nuts and stir. Add salad dressing you've made, toss to coat well, divide between plates and serve as a side salad.

Nutrition Facts Per Serving: Calories: 220; Fat: 10g; Fiber: 2g; Carbs: 7g; Protein: 6g

Roasted Beets

(Prep + Cook Time: 1 hour 10 minutes | **Servings**: 4)

Ingredients:
- 2 tbsp. balsamic vinegar
- 8 beets; cut in quarters
- 1 tbsp. melted coconut oil
- 1/4 tsp. truffle salt

Instructions:
1. In a bowl; mix beets with vinegar, oil and truffle salt, toss to coat well and spread them on a lined baking sheet.
2. Introduce beets in the oven at 350 °F and roast them for 1 hour. Divide beets between plates and serve them.

Nutrition Facts Per Serving: Calories: 150; Fat: 3g; Fiber: 3g; Carbs: 5g; Protein: 10g

Fennel Side Dish

(Prep + Cook Time: 10 minutes | **Servings**: 4)

Ingredients:
- 3 tbsp. lemon juice
- 1 lb. fennel; chopped
- A pinch of sea salt
- 2 tbsp. olive oil
- A pinch of black pepper

Instructions:
1. In a salad bowl; mix fennel with a pinch of salt and black pepper and stir.
2. In another bowl; mix oil with a pinch of salt, pepper and lemon juice and whisk well.
3. Add this to the salad bowl; toss to coat well and divide between plates. Serve as a Paleo side.

Nutrition Facts Per Serving: Calories: 100; Fat: 1g; Fiber: 1g; Carbs: 1g; Protein: 3g

Zucchini and Leeks Side Dish

(Prep + Cook Time: 20 minutes | **Servings**: 4)

Ingredients:
- 2 zucchinis, sliced
- 2 leeks, sliced lengthwise
- 1/4 cup extra virgin olive oil
- 1/3 cup walnuts, toasted and chopped
- 1/4 cup cilantro, chopped
- 1/4 cup parsley, chopped
- A pinch of sea salt
- Black pepper to the taste
- Juice of 1 lemon
- 2 garlic cloves, minced

Instructions:
1. Season leeks and zucchinis with a pinch of sea salt and pepper to the taste, arrange them on heated grill over medium-high heat and cook them for 8 minutes, flipping them from time to time.
2. Transfer veggies to a bowl; add walnuts, parsley, oil, cilantro, garlic and lemon. Toss to coat and serve as a side dish.

Nutrition Facts Per Serving: Calories: 120; Fat: 20g; Carbs: 12; Sugar: 0g; Fiber: 1g; Protein: 4g

Veggie Mix

(Prep + Cook Time: 1 hour 40 minutes | **Servings**: 8)

Ingredients:
- 1 lb. yellow squash; peeled and chopped
- 1 yellow onion; chopped
- 3 tbsp. olive oil
- 2 garlic cloves; minced
- 2 cups chicken stock
- 4 lbs. mixed sweet potatoes; parsnips and carrots, chopped
- 1 cup white wine
- A pinch of black pepper

Instructions:
1. Heat up a pan with half of the oil over medium high heat, add onion, stir; cook for 10 minutes and transfer to a baking dish.
2. Add the rest of the oil to the pan and heat up again over medium heat.
3. Add squash, stir and cook for 10 minutes more.
4. Add garlic, stir and cook for 2 minutes.
5. Add stock, wine and a pinch of black pepper, stir; cook for 10 minutes more, transfer to a blender and pulse really well.
6. Spread this over sautéed onions from the baking dish, also add mixed veggies, toss a bit, place in the oven at 400 °F and bake for 1 hour. Divide between plates and serve warm as a side dish.

Nutrition Facts Per Serving: Calories: 230; Fat: 4g; Fiber: 4g; Carbs: 6g; Protein: 12g

Sautéed Spinach Dish

(Prep + Cook Time: 43 minutes | **Servings**: 3)

Ingredients:
- 3 cups spinach; torn
- 3 yellow onions; sliced
- 3 garlic cloves; finely minced
- A pinch of sea salt
- Black pepper to the taste
- 10 mushrooms; sliced
- 1 tbsp. coconut oil
- 1 tbsp. balsamic vinegar
- 1 tbsp. ghee

Instructions:
1. Heat up a pan with the oil and ghee over medium-high heat, add garlic and onions, stir and cook for 10 minutes.
2. Reduce temperature to low and cook onions for 20 minutes, stirring from time to time.
3. Add vinegar, mushrooms, salt and pepper, stir and cook for 10 minutes. Add spinach, stir; cook for 3 minutes more, take off heat, divide among plates and serve.

Nutrition Facts Per Serving: Calories: 89; Fat: 7g; Carbs: 3.7g; Fiber: 1.4; Sugar: 0.3g; Protein: 2g

Butternut Squash

(Prep + Cook Time: 45 minutes | **Servings**: 6)

Ingredients:
- 2 lbs. butternut squash; peeled, seeded and cubed
- 2 tbsp. coconut oil; melted
- 2 tsp. thyme; chopped
- A pinch of black pepper

Instructions:
1. In a bowl; mix squash cubes with oil, thyme and pepper and toss to coat well.
2. Spread this on a lined baking sheet, place in the oven at 425 °F and bake for 35 minutes, stirring every once in a while.
3. Leave roasted squash pieces to cool down, divide between plates and serve as a Paleo side.

Nutrition Facts Per Serving: Calories: 100; Fat: 1g; Fiber: 2g; Carbs: 3g; Protein: 6g

Kale and Beets

(**Prep + Cook Time**: 40 minutes | **Servings**: 4)

Ingredients:
- 3 beets; cut into quarters and thinly sliced
- 1 tbsp. coconut oil
- 4 cups kale; torn
- 2 tbsp. water
- A pinch of cayenne pepper

Instructions:
1. Put water in a pot, add beets, bring to a boil over medium high heat, cover, reduce temperature, cook for 20 minutes and drain.
2. Heat up a pan with the oil over medium high heat, add kale and the water, stir and cook for 10 minutes.
3. Add beets and cayenne pepper, stir; cook for 2 minutes more, divide between plates and serve as a side dish!

Nutrition Facts Per Serving: Calories: 120; Fat: 2g; Fiber: 1g; Carbs: 2g; Protein: 4g

Grilled Artichokes

(**Prep + Cook Time**: 40 minutes | **Servings**: 4)

Ingredients:
- 2 artichokes; trimmed and cut into halves lengthwise
- 4 garlic cloves; chopped
- 3/4 cup extra virgin olive oil
- Juice of 1 lemon
- A pinch of sea salt
- Black pepper to the taste

Instructions:
1. Put water in a bowl; add half of the lemon juice and artichoke halves and leave aside for now.
2. Put water in a bowl; place on stove over medium high heat, bring to a boil, add artichokes, cook for 15 minutes and drain them.
3. Put artichokes in a bowl; add the rest of the lemon juice, the oil, a pinch of salt, black pepper to the taste and garlic and toss to coat.
4. Drain artichokes and reserve lemon dressing, arrange them on preheated grill over medium-high heat, grill them for 10 minutes and transfer them to a plate. Serve as a side dish with the reserved dressing drizzled on top.

Nutrition Facts Per Serving: Calories: 119; Fat: 3.8g; Carbs: 23g; Fiber: 11.4g; Protein: 6.1

Slow Cooked Mushrooms

(**Prep + Cook Time**: 4 hours 10 minutes | **Servings**: 4)

Ingredients:
- 24 oz. cremini mushrooms
- 4 garlic cloves; finely minced
- 1/4 cup coconut milk
- 1 cup veggie stock
- 1/4 tsp. thyme; dried
- 1/2 tsp. basil; dried
- 1/2 tsp. oregano; dried
- 1 bay leaf
- 2 tbsp. parsley leaves; chopped
- 2 tbsp. ghee
- Black pepper to the taste
- A pinch of sea salt

Instructions:
1. In your slow cooker, mix mushrooms with garlic, basil, oregano, thyme, parsley and bay leaf.
2. Add coconut milk, ghee, veggie stock, salt and pepper, stir; cover pot and cook on Low for 4 hours.
3. Uncover pot, discard bay leaf, transfer to plates and serve as a side dish.

Nutrition Facts Per Serving: Calories: 100; Fat: 10g; Carbs: 6; Sugar: 1g; Fiber: 1g; Protein: 5g

Pumpkin Fries

(Prep + Cook Time: 45 minutes | **Servings**: 4)

Ingredients:
- 1 big pumpkin; peeled and cut in medium fries
- 1 tbsp. sriracha sauce
- 1 tbsp. maple syrup
- 1 tbsp. coconut oil; melted

Instructions:
1. Drizzle the oil on a lined baking sheet, add pumpkin fries and toss them well.
2. Add maple syrup and sriracha, toss to coat well again, place in the oven at 400 °F and bake for 35 minutes.
3. Divide pumpkin fries between plates and serve them as a Paleo side dish.

Nutrition Facts Per Serving: Calories: 60; Fat: 2g; Fiber: 1g; Carbs: 1g; Protein: 1g

Roasted Cauliflower

(Prep + Cook Time: 40 minutes | **Servings**: 4)

Ingredients:
- 1 cauliflower head; florets separated
- 1/4 cup coconut oil; melted
- 1/4 cup parsley; chopped
- 2 tsp. lemon zest; grated
- A pinch of sea salt and black pepper
- 10 garlic cloves; minced

Instructions:
1. Spread cauliflower florets on a lined baking sheet, add oil and toss to coat.
2. Add a pinch of salt and black pepper, garlic and lemon zest, toss again to coat well, place in the oven at 450 °F and bake for 30 minutes.
3. Take cauliflower out of the oven, sprinkle parsley on top, stir gently, divide between plates and serve.

Nutrition Facts Per Serving: Calories: 100; Fat: 1g; Fiber: 2g; Carbs: 4g; Protein: 12g

Mushrooms and Thyme Side Dish

(Prep + Cook Time: 35 minutes | **Servings**: 4)

Ingredients:
- 4 garlic cloves; finely chopped
- 2 tbsp. extra virgin olive oil
- 8 thyme springs
- 16 oz. mushrooms
- A pinch of sea salt
- White pepper to the taste

Instructions:
1. Grease a baking dish with some of the oil and spread thyme on the bottom.
2. Add mushrooms, garlic, season them with a pinch of salt and pepper to the taste and drizzle the rest of the olive oil all over.
3. Introduce dish in the oven at 375 °F and bake for 25 minutes. Take mushrooms out of the oven, divide between plates, pour pan sauces over them and serve as a side dish.

Nutrition Facts Per Serving: Calories: 131; Fat: 7g; Carbs: 10g; Fiber: 3; Sugar: 2. protein 8.1

Mashed Sweet Potatoes

(Prep + Cook Time: 1 hour 25 minutes | **Servings**: 6)

Ingredients:
- 3 lbs. sweet potatoes
- 1/4 cup coconut oil
- A pinch of sea salt
- Black pepper to the taste

Instructions:
1. Wash sweet potatoes and arrange them on a lined baking sheet.
2. Place in the oven at 375 °F and bake them for 1 hour.
3. Leave potatoes to cool down, peel and transfer flesh to a baking dish.
4. Mash them well, add oil and stir very well.

5. Also, add a pinch of salt and black pepper to the taste, stir well again and bake in the oven at 375 °F for 15 minutes more. Divide between plates and serve as a side dish.

Nutrition Facts Per Serving: Calories: 240; Fat: 1g; Fiber: 4g; Carbs: 6g; Protein: 4g

Roasted Carrots

(**Prep + Cook Time**: 40 minutes | **Servings**: 4)

Ingredients:
- 1½ lbs. young carrots (yellow; purple and red ones)
- 2 tbsp. balsamic vinegar
- 2 garlic cloves; finely minced
- 2 tbsp. coconut oil; melted
- A pinch of sea salt
- 1 tbsp. honey
- Black pepper to the taste
- A handful parsley leaves; finely chopped

Instructions:
1. In a bowl; mix vinegar with oil, honey, garlic, a pinch of salt and pepper to the taste and stir very well.
2. Add carrots and toss to coat. Transfer this to a baking dish, introduce in the oven at 400 °F and bake for 30 minutes.
3. Take carrots out of the oven, sprinkle parsley on top, toss gently and serve right away as a side dish.

Nutrition Facts Per Serving: Calories: 40g; Carbs: 20g; Protein: 2; Fat: 6; Sugar: 1g; Fiber: 1

Butternut Squash Mix

(**Prep + Cook Time**: 40 minutes | **Servings**: 4)

Ingredients:
- 1½ lbs. butternut squash; peeled, seeded and cubed
- 1 green plantain; peeled and cubed
- 1/2 tsp. cinnamon powder
- 2 tbsp. red palm oil
- 2 apples; peeled, cored and cubed

Instructions:
1. In a baking dish, mix apples with plantain, squash, cinnamon and oil, toss to coat, place in the oven at 350 °F and roast for 30 minutes.
2. Leave this mix to cool down a bit before dividing on plates and serving.

Nutrition Facts Per Serving: Calories: 100; Fat: 2g; Fiber: 2g; Carbs: 4g; Protein: 10g

Pumpkin and Bok Choy

(**Prep + Cook Time**: 25 minutes | **Servings**: 4)

Ingredients:
- 4 bok choy heads; cut in quarters
- 2 garlic cloves; minced
- 1 small pumpkin; peeled, seeded and thinly sliced
- 2 tsp. sesame oil
- 2 tbsp. olive oil
- 3 tbsp. coconut aminos
- 1 inch ginger; grated
- A pinch of red pepper flakes
- 1 tbsp. sesame seeds; toasted

Instructions:
1. Heat up a pan with the sesame and olive oil over medium heat, add coconut aminos, garlic, pepper flakes and ginger, stir; cook for 1 minute and take off heat.
2. Heat up another pan, add some water, bring to a simmer over medium high heat, add pumpkin pieces, cover and cook them for 10 minutes.
3. Drain pumpkin slices really well and transfer them to a platter.
4. Add bok choy to the pan with the water, heat it up again over medium high heat, cover and cook for 5 minutes.
5. Drain this as well and add to the same platter with the pumpkin. Add sesame oil mix from the pan, add sesame seeds as well, toss everything and serve as a side dish.

Nutrition Facts Per Serving: Calories: 160; Fat: 2g; Fiber: 2g; Carbs: 4g; Protein: 5g

Side Dish

(Prep + Cook Time: 1 hour 10 minutes | **Servings**: 4)

Ingredients:
- 1½ lbs. turnips; thinly sliced
- 6 cups cauliflower florets
- 1 egg
- 2 cups chicken stock
- 1/4 cup avocado oil
- A pinch of sea salt
- Black pepper to the taste

Instructions:
1. Put stock in a pot, bring to a simmer over medium high heat, add cauliflower, stir; cover and cook for 15 minutes.
2. Transfer this to your food processor and blend well.
3. Add oil and blend well again.
4. In a bowl; whisk the egg with 1 tbsp. of the cauliflower mix.
5. Add this to cauliflower and pulse again well.
6. Add a pinch of salt and pepper and stir again.
7. Arrange turnips slices into a baking dish, pour the cauliflower purée over them, place in the oven at 375 °F and bake for 30 minutes. Divide between plates and serve.

Nutrition Facts Per Serving: Calories: 230; Fat: 3g; Fiber: 2g; Carbs: 4g; Protein: 6g

Butternut Squash Side Dish

(Prep + Cook Time: 50 minutes | **Servings**: 4)

Ingredients:
- 1 butternut squash; peeled and chopped
- 3 garlic cloves; finely minced
- 2 tbsp. coconut oil
- 1 tbsp. thyme; chopped
- A pinch of sea salt
- Black pepper to the taste

Instructions:
1. Heat up a pan with the oil over medium-high heat, add garlic, squash and thyme, stir and cook for 5-6 minutes.
2. Spread well in the pan and cook for another 5 minutes. Reduce heat, cover pan and cook for 10 more minutes, stirring from time to time.
3. Add a pinch of salt and pepper to the taste, stir again, take off heat, transfer to plates and serve as a side dish.

Nutrition Facts Per Serving: Calories: 83; Fat: 2.4g; Carbs: 16g; Fiber: 3; Sugar: 3g; Protein: 1.4

Roasted Green Beans

(Prep + Cook Time: 30 minutes | **Servings**: 4)

Ingredients:
- 1½ lbs. green beans
- 2 tbsp. lemon juice
- A pinch of sea salt
- 3 tbsp. avocado oil

Instructions:
1. In a bowl; mix green beans with a pinch of salt, oil and lemon juice, toss to coat well, spread on a lined baking sheet, place in the oven at 450 °F and roast for 20 minutes.
2. Leave green beans to cool down a bit, divide them between plates and serve.

Nutrition Facts Per Serving: Calories: 100; Fat: 3g; Fiber: 1g; Carbs: 4g; Protein: 9g

Poached Kohlrabi Dish

(**Prep + Cook Time**: 27 minutes | **Servings**: 3)

Ingredients:
- 3 kohlrabi; peeled and cubed
- 4 tbsp. ghee
- 1 tbsp. sage; chopped
- A pinch of sea salt and black pepper

Instructions:
1. Heat up a pan with the ghee over medium high heat, add kohlrabi, a pinch of salt and black pepper, stir and cook for 15 minutes.
2. Add sage, stir again, cook for 2 minutes more, divide between plates and serve.

Nutrition Facts Per Serving: Calories: 120; Fat: 2g; Fiber: 1g; Carbs: 2g; Protein: 5g

Stir Fried Side Dish

(**Prep + Cook Time**: 25 minutes | **Servings**: 4)

Ingredients:
- 1 lb. white mushrooms; sliced
- 1 bunch turnip greens; trimmed
- 2 garlic cloves; minced
- 1/2 cup raw almonds
- 1/4 cup lime juice
- 2 tbsp. coconut oil; melted
- 1 tbsp. coconut aminos
- 2 tsp. arrowroot flour
- 1 tsp. ginger; grated
- Black pepper to the taste
- A pinch of sea salt

Instructions:
1. Heat up a pan with the oil over medium high heat, add mushrooms and turnips greens, stir and cook for 2 minutes.
2. Add ginger and garlic, stir and cook for 2 minutes more.
3. Add lime juice, almonds, arrowroot, coconut aminos, a pinch of salt and black pepper, stir and cook for 10 minutes more. Stir your mix again, divide it between plates and serve.

Nutrition Facts Per Serving: Calories: 120; Fat: 2g; Fiber: 2g; Carbs: 4g; Protein: 5g

Mushrooms and Red Chard Side Dish

(**Prep + Cook Time**: 25 minutes | **Servings**: 4)

Ingredients:
- 1/2 lb. brown mushrooms; sliced
- 5 cups kale; roughly chopped
- 1½ tbsp. coconut oil
- 3 cups red chard; chopped
- 2 tbsp. water
- Black pepper to the taste

Instructions:
1. Heat up a pan with the oil over medium high heat, add mushrooms, stir and cook for 5 minutes.
2. Add red chard, kale and water, stir and cook for 10 minutes.
3. Add black pepper to the taste, stir and cook for a couple more minutes. Divide between plates and serve.

Nutrition Facts Per Serving: Calories: 100; Fat: 1g; Fiber: 1g; Carbs: 5g; Protein: 3g

Mashed Carrots

(Prep + Cook Time: 26 minutes | **Servings**: 4)

Ingredients:
- 1 lb. rutabaga; peeled and chopped
- 1 lb. carrots; chopped
- 4 tbsp. ghee
- 1 tbsp. parsley; chopped
- A pinch of sea salt
- Black pepper to the taste

Instructions:
1. Put rutabaga and carrots in a pot, add water to cover, place on stove, bring to a boil over medium-high heat, reduce temperature, cover pot and cook for 20 minutes.
2. Drain carrots and rutabaga, transfer them to a bowl; mash with a potato masher, mix with ghee, a pinch of salt and pepper to the taste, stir well and divide among plates. Sprinkle parsley on top and serve as a side dish.

Nutrition Facts Per Serving: Calories: 100; Fat: 1g; Carbs: 11g; Fiber: 3.5; Sugar: 3g; Fiber: 1.4

Spaghetti Squash

(Prep + Cook Time: 65 minutes | **Servings**: 4)

Ingredients:
- 1 spaghetti squash; cut in halves and seeded
- 12 sage leaves
- 3 tbsp. ghee
- A pinch of sea salt
- Black pepper to the taste

Instructions:
1. Place spaghetti squash on a lined baking sheet, place in the oven at 375 °F and bake for 40 minutes.
2. Take spaghetti squash out of the oven and scoop strings of flesh.
3. Heat up a pan with the ghee over medium heat, add sage, cook for 5 minutes and transfer them to paper towels.
4. Heat up the pan again over medium heat, add spaghetti squash, a pinch of sea salt and black pepper to the taste, stir and cook for 3 minutes. Crumble sage leaves, add them to spaghetti, stir; divide between plates and serve as a side.

Nutrition Facts Per Serving: Calories: 100; Fat: 6g; Fiber: 2g; Carbs: 6g; Protein: 2g

Squash and Cranberries

(Prep + Cook Time: 40 minutes | **Servings**: 2)

Ingredients:
- 2 garlic cloves; minced
- 1 small yellow onion; chopped
- 1 butternut squash; peeled and cubed
- 12 oz. canned coconut milk
- 1 tbsp. coconut oil
- 1 tsp. curry powder
- 1 tsp. cinnamon powder
- 1/2 cup cranberries

Instructions:
1. Spread squash pieces on a lined baking sheet, place in the oven at 425 °F and bake for 15 minutes.
2. Take squash out of the oven and leave aside for now.
3. Heat up a pan with the oil over medium high heat, add garlic and onion, stir and cook for 5 minutes.
4. Add roasted squash, stir and cook for 3 minutes.
5. Add coconut milk, cranberries, cinnamon and curry powder, stir and cook for 5 minutes more. Divide between plates and serve as a side dish!

Nutrition Facts Per Serving: Calories: 100; Fat: 2g; Fiber: 4g; Carbs: 8g; Protein: 2g

Mint Zucchini

(Prep + Cook Time: 17 minutes | **Servings**: 4)

Ingredients:
- 2 zucchinis; cut into halves and then slice into half moons
- 2 tbsp. mint
- 1 tbsp. coconut oil
- 1/2 tbsp. dill; chopped
- A pinch of cayenne pepper

Instructions:
1. Heat up a pan with the oil over medium high heat, add zucchinis, stir and cook for 6 minutes.
2. Add cayenne, dill and mint, stir; cook for 1 minute more, divide between plates and serve.

Nutrition Facts Per Serving: Calories: 80; Fat: 0g; Fiber: 1g; Carbs: 1g; Protein: 5g

Spicy Sweet Potatoes

(Prep + Cook Time: 50 minutes | **Servings**: 4)

Ingredients:
- 4 sweet potatoes; peeled and thinly sliced
- 2 tsp. nutmeg
- 2 tbsp. coconut oil; melted
- Cayenne pepper to the taste

Instructions:
1. In a bowl; mix sweet potato slices with nutmeg, cayenne and oil and toss to coat really well.
2. Spread these on a lined baking sheet, place in the oven at 350 °F and bake for 25 minutes.
3. Take potatoes out of the oven, flip them, put them back into the oven and bake for 15 minutes more. Serve as a tasty Paleo side dish!

Nutrition Facts Per Serving: Calories: 140; Fat: 3g; Fiber: 2g; Carbs: 4g; Protein: 10g

Chard Side Dish

(Prep + Cook Time: 20 minutes | **Servings**: 2)

Ingredients:
- 1/2 cup cashews; chopped
- 1 bunch chard; cut into thin strips
- A pinch of sea salt
- Black pepper to the taste
- 1 tbsp. coconut oil

Instructions:
1. Heat up a pan with the oil over medium heat, add chard and cashews, stir and cook for 10 minutes.
2. Add a pinch of salt and pepper to the taste, stir; cook for 1 minute more, take off heat, transfer to plates and serve as a side dish.

Nutrition Facts Per Serving: Calories: 60; Fat: 0.3g; Carbs: 2g; Fiber: 1g; Protein: 2; Sugar: 0

Basil Zucchini Spaghetti

(Prep + Cook Time: 1 hour 20 minutes | **Servings**: 4)

Ingredients:
- 1/3 cup bacon grease
- 4 zucchinis; cut with a spiralizer
- 1/2 cup walnuts; chopped
- 2 garlic cloves; minced
- 1/4 cup basil; chopped
- A pinch of sea salt
- Black pepper to the taste

Instructions:
1. In a bowl; mix zucchini spaghetti with a pinch of salt and pepper, toss to coat, leave aside for 1 hour, drain well, rinse, drain again and put in a bowl.
2. Heat up a pan with the bacon grease over medium high heat, add zucchini spaghetti and garlic, stir and cook for 5 minutes.
3. Add basil and walnuts and some black pepper, stir and cook for 3 minutes more. Divide between plates and serve.

Nutrition Facts Per Serving: Calories: 240; Fat: 1g; Fiber: 4g; Carbs: 7g; Protein: 13g

Turnips and Sauce

(Prep + Cook Time: 25 minutes | **Servings**: 4)

Ingredients:
- 16 oz. turnips; thinly sliced
- 1 tbsp. lemon juice
- Zest from 2 oranges
- 3 tbsp. coconut oil
- 1 tbsp. rosemary; chopped
- A pinch of sea salt
- Black pepper to the taste

Instructions:
1. Heat up a pan with the oil over medium high heat, add turnips, stir and cook for 4 minutes.
2. Add lemon juice, a pinch of salt, black pepper and rosemary, stir and cook for 10 minutes more. Take off heat, add orange zest, stir; divide between plates and serve.

Nutrition Facts Per Serving: Calories: 90; Fat: 1g; Fiber: 2g; Carbs: 3g; Protein: 4g

Eggplant and Mushrooms

(Prep + Cook Time: 1 hour 40 minutes | **Servings**: 4)

Ingredients:
- 2 lbs. oyster mushrooms; chopped
- 6 oz. bacon; chopped
- 1 yellow onion; chopped
- 2 eggplants; cubed
- 3 celery stalks; chopped
- 1 tbsp. parsley; chopped
- A pinch of sea salt
- Black pepper to the taste
- 1 tbsp. savory; dried
- 3 tbsp. coconut oil

Instructions:
1. Put eggplant pieces in a bowl; add a pinch of salt and black pepper, toss a bit, leave aside for 1 hour, drain well and leave aside in a bowl.
2. Heat up a pan with the oil over medium high heat, add onion, stir and cook for 4 minutes.
3. Add bacon, stir and cook for 4 more minutes.
4. Add eggplant pieces, mushrooms, celery, savory and black pepper to the taste, stir and cook for 15 minutes. Add parsley, stir again, cook for a couple more minutes, divide between plates and serve.

Nutrition Facts Per Serving: Calories: 200; Fat: 3g; Fiber: 3g; Carbs: 6g; Protein: 9g

Cauliflower and Leeks

(Prep + Cook Time: 30 minutes | **Servings**: 4)

Ingredients:
- 1½ cups leeks; chopped
- 1½ cups cauliflower florets
- 2 garlic cloves; minced
- 1½ cups artichoke hearts
- 2 tbsp. bacon grease
- Black pepper to the taste

Instructions:
1. Heat up a pan with the bacon grease over medium high heat, add garlic, leeks, cauliflower florets and artichoke hearts, stir and cook for 20 minutes. Add black pepper, stir; divide between plates and serve.

Nutrition Facts Per Serving: Calories: 110; Fat: 2g; Fiber: 2g; Carbs: 6g; Protein: 3g

Taro Dish

(Prep + Cook Time: 35 minutes | **Servings**: 4)

Ingredients:
- 2 lbs. taro
- 3 tbsp. coconut oil
- 1/2 tsp. garlic powder
- 2 tsp. rosemary; dried
- A pinch of sea salt
- Black pepper to the taste

Instructions:
1. Put taro in a steamer, steam for 15 minutes, leave them to cool down, peel them and cut into quarters.

2. Heat up a pan with the oil over medium high heat, add taro, rosemary, garlic powder, salt and pepper, toss to coat and place in preheated broiler.
3. Broil for 10 minutes, divide between plates and serve as a Paleo side dish.

Nutrition Facts Per Serving: Calories: 120; Fat: 3g; Fiber: 2g; Carbs: 4g; Protein: 7g

Roasted Brussels Sprouts

(Prep + Cook Time: 40 minutes | **Servings**: 6)

Ingredients:
- 1½ lbs. Brussels sprouts; cut in halves
- A pinch of sea salt
- Black pepper to the taste
- 1 tsp. garlic powder
- 2/3 cups pecans; chopped
- 1 cup pomegranate seeds
- 2 tbsp. extra virgin olive oil

Instructions:
1. In a bowl; mix oil with a pinch of sea salt, pepper and garlic powder and stir well.
2. Add Brussels sprouts and pecans and toss to coat. Spread this in lined baking dish, introduce in the oven at 400 °F and bake for 30 minutes.
3. Take sprouts out of the oven, transfer to plates, top with pomegranate seeds and serve as a side dish.

Nutrition Facts Per Serving: Calories: 100; Fat: 1g; Carbs: 10g; Fiber: 4; Sugar: 1g; Protein: 4g

Roasted Broccoli

(Prep + Cook Time: 40 minutes | **Servings**: 4)

Ingredients:
- 8 garlic cloves; minced
- 1/4 cup avocado oil
- 8 cups broccoli florets
- 1/4 cup parsley; chopped
- Zest from 1 lemon; grated
- Black pepper to the taste
- A pinch of sea salt

Instructions:
1. In a bowl; mix broccoli with salt, pepper, oil, garlic and lemon zest, toss to coat, spread on a lined baking sheet, place in the oven at 450 °F and bake for 30 minutes.
2. Take baked broccoli out of the oven, divide between plates, sprinkle parsley on top and serve as a side.

Nutrition Facts Per Serving: Calories: 120; Fat: 1g; Fiber: 2g; Carbs: 3g; Protein: 6g

Stuffed Artichokes

(Prep + Cook Time: 1 hour 20 minutes | **Servings**: 4)

Ingredients:
- 4 artichokes; stems cut off and hearts chopped
- 3 garlic cloves; minced
- 2 cups spinach; chopped
- 1 tbsp. coconut oil
- 1 yellow onion; chopped
- 4 oz. bacon; chopped, cooked and crumbled
- A pinch of black pepper

Instructions:
1. Put artichokes in a pot, add water to cover, bring to a boil over medium heat, cook for 30 minutes, drain them and leave them aside to cool down.
2. Heat up a pan with the oil over medium high heat, add onion, stir and cook for 10 minutes.
3. Add spinach, stir; cook for 3 minutes, take off heat and leave aside to cool down.
4. Put cooked bacon in your food processor, add artichoke insides as well and pulse really well.
5. Add this to spinach and onion mix and stir well everything.
6. Place artichoke cups on a lined baking sheet, stuff them with spinach mix, place in the oven at 375 °F and bake for 30 minutes. Arrange them on plates and serve as a side with a juicy steak.

Nutrition Facts Per Serving: Calories: 200; Fat: 3g; Fiber: 2g; Carbs: 6g; Protein: 8g

Paleo Tapioca Root Fries

(Prep + Cook Time: 1 hour 10 minutes | **Servings**: 4)

Ingredients:
- 2½ lb. tapioca root; cut in medium fries
- 1/2 cup duck fat; soft
- Black pepper to the taste
- A pinch of smoked paprika

Instructions:
1. Put some water in a pot and bring to a boil over medium high heat. Add tapioca fries, boil for 10 minutes and drain them well.
2. Spread them on a lined baking sheet, add black pepper, paprika and duck fat, toss everything to coat well, place in the oven at 375 °F and bake for 45 minutes.
3. Leave your tapioca fries to cool down a bit, divide them between plates and serve as a side.

Nutrition Facts Per Serving: Calories: 120; Fat: 2g; Fiber: 2g; Carbs: 4g; Protein: 10g

Plantain Fries

(Prep + Cook Time: 20 minutes | **Servings**: 4)

Ingredients:
- 1/2 cup duck fat
- 2 green plantains; peeled and sliced
- A pinch of sea salt
- Black pepper to the taste

Instructions:
1. Heat up a pan with the duck fat over medium high heat, season plantain slices with a pinch of salt and black pepper, add half of them to the pan, cook for 5 minutes and transfer to paper towels.
2. Fry the second batch of plantain slices, drain grease as well, divide them between plates and serve them as a side.

Nutrition Facts Per Serving: Calories: 120; Fat: 2g; Fiber: 2g; Carbs: 4g; Protein: 3g

Plantain Mash

(Prep + Cook Time: 40 minutes | **Servings**: 4)

Ingredients:
- 6 oz. bacon; chopped
- 3 green bananas; peeled, cut in halves lengthwise and cut in semi-circles
- 4 garlic cloves; minced
- 1 yellow onion; chopped
- 2 tbsp. coconut oil
- A pinch of sea salt

Instructions:
1. Put water in a pot, bring to a boil over medium high heat, add plantain slices, cover and cook them for 20 minutes.
2. Drain plantains and leave them aside for now.
3. Heat up a pan over medium high heat, add bacon, stir and cook for 5 minutes.
4. Add garlic and onion, stir; cook for 5 minutes more, drain excess grease and transfer everything to a blender.
5. Add plantains and 2 tbsp. oil and pulse really well. Add a pinch of sea salt, blend again, divide between plates and serve.

Nutrition Facts Per Serving: Calories: 200; Fat: 1g; Fiber: 4g; Carbs: 6g; Protein: 2g

Creamy Mashed Pumpkin

(Prep + Cook Time: 55 minutes | **Servings**: 4)

Ingredients:
- 1 cup unsweetened coconut; shredded
- 1 pumpkin; peeled, seeded and cubed
- 1/2 cup coconut oil
- 1 tsp. cinnamon powder
- A pinch of white pepper
- A pinch of sea salt

Instructions:
1. Put water in a pot, add pumpkin cubes, heat up over medium high heat, cover and cook for 30 minutes.
2. Drain water, add a pinch of salt and pepper, oil and coconut to the pan, stir and cook everything for 3 minutes more.
3. Mash using a potato masher, add cinnamon, stir well, cook for 2 minutes more, divide between plates and serve.

Nutrition Facts Per Serving: Calories: 100; Fat: 2g; Fiber: 2g; Carbs: 3g; Protein: 3g

Brussels Sprouts Side Dish

(Prep + Cook Time: 40 minutes | **Servings**: 4)

Ingredients:
- 4 lbs. Brussels sprouts; cut in quarters
- 1/4 cup avocado oil
- A pinch of sea salt
- Black pepper to the taste

Instructions:
1. In a bowl; mix Brussels sprouts with oil, salt and pepper, toss to coat well, spread on a lined baking sheet, place in the oven at 375 °F and bake for 30 minutes.
2. Divide between plates and serve as a Paleo side dish!

Nutrition Facts Per Serving: Calories: 120; Fat: 1g; Fiber: 1g; Carbs: 2g; Protein: 5g

Broccoli and Tasty Hazelnuts

(Prep + Cook Time: 25 minutes | **Servings**: 4)

Ingredients:
- 1 lb. broccoli florets
- 1 tbsp. olive oil
- 1 garlic clove; minced
- 1/3 cup hazelnuts
- Black pepper to the taste

Instructions:
1. Heat up a pan with the oil over medium high heat, add hazelnuts, stir and cook for 5 minutes.
2. Transfer hazelnuts to a bowl and leave them aside for now.
3. Heat up the same pan again over medium high heat, add broccoli and garlic, stir; cover and cook for 6 minutes more. Add hazelnuts and black pepper to the taste, stir; divide between plates and serve.

Nutrition Facts Per Serving: Calories: 130; Fat: 3g; Fiber: 2g; Carbs: 5g; Protein: 6g

Dill Carrots

(Prep + Cook Time: 40 minutes | **Servings**: 4)

Ingredients:
- 1 lb. baby carrots
- 1 tbsp. coconut oil; melted
- 2 tbsp. dill; chopped
- 1 tbsp. honey
- A pinch of black pepper

Instructions:
1. Put carrots in a pot, add water to cover, bring to a boil over medium high heat, cover and simmer for 30 minutes.
2. Drain well, put carrots in a bowl; add melted oil, black pepper, dill and honey, stir very well, divide between plates and serve.

Nutrition Facts Per Serving: Calories: 120; Fat: 2g; Fiber: 3g; Carbs: 5g; Protein: 6g

Kale Dish

(Prep + Cook Time: 30 minutes | **Servings**: 4)

Ingredients:
- 2 celery stalks; chopped
- 5 cups kale; torn
- 1 small red bell pepper; chopped
- 3 tbsp. water
- 1 tbsp. coconut oil

Instructions:
1. Heat up a pan with the oil over medium high heat, add celery, stir and cook for 10 minutes.
2. Add kale, water and bell pepper, stir and cook for 10 minutes more. Divide between plates and serve really soon!

Nutrition Facts Per Serving: Calories: 90; Fat: 1g; Fiber: 2g; Carbs: 2g; Protein: 6g

Soups & Stews Recipes

Veggie and Chorizo Stew

(Prep + Cook Time: 40 minutes | **Servings**: 3)

Ingredients:
- 1 yellow onion; chopped
- 1 tbsp. coconut oil
- 2 chorizo sausages; skinless and thinly sliced
- 1 red bell pepper; chopped
- 1 carrot; thinly sliced
- 1 celery stick; chopped
- 1 tomato; chopped
- 2 garlic cloves; finely minced
- 2 cups chicken broth
- 1 tbsp. lemon juice
- Black pepper to the taste
- 1 zucchini; chopped
- A handful parsley leaves; finely chopped

Instructions:
1. Heat up a pan with the oil over medium-high heat, add chorizo, onion, celery and carrot, stir and cook for 3 minutes.
2. Add red bell pepper, tomatoes and garlic, stir and cook 1 minute.
3. Add lemon juice, stock and pepper, stir; bring to a boil, cover pan, reduce heat to medium and cook for 10 minutes.
4. Add zucchini, stir; cover again and cook for 10 more minutes.
5. Uncover pan, cook the stew for 2 minutes more stirring often. Add parsley, stir; take off heat, transfer to dishes and serve.

Nutrition Facts Per Serving: Calories: 420; Fat: 12g; Carbs: 45g; Fiber: 11; Sugar: 5g; Protein: 33.2

Coconut and Zucchini Soup

(Prep + Cook Time: 25 minutes | **Servings**: 2)

Ingredients:
- 1 brown onion; chopped
- 2 zucchinis; cubed
- 1 tbsp. coconut oil
- A pinch of sea salt
- White pepper to the taste
- 2 tsp. turmeric powder
- 3 garlic cloves; chopped
- 1 tsp. curry powder
- 1 cup coconut milk
- 1 cup veggie stock
- 2 tbsp. lime juice
- Some chopped cilantro for serving

Instructions:
1. Heat up a pot with the oil over medium heat, add onion, stir and cook for 4 minutes.
2. Add garlic, salt, pepper and zucchinis, stir and cook for 1 minute.
3. Add turmeric and curry powder, stir well and cook for 1 minute more.
4. Add coconut milk and stock, stir; bring to a boil, cover pot and simmer soup for 10 minutes. Add lime juice and cilantro, stir; ladle into bowls and serve.

Nutritional value: Calories: 140; Fat: 1g; Fiber: 1g; Carbs: 2g; Protein: 1g

Healthy Veggie Stew

(Prep + Cook Time: 1 hour 10 minutes | **Servings**: 6)

Ingredients:
- 4 lbs. mixed root vegetables (parsnips; carrots, rutabagas, beets, celery root, turnips), chopped
- 6 tbsp. extra virgin olive oil
- 1 garlic head; cloves separated and peeled
- 1/2 cup yellow onion; chopped
- Black pepper to the taste
- 28 oz. canned tomatoes; peeled and chopped
- 1 tbsp. tomato paste
- 2 cups kale leaves; torn
- 1 tsp. oregano; dried
- Tabasco sauce for serving

Instructions:
1. In a baking dish, mix all root vegetables with black pepper, half of the oil and garlic, toss to coat, introduce in the oven at 450 degrees G and roast them for 45 minutes.
2. Heat up a pot with the rest of the oil over medium-high heat, add onions and cook for 2-3 minutes stirring often.
3. Add tomato paste, stir and cook 1 more minute.
4. Add tomatoes and their liquid, some salt and pepper and the oregano, stir; bring to a simmer, reduce heat to low and cook until veggies become roasted.
5. Take root veggies out of the oven, add them to the pot and stir.
6. Add kale, stir and cook for 5 minutes. Add Tabasco sauce to the taste, stir; transfer to bowls and serve.

Nutrition Facts Per Serving: Calories: 150; Fat: 7g; Carbs: 17.2g; Fiber: 3.7; Sugar: 5g; Protein: 2.4

Veggie Soup

(Prep + Cook Time: 55 minutes | **Servings**: 4)

Ingredients:
- 2 sweet potatoes; peeled and chopped
- 2 yellow onions; cut into eighths
- 2 lbs. carrots; diced
- 4 tbsp. coconut oil
- 2 cups chicken stock
- 3 tbsp. maple syrup
- 1 head garlic; cloves peeled
- A pinch of sea salt
- Black pepper to the taste

Instructions:
1. Put onions, carrots, sweet potatoes and garlic in a baking dish, add coconut oil, a pinch of sea salt and pepper to the taste, toss to coat, introduce in the oven at 425 °F and bake for 35 minutes.
2. Take veggies out of the oven, transfer to a pot, add chicken stock and heat everything up on the stove on medium-high heat.
3. Bring soup to a boil, reduce heat to medium, cover and simmer for 10 minutes. Transfer soup to your blender, add more pepper and the maple syrup, pulse well to obtain a cream, pour into soup bowls and serve.

Nutrition Facts Per Serving: Calories: 130; Fat: 3g; Carbs: 12g; Fiber: 3.5; Sugar: 6g; Protein: 3g

Cauliflower Cream

(Prep + Cook Time: 30 minutes | **Servings**: 2)

Ingredients:
- 1 yellow onion; chopped
- 2 tbsp. olive oil
- 1 cauliflower head; florets separated and chopped
- 3 cups veggie stock
- 3 garlic cloves; minced
- Black pepper to the taste
- A pinch of sea salt
- 3/4 cup bacon; chopped
- 1 tsp. coconut oil
- 1 egg
- 2 tbsp. cilantro; chopped

Instructions:
1. Heat up a pot with the olive oil over medium heat, add onion, stir and cook for 4 minutes.
2. Add stock, cauliflower and garlic, stir and bring to a boil.
3. Reduce heat to medium-low, season with a pinch of salt and black pepper to the taste, cover pot and simmer soup for 10 minutes.
4. Meanwhile; heat up a pan with the coconut oil over medium heat, add bacon, cook until it's crispy, transfer to paper towels, drain grease and leave aside for now.
5. Meanwhile; put water in a pot and bring to a boil.
6. Place a bowl on top of boiling water, crack the egg into the bowl; whisk it for 3 minutes and take off heat.
7. Take your cauliflower soup off the heat, blend it using an immersion blender, add whisked egg and blend some more. Ladle into bowls, sprinkle crumbled bacon and cilantro on top and serve.

Nutrition Facts Per Serving: Calories: 200; Fat: 3g; Fiber: 2g; Carbs: 4g; Protein: 7g

Beef and Plantain Stew

(Prep + Cook Time: 5 hours 10 minutes | **Servings**: 4)

Ingredients:
- 6 plantains; skinless and cubed
- 2 lbs. beef meat; cubed
- 3 cups collard greens; chopped
- A pinch of sea salt
- Black pepper to the taste
- 3 cups water
- 1/2 cup sweet paprika
- 3 tbsp. allspice
- 1/4 cup garlic powder
- 1 tsp. chili powder
- 1 tsp. cayenne pepper

Instructions:
1. In your slow cooker, mix beef with plantains, collard greens, water, paprika, garlic powder, allspice, chili powder, cayenne, a pinch of salt and pepper to the taste.
2. Stir, cover pot and cook on High for 5 hours. Uncover slow cooker, leave stew to cool down for a few minutes, transfer to bowls and serve.

Nutrition Facts Per Serving: Calories: 410; Fat: 11g; Carbs: 39g; Fiber: 10g; Protein: 34; Sugar: 5

Lemon and Garlic Soup

(Prep + Cook Time: 20 minutes | **Servings**: 4)

Ingredients:
- 6 cups shellfish stock
- 1 tbsp. garlic; finely minced
- 1 tbsp. coconut oil; melted
- 2 eggs
- 1/2 cup lemon juice
- A pinch of sea salt
- White pepper to the taste
- 1 tbsp. arrowroot powder
- Cilantro; finely chopped for serving

Instructions:
1. Heat up a pot with the oil over medium high heat, add garlic, stir and cook for 2 minutes.
2. Add stock but reserve 1/2 cup, stir and bring to a simmer.
3. Meanwhile; in a bowl, mix eggs with sea salt, pepper, reserved stock, lemon juice and arrowroot and whisk very well.
4. Pour this into soup, stir and cook for a few minutes. Ladle into bowls and serve with chopped cilantro on top.

Nutrition Facts Per Serving: Calories: 135; Fat: 3g; Carbs: 12g; Fiber: 1g; Protein: 8; Sugar: 0

Chicken Stew

(Prep + Cook Time: 8 hours 15 minutes | **Servings**: 6)

Ingredients:
- 5 garlic cloves; finely chopped
- 2 celery stalks; chopped
- 2 yellow onions; chopped
- 2 carrots; chopped
- 30 oz. canned pumpkin puree
- 2 quarts chicken stock
- 2 cups chicken meat; chopped
- 1/4 cup coconut flour
- Black pepper to the taste
- 1/2 lb. baby spinach
- 1/4 tsp. cayenne pepper

Instructions:
1. In your slow cooker, mix chicken meat with onions, carrots, celery, garlic, pumpkin puree, chicken stock, black pepper, flour and cayenne, stir well, cover and cook on low for 7 hours and 50 minutes.
2. Uncover slow cooker, add spinach, cover again and cook for 10 more minutes. Transfer to bowls and serve hot.

Nutrition Facts Per Serving: Calories: 244; Fat: 2g; Carbs: 38g; Fiber: 6; Sugar: 4g; Protein: 20g

Brussels Sprouts Soup

(Prep + Cook Time: 30 minutes | **Servings**: 4)

Ingredients:
- 2 lbs. Brussels sprouts; trimmed and halved
- 2 tbsp. olive oil
- 1 yellow onion; chopped
- 4 cups chicken stock
- 1/4 cup coconut cream
- A pinch of black pepper

Instructions:
1. Heat up a pot with the oil over medium high heat, add onion, stir and cook for 3 minutes.
2. Add Brussels sprouts, stir and cook for 2 minutes.
3. Add stock and black pepper, stir; bring to a simmer and cook for 20 minutes.
4. Use an immersion blender to make your cream, add coconut cream, stir well and ladle into bowls. Serve right away and serve.

Nutrition Facts Per Serving: Calories: 200; Fat: 11g; Fiber: 3g; Carbs: 6g; Protein: 11g

Tasty Turkey Soup

(Prep + Cook Time: 40 minutes | **Servings**: 4)

Ingredients:
- 3½ cups chicken stock
- 3 celery stalks; chopped
- 2 carrots; chopped
- 1 sweet potato; peeled and cubed
- 2 cups turkey meat; cooked and shredded
- 1 yellow onion; chopped
- 3 tbsp. coconut oil
- 1 cup coconut cream
- 1 tbsp. sage; chopped
- 1 tsp. thyme; dried
- A handful parsley; chopped
- Black pepper to the taste
- A pinch of sea salt

Instructions:
1. Heat up a pot with the oil over medium heat, add celery, onions, sweet potato and carrots, stir and cook for 5 minutes.
2. Add stock, a pinch of salt, black pepper to the taste, stir; bring to a simmer and cook for 20 minutes.
3. Add turkey, coconut cream, sage, parsley and thyme, stir; cook for 2 minutes more, ladle into bowls and serve.

Nutrition Facts Per Serving: Calories: 180; Fat: 3g; Fiber: 2g; Carbs: 3g; Protein: 5g

Chicken Soup

(Prep + Cook Time: 1 hour 15 minutes | **Servings**: 4)

Ingredients:
- 3 carrots; chopped
- 1 yellow onion; chopped
- 1 zucchini; chopped
- 12 oz. canned mushrooms; chopped
- 1/4 butternut squash; cubed
- 4 cups chicken meat; already cooked and shredded
- 2 tsp. coconut oil
- 2 tsp. rosemary; dried
- 1 tsp. thyme; dried
- 1 tbsp. apple cider vinegar
- 1 tsp. cumin
- 2½ cups chicken stock
- A pinch of sea salt
- Black pepper to the taste

Instructions:
1. Heat up a pot with the coconut oil over medium heat, add carrots and onion, stir and cook for 5 minutes.
2. Add zucchini, mushrooms and squash, stir and cook for 5 more minutes.
3. Add chicken meat, rosemary, thyme, vinegar, cumin and chicken stock.
4. Stir, bring to a boil, reduce heat to medium-low and simmer for 40 minutes. Add a pinch of salt and pepper to the taste, stir again, take off heat and pour into soup bowls.

Nutrition Facts Per Serving: Calories: 390; Fat: 2g; Carbs: 34g; Protein: 6; Sugar: 0g; Fiber: 4

Delicious Paleo Soup

(Prep + Cook Time: 55 minutes | **Servings**: 6)

Ingredients:
- 1 lb. sausage; chopped
- 28 oz. canned tomatoes; chopped
- 6 oz. tomato paste
- 3 garlic cloves; finely minced
- 14 oz. beef stock
- 6 mushrooms; chopped
- 1 small red bell pepper; chopped
- 5 oz. pepperoni
- 2.5 oz. black olives; chopped
- 1/4 cup water
- 1 yellow onion; finely chopped
- 1 tbsp. avocado oil
- 3 thyme springs; chopped
- A pinch of red pepper flakes

Instructions:
1. Heat up a pot with the oil over medium high heat and melt it.
2. Add half of the onion, garlic and thyme, stir and cook for 5 minutes.
3. Add tomatoes, tomato paste and water, stir; bring to a boil, reduce heat to medium-low and simmer for 20 minutes.
4. Pour this into your blender, pulse well and leave aside for now.
5. Heat up a pot over medium-high heat, add sausage, stir and cook for a few minutes, breaking into small pieces with a fork.
6. Add the rest of the onion, mushrooms and the bell pepper, stir and cook for 5 minutes.
7. Add tomato soup you've blended and beef stock, stir and cook for 5 more minutes.
8. Heat up a pan over medium high heat, add pepperoni slices, stir and cook until they brown. Pour soup into bowls, top with red pepper flakes, olives and pepperoni.

Nutrition Facts Per Serving: Calories: 224; Fat: 16g; Carbs: 8g; Fiber: 3; Sugar: 5.5g; Protein: 7g

Clam Soup

(Prep + Cook Time: 40 minutes | **Servings**: 6)

Ingredients:
- 20 oz. canned clams
- 1 small cauliflower head; florets separated
- 2 carrots; chopped
- 1 onion; chopped
- 2 sweet potatoes; chopped
- 1 celery rib; chopped
- 1 cup coconut milk
- 2 tbsp. coconut oil
- 2 cups chicken stock
- A pinch of sea salt
- Black pepper to the taste

Instructions:
1. Heat up a pot with half of the oil over medium high heat, add half of the onion, cauliflower and stock, stir; bring to a boil and cook for 10 minutes.
2. Use an immersion blender to make cream, transfer this to a bowl and leave aside for now.
3. Heat up the same pot with the rest of the oil over medium high heat, add the rest of the onion, celery, carrot, a pinch of sea salt and black pepper to the taste, stir and cook for 10 minutes.
4. Add potato, 2 cups of the cauliflower cream, stir; bring to a boil and simmer for 10 minutes.
5. Add coconut milk, clams and the rest of the cauliflower cream, stir and cook for 2 minutes more. Ladle into soup bowls and serve.

Nutrition Facts Per Serving: Calories: 250; Fat: 13g; Fiber: 3g; Carbs: 6g; Protein: 12g

Tomato and Basil Soup

(Prep + Cook Time: 45 minutes | **Servings**: 4)

Ingredients:
- 56 oz. canned tomatoes; crushed
- 2 cups tomato juice
- 2 cups chicken stock
- 1/4 lb. coconut butter
- 14 basil leaves; torn
- 1 cup coconut milk
- Salt and black pepper to the taste

Instructions:
1. Put tomatoes, tomato juice and stock in a pot, heat up over medium-high heat, bring to a boil, reduce heat, stir and simmer for 30 minutes.
2. Pour this into your blender, add basil, pulse very well and return to pot.
3. Heat up soup again, add butter and coconut milk, stir and cook on low heat for a few more minutes. Add salt and pepper to the taste, stir well, pour into soup bowls and serve.

Nutrition Facts Per Serving: Calories: 170; Fat: 10g; Carbs: 14g; Protein: 2; Sugar: 1

Beef Soup

(Prep + Cook Time: 1 hour 10 minutes | **Servings**: 6)

Ingredients:
- 1 lb. organic beef; ground
- 1 lb. sausage; sliced
- 4 cups beef stock
- 30 oz. canned tomatoes; diced
- 1 green bell pepper; chopped
- 3 zucchinis; chopped
- 1 cup celery; chopped
- 1 tsp. Italian seasoning
- 1/2 yellow onion; chopped
- 1/2 tsp. oregano; dried
- 1/2 tsp. basil; dried
- 1/4 tsp. garlic powder
- A pinch of sea salt
- Black pepper to the taste

Instructions:
1. Heat up a pot over medium heat, add sausage and beef, stir; cook until it browns and drains excess fat.
2. Add tomatoes, zucchini, bell pepper, celery, onion, Italian seasoning, basil, oregano, garlic powder, sea salt, pepper to the taste and the stock.

3. stir; bring to a boil, reduce heat to medium-low and simmer for 1 hour. Pour into soup bowls and serve right away.

Nutrition Facts Per Serving: Calories: 370; Fat: 17g; Carbs: 35g; Fiber: 10g; Protein: 25g

Cauliflower Soup

(**Prep + Cook Time**: 1 hour 10 minutes | **Servings**: 6)

Ingredients:
- 2 lbs. cauliflower florets
- 1 yellow onion; finely chopped
- 2 tbsp. extra virgin olive oil
- A pinch of sea salt
- Black pepper to the taste
- 20 saffron threads
- 2 garlic cloves; minced
- 5 cups veggie stock

Instructions:
1. Heat up a pot with the oil over medium heat, add onion and garlic, stir and cook for 10 minutes.
2. Add cauliflower, a pinch of sea salt and pepper to the taste, stir and cook for 12 more minutes.
3. Add stock, stir; bring to a boil, reduce heat to medium and simmer for 25 minutes.
4. Take soup off the heat, add saffron, cover pot and leave it aside for 20 minutes.
5. Transfer soup to your blender and pulse very well. Pour into soup bowls and serve right away.

Nutrition Facts Per Serving: Calories: 170; Fat: 11g; Carbs: 5g; Fiber: 2; Sugar: 0.1g; Protein: 7g

Sweet Potato Soup

(**Prep + Cook Time**: 35 minutes | **Servings**: 2)

Ingredients:
- 5 garlic cloves; minced
- 14 oz. veggie stock
- 1 sweet potato; chopped
- 4 lemon peels
- 4 tbsp. olive oil
- 1/2 tsp. cumin seeds
- Black pepper to the taste
- A pinch of sea salt
- 4 tbsp. pine nuts

Instructions:
1. Heat up a pot with the oil over medium heat, add garlic, stir and cook for 4 minutes.
2. Add lemon peel, sweet potato, stock, cumin, a pinch of salt and black pepper to the taste, stir; bring to a boil and cook for 15 minutes.
3. Heat up a pan over medium high heat, add pine nuts, stir and cook for 4 minutes.
4. Discard lemon peel from soup, blend it using an immersion blender and mix with half of the pine nuts. Blend again, ladle into bowls and sprinkle the rest of the pine nuts on top.

Nutrition Facts Per Serving: Calories: 150; Fat: 2g; Fiber: 2g; Carbs: 7g; Protein: 3g

Seafood Soup

(**Prep + Cook Time**: 2 hours 40 minutes | **Servings**: 4)

Ingredients:
- 1 lb. cod fillets; cubed
- 10 cherry tomatoes; halved
- 1 lb. mussels; scrubbed
- 1 lb. shrimp; peeled and deveined
- 10 garlic cloves; minced
- 1/4 cup parsley; chopped
- 1 yellow onion; chopped
- 2 tomatoes; chopped
- 3 tbsp. olive oil
- 1 tbsp. lemon juice
- 1 tbsp. tomato paste
- 2 bay leaves
- 2½ cups water
- A pinch of sea salt
- Black pepper to the taste

Instructions:
1. In a bowl; mix 6 garlic cloves with 2 tbsp. oil, parsley and lemon juice and stir.
2. Add fish cubes, toss to coat, cover bowl and keep in the fridge for 2 hours.

3. Heat up a pot with the rest of the oil over medium high heat, add onion, stir and cook for 2 minutes.
4. Add the rest of the garlic, stir and cook for 1 minute.
5. Add tomatoes, tomato paste, bay leaves, water, salt, pepper and marinated fish, stir; bring to a simmer and cook for 10 minutes.
6. Add shrimp, cherry tomatoes and mussels, stir and cook for 6 minutes more. Discard unopened mussels, ladle soup into bowls and serve.

Nutrition Facts Per Serving: Calories: 160; Fat: 2g; Fiber: 2g; Carbs: 4g; Protein: 7g

Easy Paleo Soup

(**Prep + Cook Time**: 10 minutes | **Servings**: 3)

Ingredients:
- 1 avocado; pitted and chopped
- 1 cucumber; chopped
- 2 bunches spinach
- 1½ cups watermelon; chopped
- 1 bunch cilantro; roughly chopped
- Juice from 2 lemons
- 1/2 cup coconut aminos
- 1/2 cup lime juice

Instructions:
1. In your kitchen blender, mix cucumber with avocado and pulse well.
2. Add cilantro, spinach and watermelon and blend again well.
3. Add lemon and lime juice and coconut amino and pulse a few more times. Transfer to soup bowls and enjoy!

Nutrition Facts Per Serving: Calories: 100; Fat: 7g; Carbs: 6.5g; Fiber: 3.5; Sugar: 2.4g; Protein: 2.3

Oxtail Stew

(**Prep + Cook Time**: 6 hours 15 minutes | **Servings**: 8)

Ingredients:
- 4½ lbs. oxtail; cut into medium chunks
- A drizzle of extra virgin olive oil
- 1 tbsp. extra virgin olive oil
- 2 leeks; chopped
- 4 carrots; chopped
- 2 celery sticks; chopped
- 4 thyme springs; chopped
- 4 rosemary springs; chopped
- 4 cloves
- 4 bay leaves
- Black pepper to the taste
- 2 tbsp. coconut flour
- 28 oz. canned plum tomatoes; chopped
- 9 oz. red wine
- 1-quart beef stock

Instructions:
1. In a roasting pan, mix oxtail with black pepper and a drizzle of oil.
2. Toss to coat, introduce in the oven at 425 °F and bake for 20 minutes.
3. Heat up a pot with 1 tbsp. oil over medium heat, add leeks, celery and carrots, stir and cook for 4 minutes.
4. Add thyme, rosemary and bay leaves, stir and cook everything for 20 minutes.
5. Take oxtail out of the oven and leave aside for a few minutes.
6. Add flour and cloves to veggies and stir.
7. Also add tomatoes, wine, oxtail and its juices and stock, stir; increase heat to high and bring to a boil.
8. Introduce pot in the oven at 325 °F and bake for 5 hours.
9. Take stew out of the oven, leave aside for 10 minutes, take oxtail out of the pot and discard bones. Return meat to pot, add more pepper to the taste, stir; transfer to plates and serve.

Nutrition Facts Per Serving: Calories: 523; Fat: 38g; Carbs: 12; Sugar: 6.5g; Fiber: 2.6g; Protein: 28g

Beef Stew

(**Prep + Cook Time**: 2 hours 10 minutes | **Servings**: 4)

Ingredients:
- 2 lbs. beef fillet; cubed
- 1 red chili; seeded and chopped
- 1-star anise
- 2 celery stick; chopped
- 2 carrots; thinly sliced
- 1-quart beef stock
- 6 button mushrooms; chopped
- 1 brown onion; finely chopped
- 1/2 cup dried mushrooms
- 1/2 cup white wine
- 1 tsp. ghee
- 2 tbsp. extra virgin olive oil
- A pinch of sea salt
- Black pepper to the taste
- 2/3 tsp. nutmeg
- 2 tbsp. Worcestershire sauce; gluten free
- 1 garlic clove; minced
- 1/2 tbsp. dry sherry
- 1 tsp. rosemary; dry
- 4 thyme springs
- 1/4 tsp. fennel seeds
- 2 tbsp. almond flour
- 1 sweet potato; chopped

Instructions:
1. Heat up a pot with the ghee and the olive oil over medium-high heat, add onion, chili, some sea salt and pepper, stir and cook for 2-3 minutes.
2. Add meat, stir and brown it for 5 minutes.
3. Add Worcestershire sauce, wine, sherry, dried mushrooms, garlic, stock, thyme, fennel, rosemary, nutmeg and star anise, stir; bring to a boil, cover, reduce heat to low and cook for 1 hour and 10 minutes.
4. Add celery, carrots, fresh mushrooms, potato, stir; cover and cook for 15 minutes.
5. Increase heat to medium, uncover the pot and cook the stew for 15 minutes.
6. In a bowl; mix the flour with a cup of liquid from the stew, stir well, pour over stew and cook for 15 more minutes. Transfer to bowls and serve hot.

Nutrition Facts Per Serving: Calories: 313; Fat: 8g; Carbs: 21g; Fiber: 3; Sugar: 7g; Protein: 38

Asparagus Soup

(**Prep + Cook Time**: 35 minutes | **Servings**: 3)

Ingredients:
- 2 lbs. asparagus; trimmed and roughly chopped
- 1 celery stick; chopped
- 1 zucchini; chopped
- 1 yellow onion; chopped
- 2 garlic cloves; minced
- Grated lemon peel from 1/2 lemon
- Black pepper to the taste
- 2 cups water
- 1 tbsp. olive oil

Instructions:
1. Place asparagus, zucchini, celery, onion, lemon peel and garlic on a lined baking sheet, drizzle the oil, season with black pepper, place in the oven at 400 °F and bake for 25 minutes.
2. Transfer these to a food processor, add the water and pulse really well.
3. Transfer soup to a pot and heat up over medium high heat. Ladle into bowls and serve right away.

Nutrition Facts Per Serving: Calories: 160; Fat: 3g; Fiber: 2g; Carbs: 6g; Protein: 6g

Mushroom Cream

(Prep + Cook Time: 30 minutes | **Servings**: 4)

Ingredients:
- 1 oz. dried porcini mushrooms
- 3 cups veggie stock
- 1 sweet potato; peeled and chopped
- 2 bay leaves
- 1 leek; chopped
- 2 tbsp. olive oil
- 1 celery stick; chopped
- 3 garlic cloves; chopped
- 14 brown mushrooms; chopped
- 1 tbsp. thyme; chopped
- 1/2 tsp. Dijon mustard
- 1 tsp. lemon zest; grated
- 1/2 tsp. black pepper
- 1 tbsp. lemon juice
- 3 tbsp. sunflower seed butter

Instructions:
1. Put dried mushrooms in a small bowl; cover with boiling water, leave aside for 10 minutes, strain, reserve water and chop them.
2. Heat up a pot with the oil over medium heat, add celery and leek, stir and cook for 5 minutes.
3. Add mushrooms, thyme, garlic and sweet potatoes, stir and cook for 1 minute.
4. Add dried mushrooms and half of their liquid, stock, bay leaves, mustard, black pepper and lemon zest, stir; cover pot and simmer soup over medium heat for 15 minutes.
5. Discard bay leaves, use an immersion blender to make your mushroom cream, add lemon juice and sunflower seed butter, stir well, ladle into bowls and serve.

Nutrition Facts Per Serving: Calories: 100; Fat: 2g; Fiber: 1g; Carbs: 4g; Protein: 3g

Gazpacho

(Prep + Cook Time: 12 minutes | **Servings**: 4)

Ingredients:
- 8 tomatoes
- 1 red onion; chopped
- 1 cucumber; peeled and chopped
- 1 red bell pepper; chopped
- 1 green bell pepper; chopped
- 1 red chili pepper; chopped
- 3 garlic cloves
- 1 cup tomato juice
- 1 cup water
- 2 tbsp. apple cider vinegar
- Zest from 1/2 orange
- 3/4 cup olive oil
- A pinch of sea salt
- Black pepper to the taste

Instructions:
1. Put some water in a pot and bring to a boil over medium high heat.
2. Add tomatoes, leave them in boiling water for 2 minutes, drain and rinse them.
3. Peel, chop and put them in your food processor.
4. Add red onion, cucumber, red bell pepper, green bell pepper, chili pepper, garlic, tomato juice, water, vinegar, orange zest, olive oil, a pinch of salt and black pepper to the taste and pulse really well until you obtain cream. Ladle into soup bowls and serve cold.

Nutrition Facts Per Serving: Calories: 140; Fat: 1g; Fiber: 1g; Carbs: 3g; Protein: 2g

French Chicken Stew

(Prep + Cook Time: 2 hours 15 minutes | **Servings**: 4)

Ingredients:
- 10 garlic cloves; peeled
- 30 black olives; pitted
- 2 lbs. chicken pieces
- 2 cups chicken stock
- 28 oz. canned tomatoes; chopped
- 2 tbsp. rosemary; chopped
- 2 tbsp. parsley leaves; chopped
- 2 tbsp. basil leaves; chopped
- A pinch of sea salt
- Black pepper to the taste
- A drizzle of extra virgin olive oil

Instructions:
1. Heat up a pot with some olive oil over medium-high heat, add chicken pieces, a pinch of sea salt and pepper to the taste and cook for 4 minutes, stirring often.
2. Add garlic, stir and brown for 2 minutes.
3. Add chicken stock, tomatoes, olives, thyme and rosemary, stir; cover pot and bake in the oven at 325 °F for 1 hour.
4. Add parsley and basil, stir; introduce in the oven again and bake for 45 more minutes. Leave stew to cool down for a few minutes, transfer to plates and serve.

Nutrition Facts Per Serving: Calories: 300; Fat: 48g; Carbs: 16; Sugar: 0g; Protein: 61

Beef Stew

(Prep + Cook Time: 2 hours 10 minutes | **Servings**: 4)

Ingredients:
- 2 lbs. organic beef steak; cubed
- 1 tbsp. coconut oil
- A pinch of sea salt
- Black pepper to the taste
- 1 red chili pepper; chopped
- 1 yellow onion; chopped
- 4 cups beef stock
- 2 carrots; chopped
- 1 sweet potato; chopped
- 6 white mushrooms; chopped
- 2 celery; sticks, chopped
- 1 tbsp. coconut aminos
- 1/2 cup white wine
- 1 tbsp. lemon juice
- A pinch of nutmeg; ground
- 2 garlic cloves; minced
- 1 tsp. thyme; dried
- 1/4 tsp. fennel seeds
- 1-star anise
- 1 tsp. rosemary; dried
- 1½ tbsp. arrowroot flour

Instructions:
1. Heat up a pot with the oil over medium heat, add onion, stir and cook for 5 minutes.
2. Add a pinch of sea salt, black pepper to the taste and the chili pepper, stir and cook for 1-2 minutes more.
3. Add beef, stir and cook for 5 minutes.
4. Add coconut aminos, wine, lemon juice, garlic, thyme, rosemary, fennel, nutmeg, star anise and stock, stir and bring to a boil.
5. Cover the pot, cook for 1 hour and 15 minutes and then mix with celery, sweet potato, carrots and mushrooms.
6. Stir, cover pot again and cook for 10 minutes more.
7. Uncover pot, stir and cook everything for 15 minutes.
8. In a bowl; mix 2 tbsp. cooking liquid from the pot with the arrowroot flour and stir very well. Add this to the stew, stir; cook for a couple more minutes, divide into bowls and serve.

Nutrition Facts Per Serving: Calories: 313; Fat: 7g; Fiber: 3g; Carbs: 10g; Protein: 23g

Broccoli Soup

(Prep + Cook Time: 30 minutes | **Servings**: 4)

Ingredients:
- 1 yellow onion; chopped
- 2 tbsp. olive oil
- 1 celery stick; chopped
- Zest from 1/2 lemon
- 1-quart veggie stock
- 17 oz. water
- 1 tsp. cumin; ground
- 1 broccoli head; florets separated
- Black pepper to the taste
- 3 garlic cloves; minced
- 2 bay leaves
- Juice of 1/2 lemon
- A pinch of sea salt

For the pesto:
- 1/2 cup almonds; chopped
- 1 garlic clove
- 2 tbsp. lemon juice
- 2 tbsp. olive oil
- 4 tbsp. green olives; pitted and chopped

Instructions:
1. Heat up a pot with 2 tbsp. olive oil over medium high heat, add onion, lemon zest and a pinch of salt, stir and cook for 3 minutes.
2. Add celery and 3 garlic cloves, stir and cook for 1 minute more.
3. Add stock, cumin, water and black pepper, stir; cover, bring to a boil and simmer for 10 minutes.
4. Add bay leaves and broccoli, stir; cover again and cook for 6 minutes more.
5. Take soup off the heat, discard bay leaves, transfer to your blender and pulse really well.
6. Add juice from 1/2 lemon, pulse again, return to the pot and heat up again over medium-low heat.
7. Meanwhile; in your food processor, blend well almond with 1 garlic clove, 2 tbsp. lemon juice, 2 tbsp. olive oil and green olives. Divide soup into bowls, top with the pesto you've just made and serve hot.

Nutrition Facts Per Serving: Calories: 139; Fat: 2g; Fiber: 1g; Carbs: 4g; Protein: 1g

Root Soup

(Prep + Cook Time: 1 hour 40 minutes | Servings: 8)

Ingredients:
- 1 sweet onion; chopped
- 2 tbsp. ghee
- 5 carrots; chopped
- 3 parsnips; chopped
- 3 beets; chopped
- 3 bacon slices
- 1-quart chicken stock
- A pinch of sea salt
- Black pepper to the taste
- 2 quarts water
- 1/2 tsp. chili flakes
- 1 tbsp. mixed thyme and rosemary

Instructions:
1. Heat up a Dutch oven with the ghee over medium-high heat, add onion, stir and cook for 5 minutes.
2. Add carrots, parsnips, beets, bacon, chicken stock and water and stir.
3. Also add sea salt, pepper to the taste, chili flakes, thyme and rosemary, stir again, bring to a boil, reduce heat to medium-low and simmer for 1 hour and 30 minutes. Pour into soup bowls and serve hot.

Nutrition Facts Per Serving: Calories: 180; Fat: 2g; Carbs: 4g; Fiber: 1; Sugar: 0.5g; Protein: 3.5

Pork Stew

(Prep + Cook Time: 8 hours 10 minutes | Servings: 8)

Ingredients:
- 2 lbs. pork loin; cubed and marinated in some beer in the fridge for 1 day
- 2 yellow onions; chopped
- 1 small cabbage head; finely chopped
- 5 small sweet potatoes; chopped
- 30 oz. canned tomatoes; chopped
- 3 cups beef stock
- 1 tbsp. coconut oil
- 3 garlic cloves; minced
- 1 cup arrowroot flour
- 6 carrots; chopped
- Black pepper to the taste
- A pinch of sea salt

Instructions:
1. In a bowl mix arrowroot flour with marinated pork cubes and rub them well.
2. Heat up a pan with the oil over medium high heat, add pork cubes, brown them on all sides and transfer to your slow cooker.
3. Add garlic, carrots, a pinch of salt, black pepper, onion, cabbage, sweet potatoes, tomatoes and stock, stir; cover pot and cook your stew on Low for 8 hours. Uncover pot, stir stew again, divide into bowls and serve.

Nutrition Facts Per Serving: Calories: 260; Fat: 6g; Fiber: 4g; Carbs: 7g; Protein: 14g

Chicken Soup

(**Prep + Cook Time**: 45 minutes | **Servings**: 6)

Ingredients:
- 2 carrots; chopped
- 1/2 cup arrowroot
- 6 cups chicken stock
- 1½ cups coconut milk
- 3 cups organic chicken meat; already cooked and cubed
- 2 celery stalks; chopped
- 1/2 cup coconut oil
- 1 tsp. dry parsley
- 1/2 cup water
- 1 bay leaf
- A pinch of sea salt
- Black pepper to the taste
- 1/2 tsp. dry thyme

Instructions:
1. Heat up a soup pot with the oil over medium-high heat, add carrots and celery, stir and cook for 10 minutes.
2. Add stock, stir and bring to a boil.
3. In a bowl; mix arrowroot with 1/2 cup water and whisk well.
4. Add this to soup and also add parsley, sea salt, pepper to the taste, bay leaf and thyme.
5. Stir and cook everything for 15 minutes. Add chicken meat and coconut milk, stir; cook 1 more minute, take off heat, pour into soup bowls and serve.

Nutrition Facts Per Serving: Calories: 412; Fat: 31g; Carbs: 8g; Fiber: 2g; Protein: 27; Sugar: 4

Chicken Soup

(**Prep + Cook Time**: 25 minutes | **Servings**: 2)

Ingredients:
- 1 red bell pepper; chopped
- 1½ cups chicken breast; cooked and shredded
- 2½ cups chicken stock
- 2 cups kale; torn
- 1 yellow onion; chopped
- 1/4 cup pickled jalapeno peppers; chopped
- 2 garlic cloves; minced
- 1 tsp. coconut oil
- 1 tbsp. ghee
- 1 tsp. cumin; ground
- 1 tsp. coriander; ground
- 1 tsp. oregano; dried
- Zest from 1 lime; grated
- Juice from 1 lime
- A pinch of sea salt
- 2 tbsp. spring onions; chopped
- 3 tbsp. pumpkin seeds; chopped
- 1 avocado; peeled, pitted and sliced
- 15 oz. canned tomatoes; chopped
- 1 tsp. sweet paprika
- 3 tbsp. coriander; chopped

Instructions:
1. Heat up a pot with the oil over medium heat, add onion, stir and cook for 2 minutes.
2. Add red bell peppers, stir and cook for 1 minute. Add garlic, jalapenos, oregano, cumin, coriander and ghee, stir and cook for 1 minute more.
3. Add tomatoes, kale, chicken, lime zest, stock, lime juice and a pinch of salt, stir; bring to a boil, cook for 5 minutes and take off heat.
4. Heat up a pan over medium heat, add pumpkin seeds, toast them for 2 minutes and take off heat.
5. Ladle soup into bowls, top with pumpkin seeds, green onion, paprika, chopped coriander and avocado and serve.

Nutrition Facts Per Serving: Calories: 170; Fat: 2g; Fiber: 3g; Carbs: 4g; Protein: 7g

Zucchini Soup

(**Prep + Cook Time**: 30 minutes | **Servings**: 4)

Ingredients:
- 3 zucchinis; cut into medium chunks
- 1 onion; chopped
- 2 tbsp. coconut milk
- 2 garlic cloves; minced
- 4 cups chicken stock
- 2 tbsp. coconut oil
- A pinch of sea salt
- Black pepper to the taste

Instructions:
1. Heat up a pot with the oil over medium heat, add zucchinis, garlic and onion, stir and cook for 5 minutes.
2. Add stock, salt, pepper, stir; bring to a boil, cover pot, simmer soup for 20 minutes and take off heat. Add coconut milk, blend using an immersion blender, ladle into bowls and serve.

Nutrition Facts Per Serving: Calories: 160; Fat: 2g; Fiber: 2g; Carbs: 4g; Protein: 7g

Nettles Soup

(**Prep + Cook Time**: 30 minutes | **Servings**: 3)

Ingredients:
- 1 cup sweet potato; chopped
- 1 yellow onion; chopped
- 1/2 broccoli head; florets separated
- 1/2 cauliflower head; florets separated
- 5 thyme springs; leaves separated
- 4 bacon slices; cooked and crumbled
- 1/2 cup coconut cream
- 1 tbsp. coconut oil
- 1 bay leaf
- 3 garlic cloves; minced
- Zest from 1 lemon; grated
- 1 tsp. Dijon mustard
- 3½ cups veggie stock
- Black pepper to the taste
- A pinch of sea salt
- 4 cups nettles
- Juice of 1 lemon

Instructions:
1. Heat up a pot with the coconut oil over medium heat, add sweet potato, onion, broccoli and cauliflower, stir and cook for 6 minutes.
2. Add bay leaf, garlic, veggie stock, lemon zest, salt, pepper and mustard, stir and bring to a boil.
3. Reduce heat, cover pot and cook for 10 minutes.
4. Meanwhile; put water in a pot and bring to a boil.
5. Cut nettles leaves with scissors, add leaves to water, leave there for 2 minutes, drain them and transfer them to the pot with the soup.
6. Cook for 3 minutes more, add lemon juice, blend using an immersion blender and then heat up the soup again.
7. Add thyme and coconut cream, stir; cook for 1 minute and ladle into soup bowls. Top with bacon and serve.

Nutrition Facts Per Serving: Calories: 170; Fat: 2g; Fiber: 2g; Carbs: 2g; Protein: 8g

Roasted Veggie Stew

(**Prep + Cook Time**: 1 hour 10 minutes | **Servings**: 6)

Ingredients:
- 4 lbs. mixed parsnips; carrots, turnips and celery root, peeled and roughly chopped
- 1 garlic head; cloves peeled
- 1/2 cup yellow onion; chopped
- 6 tbsp. olive oil
- 1 tbsp. tomato paste
- 28 oz. canned tomatoes; chopped
- A pinch of sea salt
- Black pepper to the taste
- 2 cups kale; chopped
- 1 tsp. oregano; dried

Instructions:
1. In a big baking dish, mix root veggies with garlic cloves, half of the oil, a pinch of salt and pepper, toss to coat, place in the oven at 450 °F and roast for 45 minutes.
2. Heat up a pan with the rest of the oil over medium high heat, add onion, stir and cook for 3 minutes.
3. Add tomato paste, stir and cook for 1 minute.
4. Add canned tomatoes, oregano and some black pepper, stir; bring to a simmer and cook for a few minute more.
5. Take veggies out of the oven and add them to the pot with the tomatoes.
6. Also add kale, stir and cook everything for 5 minutes. Divide into bowls and serve.

Nutrition Facts Per Serving: Calories: 200; Fat: 3g; Fiber: 3g; Carbs: 5g; Protein: 5g

Oxtail Stew

(**Prep + Cook Time**: 6 hours 10 minutes | **Servings**: 8)

Ingredients:
- 5 lbs. oxtail; cut into medium chunks
- 4 bay leaves
- 28 oz. canned tomatoes; chopped
- 2 celery stick; chopped
- 2 leeks; chopped
- A pinch of sea salt
- Black pepper to the taste
- 2 tbsp. avocado oil
- 3 thyme springs
- 4 carrots; chopped
- 3 rosemary springs
- 2 tbsp. coconut flour
- 4 cloves
- 1-quart beef stock

Instructions:
1. Place oxtail in a roasting pan, season with a pinch of salt and black pepper, drizzle half of the avocado oil, rub well, place in the oven at 425 °F and roast for 20 minutes.
2. Heat up a pan with the rest of the oil over medium heat, add leeks, carrots, celery, thyme, rosemary and bay leaf, stir and cook for 20 minutes.
3. Add coconut flour, cloves, tomatoes and stock and stir.
4. Add oxtail, stir; cover pan and cook on low heat for 5 hours. Take oxtail out of the pot, discard bones, return them to the pot, stir; divide into bowls and serve.

Nutrition Facts Per Serving: Calories: 435; Fat: 23g; Fiber: 3g; Carbs: 7g; Protein: 30g

Paleo Stew

(**Prep + Cook Time**: 8 hours 10 minutes | **Servings**: 6)

Ingredients:
- 3 lbs. osso buco; bones in
- 1 cup carrots; chopped
- 1 cup celery; chopped
- 2 cups onions; chopped
- 4 garlic cloves; minced
- 6 tsp. baharat
- A pinch of black pepper
- 2 cups beef stock
- A handful parsley; chopped
- 1 kale; chopped

Instructions:
1. In your slow cooker, mix osso buco with carrots, celery, onions, garlic, baharat, black pepper and stock, stir; cover and cook on Low for 7 hours and 30 minutes.
2. Uncover your slow cooker, add kale and parsley, cover again and cook for 30 minutes more. Divide stew into bowls and serve.

Nutrition Facts Per Serving: 340; Fat: 2g; Fiber: 3g; Carbs: 4g; Protein: 10g

Beef Stew

(Prep + Cook Time: 8 hours 10 minutes | **Servings**: 4)

Ingredients:
- 2½ lbs. beef chuck; cubed
- 5 green plantains; peeled and cubed
- 3 cups collard greens
- 3 cups water
- 3 tbsp. allspice
- 1/4 cup garlic powder
- 1/3 cup sweet paprika
- 1 tsp. cayenne pepper
- 1 tsp. chili powder

Instructions:
1. In your slow cooker, mix beef with greens, plantains, water, allspice, garlic powder, paprika, cayenne and chili powder, stir well, cover and cook on Low for 8 hours.
2. Keep stirring from time to time. Divide into bowls and serve.

Nutrition Facts Per Serving: Calories: 250; Fat: 4g; Fiber: 3g; Carbs: 5g; Protein: 9g

Kale and Sausage Soup

(Prep + Cook Time: 45 minutes | **Servings**: 4)

Ingredients:
- 1 yellow onion; chopped
- 16 oz. sausage; chopped
- 3 sweet potatoes; chopped
- 4 cups chicken stock
- 1 lb. kale; chopped
- A pinch of sea salt and black pepper

Instructions:
1. Heat up a pot over medium heat, add sausage, stir; brown on both sides and transfer to a bowl.
2. Heat up the pot again over medium heat, add onion, stir and cook for 5 minutes.
3. Add stock and sweet potatoes, stir; bring to a simmer and cook for 20 minutes.
4. Use an immersion blender to blend your soup, add kale, a pinch of salt and black pepper and simmer everything for 2 minutes more. Ladle soup into bowls, top with sausage pieces and serve.

Nutrition Facts Per Serving: Calories: 200; Fat: 2g; Fiber: 2g; Carbs: 6g; Protein: 8g

Squash Soup

(Prep + Cook Time: 60 minutes | **Servings**: 4)

Ingredients:
- 14 oz. coconut milk
- 1 butternut squash; cut in halves lengthwise and deseeded
- A pinch of sea salt
- Black pepper to the taste
- A handful parsley; chopped
- A pinch of nutmeg; ground

Instructions:
1. Place butternut squash halves on a lined baking sheet, place in the oven at 350 °F and bake for 45 minutes.
2. Leave squash to cool down, scoop flesh and transfer it to pot. Add half of the coconut milk and blend everything using an immersion blender.
3. Heat this soup up over medium-low heat, add the rest of the coconut milk, a pinch of sea salt, black pepper to the taste, nutmeg and parsley, blend using your immersion blender for a few seconds, cook for about 4 minutes, divide into soup bowls and serve.

Nutrition Facts Per Serving: Calories: 144; Fat: 10g; Fiber: 2g; Carbs: 7g; Protein: 2g

Onion Soup

(**Prep + Cook Time**: 3 hours 10 minutes | **Servings**: 4)

Ingredients:
- 5 yellow onions; cut into halves and then slice
- 5 cups beef stock
- 2 tbsp. avocado oil
- Black pepper to the taste
- 3 thyme springs
- 1 tbsp. tomato paste

Instructions:
1. Heat up a pot with the oil over medium high heat, add onions and thyme, stir; reduce heat to low, cover and cook for 30 minutes.
2. Uncover the pot and cook onions for 1 hour and 30 minutes more stirring often.
3. Add tomato paste and stock, stir and simmer soup for 1 hour more. Ladle soup into bowls and serve.

Nutrition Facts Per Serving: Calories: 200; Fat: 4g; Fiber: 4g; Carbs: 6g; Protein: 8g

Chorizo Stew

(**Prep + Cook Time**: 40 minutes | **Servings**: 3)

Ingredients:
- 2 chorizo sausages; chopped
- 1 carrot; chopped
- 1 red bell pepper; chopped
- 1 celery stick; chopped
- 2 sweet potatoes; chopped
- 2 garlic cloves; minced
- 1 tomato; chopped
- 1 zucchini; chopped
- 2 cups chicken stock
- 1 yellow onion; chopped
- 1 tbsp. coconut oil
- A handful parsley; chopped
- 1 tbsp. lemon juice
- A pinch of sea salt
- Black pepper to the taste

Instructions:
1. Heat up a pan with the oil over medium high heat, add carrot, onion, chorizo and celery, stir and cook for 3 minutes.
2. Add sweet potatoes, garlic, tomato and red bell pepper, stir and cook for 1 minute more.
3. Add lemon juice, a pinch of salt, black pepper and stock, stir; cover, bring to a simmer and cook for 10 minutes.
4. Add zucchini, stir and cook for 12 minutes more. Add parsley, stir well, divide into bowls and serve.

Nutrition Facts Per Serving: Calories: 270; Fat: 8g; Fiber: 3g; Carbs: 5g; Protein: 8g

Eggplant Stew

(**Prep + Cook Time**: 35 minutes | **Servings**: 3)

Ingredients:
- 2 big tomatoes; chopped
- 1 eggplant; chopped
- 1 cup tomato paste
- 1 yellow onion; chopped
- A pinch of cayenne pepper
- 1 tsp. cumin powder
- A pinch pink salt
- 1/2 cup water

Instructions:
1. Put the water in a small pot and heat up over medium heat.
2. Add tomato paste, cayenne and a pinch of salt and stir well.
3. Add tomatoes, eggplant and onion, stir and bring to a simmer.
4. Cover the pot and cook the stew for 25 minutes. Divide into bowls and serve.

Nutrition Facts Per Serving: Calories: 170; Fat: 2g; Fiber: 3g; Carbs: 4g; Protein: 6g

Shrimp and Chicken Soup

(Prep + Cook Time: 40 minutes | **Servings**: 4)

Ingredients:
- 1 lb. shrimp; peeled and deveined
- 1½ cups coconut milk
- 1/2 cup coconut cream
- 5 Chinese broccoli leaves; chopped
- 1 zucchini; chopped
- 1 carrot; chopped
- 1 cucumber; chopped
- 5 tbsp. curry paste
- 1 tbsp. coconut oil
- 1 big chicken breast; cut into thin strips
- 4 tbsp. coconut aminos
- 2 cups chicken stock
- Juice from 1 lime
- A small broccoli head; florets separated
- Some chopped cilantro; chopped for serving

Instructions:
1. Heat up a pot with the oil over medium heat, add curry paste, stir and cook for 1 minute.
2. Add chicken, stir and cook for 1 minute more.
3. Add stock and lime juice, stir and cook for 2 minutes.
4. Add coconut cream, aminos and coconut milk, stir and cook for 10 minutes.
5. Add broccoli leaves, broccoli florets and carrots, stir and cook for 3 minutes.
6. Add shrimp and zucchini, stir and cook for 2 minutes. Ladle into bowls, top with cilantro and cucumber pieces and serve.

Nutritional value: Calories: 160; Fat: 3g; Fiber: 2g; Carbs: 6g; Protein: 8g

Celery Soup

(Prep + Cook Time: 30 minutes | **Servings**: 2)

Ingredients:
- 1 yellow onion; chopped
- 13 oz. celery; chopped
- 17 oz. veggie stock
- A pinch of sea salt
- 2 tbsp. cashews; chopped
- Black pepper to the taste
- 1½ tbsp. olive oil

Instructions:
1. Heat up a pot with the oil over medium high heat, add onion and celery, stir and cook for 5 minutes.
2. Add stock, a pinch of salt and black pepper to the taste, stir; bring to a simmer and cook for 10 minutes.
3. Add cashews, stir and cook for 5 minutes more. Transfer this to your blender, pulse really well until you obtain cream, divide into bowls and serve.

Nutrition Facts Per Serving: Calories: 150; Fat: 2g; Fiber: 2g; Carbs: 4g; Protein: 7g

Slow Cooker Stew

(Prep + Cook Time: 32 hours | **Servings**: 6)

Ingredients:
- 2 lbs. beef stew meat; cubed
- 3 cups dark beer
- 4 carrots; chopped
- 1 cup coconut flour
- 2 yellow onions; finely chopped
- 1/2 head cabbage; finely chopped
- 30 oz. canned tomatoes; diced
- 2 cups reserved beef marinade
- 3 cups beef stock
- 7 garlic cloves; finely minced
- A pinch of sea salt
- Black pepper to the taste

Instructions:
1. In a bowl; mix beef with beer and 3 garlic cloves, toss to coat and keep in the fridge for 1 day.
2. In a bowl; mix coconut flour with a pinch of sea salt and pepper to the taste and stir.
3. Drain meat and reserve the 2 cups of the marinade.
4. Add meat to tapioca bowls and toss to coat.
5. Heat up a pan over medium-high heat, add meat, stir and brown it for 2-3 minutes.

6. Transfer meat to your slow cooker.
7. Add reserved marinade, carrots, cabbage, onions, tomatoes, 4 garlic cloves, beef stock, salt and pepper to the taste, cover pot and cook stew on Low for 8 hours. Uncover pot, transfer stew to bowls and serve.

Nutrition Facts Per Serving: Calories: 247; Fat: 4.5g; Carbs: 25g; Fiber: 4.2; Sugar: 4g; Protein: 24.2

Eggplant Stew

(Prep + Cook Time: 40 minutes | **Servings**: 3)

Ingredients:
- 1 eggplant; chopped
- 1 yellow onion; chopped
- 2 tomatoes; chopped
- 1 tsp. cumin powder
- A pinch of sea salt
- Black pepper to the taste
- 1 cup tomato paste
- A pinch of cayenne pepper
- 1/2 cup water

Instructions:
1. Heat up a pan over medium-high heat, add water, tomato paste, a pinch of salt and pepper, cayenne and cumin and stir well.
2. Add the eggplant, tomato and onion, stir; bring to a boil, reduce heat to medium and cook for 30 minutes.
3. Take stew off heat, add a black pepper if needed, transfer to plates and serve.

Nutrition Facts Per Serving: Calories: 82; Fat: 0g; Carbs: 16g; Fiber: 1; Sugar: 0.5g; Protein: 5g

Chicken Stew

(Prep + Cook Time: 8 hours 10 minutes | **Servings**: 6)

Ingredients:
- 1/2 lb. baby spinach
- 2 celery sticks; chopped
- 2 onions; chopped
- 2 sweet potatoes; cubed
- 30 oz. canned pumpkin puree
- 2 quarts chicken stock
- 2 cups chicken meat; skinless, boneless and shredded
- 2 carrots; chopped
- 5 garlic cloves; minced
- A pinch of sea salt
- Black pepper to the taste
- 1/4 tsp. cayenne pepper
- 1/4 cup arrowroot powder

Instructions:
1. In your slow cooker, mix carrots with garlic, celery, onion, sweet potatoes, pumpkin puree, chicken, stock, salt, pepper, cayenne and arrowroot powder, stir; cover and cook on Low for 7 hours and 40 minutes.
2. Uncover slow cooker, add spinach, cover again and cook on Low for 20 minutes more. Divide into bowls and serve.

Nutrition Facts Per Serving: Calories: 280; Fat: 3g; Fiber: 3g; Carbs: 6g; Protein: 7g

African Style Stew

(Prep + Cook Time: 55 minutes | **Servings**: 4)

Ingredients:
- 4 chicken thighs
- 1 small brown onion; chopped
- 1/2 tbsp. coconut oil
- A pinch of sea salt
- Black pepper to the taste
- 1 tbsp. ginger; grated
- 1 tbsp. garlic; minced
- 1/2 tsp. paprika
- 1/2 tbsp. coriander
- 1/2 tsp. chili powder
- 2 cloves
- 2 bay leaves
- 1½ cups canned tomatoes; chopped
- 2½ tbsp. cashew butter

- 1/4 cup water
- 1 tbsp. parsley; chopped
- 1/4 tsp. vanilla extract

Instructions:
1. Heat up a pan with the oil over medium high heat, add chicken pieces, season with a pinch of salt and black pepper to the taste, stir; brown for 4 minutes on each side and transfer them to a bowl.
2. Heat up the same pan over medium heat, add ginger and onion, stir and cook for 6 minutes.
3. Add garlic, paprika, coriander, bay leaves, cloves and chili powder, stir and cook for 1 minute.
4. Add water, tomatoes and chicken pieces, stir; cover, bring to a boil and simmer for 25 minutes.
5. Take chicken out of the pot, add cashew butter and vanilla, stir and cook for 2 minutes more. Divide chicken into bowls, add stew on top, sprinkle parsley and serve hot.

Nutrition Facts Per Serving: Calories: 200; Fat: 4g; Fiber: 2g; Carbs: 5g; Protein: 8g

Veggie Soup

(**Prep + Cook Time**: 25 minutes | **Servings**: 4)

Ingredients:
- 1 yellow onion; chopped
- 2 carrots; chopped
- 6 mushrooms; chopped
- 1 red chili pepper; chopped
- 2 celery sticks; chopped
- 1 tbsp. coconut oil
- A pinch of sea salt
- Black pepper to the taste
- A handful dried porcini mushrooms
- 4 garlic cloves; minced
- 4 oz. kale; chopped
- 1 cup canned tomatoes; chopped
- 1 zucchini; chopped
- 1-quart veggie stock
- 1 bay leaf
- Some lemon zest; grated for serving
- A handful parsley; chopped for serving

Instructions:
1. Set your instant pot on Sauté mode, add oil and heat it up.
2. Add celery, carrots, onion, a pinch of salt and black pepper, stir and cook for 2 minutes.
3. Add chili pepper, garlic, dried mushrooms and mushrooms, stir and cook for 2 minutes.
4. Add tomatoes, stock, bay leaf, kale and zucchinis, stir; cover pot and cook on High for 10 minutes. Release pressure, stir soup again, ladle into bowls, top with lemon zest and parsley and serve.

Nutrition Facts Per Serving: Calories: 150; Fat: 2g; Fiber: 2g; Carbs: 4g; Protein: 6g

Lamb and Coconut Stew

(**Prep + Cook Time**: 2 hours 5 minutes | **Servings**: 4)

Ingredients:
- 1½ lbs. lamb meat; diced
- 1/2 red chili; seedless and chopped
- 1 brown onion; chopped
- 2 carrots; chopped
- A handful parsley leaves; finely chopped
- 14 oz. canned coconut milk
- 3 garlic cloves; minced
- 2 celery sticks; chopped
- 1 cup water
- 1 tbsp. coconut oil
- 2½ tsp. garam masala powder
- 1 tsp. fennel seeds
- A pinch of sea salt
- Black pepper to the taste
- 1¼ tsp. turmeric
- 1½ tsp. ghee
- 1 tbsp. lemon juice

Instructions:
1. Heat up a pan with the oil over medium-high heat, add lamb, stir and brown for 4 minutes.
2. Add celery, chili and onion, stir and cook 1 minute.
3. Reduce heat to medium, add garam masala, garlic, ghee, fennel and turmeric, stir and cook 1 minute.
4. Add a pinch of sea salt, pepper to the taste, tomato paste, coconut milk and water, stir; bring to a boil, reduce heat to low, cover and cook for 1 hour.

5. Add carrots and cook for 40 minutes more, stirring from time to time. Add lemon juice and parsley, stir; take off heat, transfer to bowls and serve.

Nutrition Facts Per Serving: Calories: 450; Fat: 31g; Carbs: 40g; Fiber: 1; Sugar: 2g; Protein: 50

Mexican Paleo Stew

(Prep + Cook Time: 60 minutes **| Servings:** 4)

Ingredients:
- 1 lb. beef meat; cubed
- 1 cup chicken stock
- 1/2 cup tomato sauce
- 1 brown onion; chopped
- 1 bay leaf
- 1 Serrano pepper; chopped
- 2 tbsp. avocado oil
- 1 tbsp. garlic; minced
- 1 tsp. chili powder
- 1 tsp. cumin; ground
- 1 tsp. paprika
- Black pepper to the taste
- 1/2 tsp. oregano; dried
- 1/2 tsp. chipotle powder
- 1 tbsp. tapioca flour

Instructions:
1. Set you pressure cooker on Sauté mode, add oil, heat it up, add beef, stir and brown for a few minutes on each side.
2. Add garlic, Serrano pepper, onion, bay leaf, black pepper, paprika, chili powder, cumin, oregano and chipotle powder, stir and cook for 4 minutes more.
3. Add stock, tapioca flour and tomato sauce, stir; cover pot and cook on High for 35 minutes. Release the pressure, uncover, stir you stew one more time and serve right away.

Nutrition Facts Per Serving: Calories: 300; Fat: 12g; Fiber: 3g; Carbs: 6g; Protein: 17g

Cucumber Soup

(Prep + Cook Time: 2 hours 10 minutes **| Servings:** 2)

Ingredients:
- 2 cucumbers; chopped
- 1 cup coconut cream
- 1 garlic clove; minced
- 1 tbsp. olive oil
- 3 tbsp. lemon juice
- A pinch of sea salt
- Black pepper to the taste

Instructions:
1. In your food processor, blend cucumber with a pinch of sea salt and black pepper, coconut cream, garlic, oil and lemon juice and pulse really well. Divide into soup bowls and serve cold.

Nutrition Facts Per Serving: Calories: 120; Fat: 1g; Fiber: 1g; Carbs: 3g; Protein: 1g

Green Soup

(Prep + Cook Time: 35 minutes **| Servings:** 6)

Ingredients:
- 2 leeks; chopped
- 4 celery sticks; chopped
- 4 garlic cloves; minced
- 2 broccoli heads; florets separated
- 1 small cauliflower head; florets separated
- 2 handfuls spinach; chopped
- 1 handful parsley; chopped
- 8 cups veggie stock
- 2 tbsp. ghee
- 1 tbsp. coconut cream
- A pinch of nutmeg; ground
- Black pepper to the taste

Instructions:
1. Heat up a pot with the ghee over medium heat, add garlic and leeks, stir and cook for 3 minutes.
2. Add broccoli, celery and cauliflower, stir and cook for 5 minutes,
3. Add stock, bring to a boil, cover pot and cook for 15 minutes.

4. Add parsley and spinach, stir and blend using an immersion blender. Add black pepper and nutmeg, stir; ladle soup into bowls and serve with some coconut cream on top.

Nutrition Facts Per Serving: Calories: 103; Fat: 4g; Fiber: 3g; Carbs: 10g; Protein: 4g

Vietnamese Stew

(**Prep + Cook Time**: 3 hours 30 minutes | **Servings**: 6)

Ingredients:
- 2½ lbs. organic beef brisket; cut into medium chunks
- 1 lb. carrots; chopped
- 1 lemongrass stalk; chopped
- 1½ tsp. curry powder
- 2½ tbsp. ginger; grated
- 2 tbsp. unsweetened applesauce
- 3 tbsp. ghee
- 1 bay leaf
- 1 yellow onion; chopped
- 2-star anise
- 2 cups canned tomatoes; chopped
- 3 cups water
- 1/4 cup cilantro; chopped
- A pinch of sea salt
- Black pepper to the taste

Instructions:
1. In a bowl; mix applesauce with lemongrass, curry powder, bay leaf, ginger and beef, toss to coat well and leave aside for 30 minutes.
2. Heat up a pot with the ghee over medium high heat, add beef, stir; brown on all sides and transfer to a plate.
3. Add marinade to browned beef and toss again.
4. Return pot to medium heat, add onion, stir and cook for a few minutes.
5. Add a pinch of salt, black pepper and tomatoes, stir and cook for 15 minutes.
6. Add beef and its marinade and star anise, stir and cook for 5 minutes.
7. Add carrots and water, stir; bring to a boil, cover, place in the oven at 300 degrees and bake for 2 hours and 30 minutes.
8. Discard bay leaf and star anise, stir the stew, divide into bowls, sprinkle cilantro on top and serve.

Nutrition Facts Per Serving: Calories: 300; Fat: 4g; Fiber: 3g; Carbs: 6g; Protein: 12g

Beef and Sweet Potatoes Stew

(**Prep + Cook Time**: 45 minutes | **Servings**: 4)

Ingredients:
- 1 lb. beef; ground
- 3 cups sweet potatoes; peeled and cubed
- 1½ cups veggie stock
- 1 carrot; chopped
- 2/3 cup canned tomatoes; chopped
- 1/4 cup parsley; chopped
- 1 red onion; chopped
- 1 tbsp. balsamic vinegar
- 2 tbsp. coconut oil
- A pinch of sea salt
- 1/4 cup pine nuts
- 3 garlic cloves; minced
- 2/3 tsp. ginger; grated
- 1 tsp. coriander seeds
- 1 tsp. cumin; ground
- 1 tsp. paprika
- Zest from 1 lemon; grated

Instructions:
1. Heat up a pot with the oil over medium heat, add onion and a pinch of salt, stir and cook for 10 minutes.
2. Add vinegar, stir and cook for 1 minute more.
3. Heat up another pan over medium heat, add pine nuts, stir; toast for 2 minutes and transfer to a bowl.
4. Add ginger and meat to onions, stir and cook for 2 minutes.
5. Add garlic, coriander, cumin and paprika, stir and cook for 2 minutes.
6. Add pine nuts, stock, carrot, tomatoes and lemon zest, stir; cover and cook for 20 minutes. Add parsley, stir; cook for 2 minutes more, divide into bowls and serve.

Nutrition Facts Per Serving: Calories: 200; Fat: 5g; Fiber: 3g; Carbs: 6g; Protein: 10g

Lamb Stew

(**Prep + Cook Time**: 2 hours | **Servings**: 4)

Ingredients:
- 1½ lbs. lamb meat; cubed
- 1 small red chili pepper; chopped
- 1 yellow onion; chopped
- 3 garlic cloves; minced
- 2 celery sticks; chopped
- 1 tbsp. coconut oil
- 2½ tsp. garam masala
- 1 tsp. fennel seeds
- 1¼ tsp. turmeric
- 1½ cups coconut milk
- 1½ tsp. ghee
- 1½ tbsp. tomato paste
- 2 carrots; chopped
- 1 cup water
- A pinch of sea salt
- 1 tbsp. lemon juice
- Chopped parsley for serving

Instructions:
1. Heat up a pot with the oil over medium high heat, add lamb, stir and cook for 4 minutes.
2. Add celery, chili and onion, stir and cook for 1 minute.
3. Reduce heat to medium, add turmeric, garam masala, garlic, ghee and fennel seeds, stir and cook for 2 minutes more.
4. Add tomato paste, coconut milk, water and a pinch of sea salt, stir; bring to a boil, cover and cook for 1 hour.
5. Add carrots, stir; cover pot again and cook for 40 minutes more. Add lemon juice and parsley, stir; divide into bowls and serve hot.

Nutrition Facts Per Serving: Calories: 360; Fat: 7g; Fiber: 2g; Carbs: 8g; Protein: 20

Slow Cooked Paleo Stew

(**Prep + Cook Time**: 7 hours 10 minutes | **Servings**: 4)

Ingredients:
- 1½ lbs. beef meat; cubed
- 8 carrots; chopped
- 2 parsnips; chopped
- 1 yellow onion; chopped
- 1/4 cup tapioca flour
- 2 bay leaves
- 1/2 tsp. peppercorns
- 2 tbsp. olive oil
- 1 tbsp. thyme; chopped
- 2 tbsp. water
- 4 cups beef stock
- A pinch of sea salt
- Black pepper to the taste

Instructions:
1. Heat up a pan with the oil over medium high heat, add beef, stir; brown for 4 minutes on all sides and transfer to your slow cooker.
2. Add peppercorns, parsnips, carrots, onion, bay leaves, thyme, stock, a pinch of salt and black pepper, stir; cover and cook on High for 6 hours and 30 minutes.
3. Uncover slow cooker, add tapioca mixed with the water, stir; cover again and cook on High for 30 minutes more. Uncover pot again, discard bay leaves, divide stew into bowls and serve.

Nutrition Facts Per Serving: Calories: 200; Fat: 5g; Fiber: 3g; Carbs: 4g; Protein: 8g

French Chicken Stew

(Prep + Cook Time: 2 hours 10 minutes | **Servings**: 4)

Ingredients:
- 2 lbs. chicken pieces
- 10 garlic cloves
- 30 oz. canned tomatoes; chopped
- 30 black olives; pitted and chopped
- 2 cups chicken stock
- 2 tbsp. parsley; chopped
- 2 tbsp. thyme; chopped
- 2 tbsp. basil; chopped
- 2 tbsp. coconut oil
- A pinch of sea salt
- Black pepper to the taste
- 2 tbsp. rosemary; chopped

Instructions:
1. Heat up a pot with the oil over medium high heat, add chicken pieces, season with a pinch of salt and black pepper to the taste, stir and brown them for 2 minutes on each side.
2. Add garlic, stock, thyme, tomatoes, olives, rosemary, basil and parsley, stir; cover, place in the oven at 325 °F and bake for 2 hours. Divide into bowls and serve.

Nutrition Facts Per Serving: Calories: 240; Fat: 10g; Fiber: 4g; Carbs: 6g; Protein: 24g

Hearty Meat Stew

(Prep + Cook Time: 4 hours 10 minutes | **Servings**: 8)

Ingredients:
- 1 lb. beef chuck; cubed
- 1 lb. lamb shoulder; cubed
- 1 lb. pork butt; cubed
- 3 sweet potatoes; cubed
- 1 tbsp. coconut oil
- 3 bacon slices
- 2 leeks; chopped
- 2 yellow onions; chopped
- 2 bay leaves
- 1 carrot; chopped
- 3 garlic cloves; minced
- 1½ tsp. thyme; chopped
- 3 cups veggie stock
- 1 tbsp. lemon juice
- 3 tbsp. parsley; chopped
- Black pepper to the taste
- A pinch of sea salt

Instructions:
1. In a Dutch oven, mix leeks with onions, bay leaves, carrot, garlic, thyme, parsley, lemon juice, beef, pork, lamb, a pinch of salt and black pepper to the taste and toss to coat
2. Add oil, potatoes and top with bacon, place in the oven at 350 °F and bake for 4 hours. Divide into bowls and serve.

Nutrition Facts Per Serving: Calories: 340; Fat: 9g; Fiber: 5g; Carbs: 7g; Protein: 15g

Beef Stew

(Prep + Cook Time: 2 hours 40 minutes | **Servings**: 4)

Ingredients:
- 2 lbs. beef meat; cubed
- 1/3 cup ghee
- 2 cups beef stock
- 3 garlic cloves; minced
- Zest from 1 lemon; grated
- 1 butternut squash; peeled, seeded and cubed
- 1 bunch cilantro; chopped
- 3 yellow onions; chopped
- Black pepper to the taste
- 2 tbsp. Moroccan spices
- 1 lemon; sliced
- Juice of 1 lemon

Instructions:
1. Heat up a Dutch ovenn with the ghee over medium heat, add beef, onions, spices, black pepper, garlic, lemon slices, lemon juice and zest and stock, stir; place in the oven at 300 °F and cook for 2 hours.
2. Add cilantro and squash, stir and cook in the oven for 30 minutes more. Divide into bowls and serve.

Nutrition Facts Per Serving: Calories: 300; Fat: 12g; Fiber: 3g; Carbs: 6g; Protein: 17g

Seafood & Fish Recipes

Grilled Calamari

(Prep + Cook Time: 15 minutes | **Servings**: 4)

Ingredients:
- 2 lbs. calamari; tentacles andtubes sliced into rings
- 1 lime; sliced
- 1 lemon; sliced
- 1 orange; sliced
- 2 tbsp. parsley; chopped
- A pinch of sea salt
- Black pepper to the taste
- 3 tbsp. lemon juice
- 1/4 cup extra virgin olive oil
- 2 garlic cloves; minced

Instructions:
1. In a bowl; mix calamari with sliced lemon, lime, orange, lemon juice, a pinch of sea salt, pepper, parsley, garlic and olive oil and toss to coat.
2. Heat up your kitchen grill over medium high heat, add calamari and fruits slices, cook for 5 minutes, divide between plates and serve.

Nutrition Facts Per Serving: Calories: 90; Fat: 3g; Carbs: 0.2g; Fiber: 0g; Protein: 15g

Shrimp and Cauliflower Rice

(Prep + Cook Time: 25 minutes | **Servings**: 4)

Ingredients:
- 1 lb. shrimp; peeled and deveined
- 2 garlic cloves; minced
- 8 oz. mushrooms; sliced
- 4 bacon slices
- 1 cauliflower head; florets separated
- 1/4 cup coconut milk
- 1 tbsp. ghee
- A pinch of red pepper flakes
- A handful mixed parsley and chives; chopped
- 1/2 cup beef stock
- Black pepper to the taste

Instructions:
1. Heat up a pan over medium high heat, add bacon slices, cook until they are crispy, drain grease on paper towels and leave them aside for now.
2. Put cauliflower florets in your food processor, blend until you obtain your "rice" and transfer to a heated pan over medium high heat.
3. Cook cauliflower rice for 5 minutes stirring often.
4. Add coconut milk and 1 tbsp. ghee, stir and cook for a couple more minutes.
5. Blend everything using an immersion blender, add black pepper to the taste, stir; reduce heat to low and continue cooking for a few minutes more.
6. Heat up the pan where you cooked the bacon over medium high heat, add shrimp, cook for 2 minutes on each side and transfer them to a plate.
7. Heat up the pan again, add mushrooms, stir and cook for a few minutes as well.
8. Add garlic, pepper flakes and some black pepper, stir and cook for 1 minute. Add stock, return shrimp to pan, stir and cook until stock evaporates.
9. Divide cauliflower rice on plates, top with shrimp and mushrooms mix, top with crispy bacon and sprinkle parsley and chives.

Nutrition Facts Per Serving: Calories: 140; Fat: 2g; Fiber: 2g; Carbs: 4g; Protein: 9g

Lobster with Sauce

(Prep + Cook Time: 20 minutes | **Servings**: 4)

Ingredients:
- 1/4 cup ghee; melted
- 4 lobster tails
- A pinch of sea salt
- Black pepper to the taste
- 2 tbsp. Sriracha sauce
- 1 tbsp. lime juice
- 1 tbsp. chives; chopped
- Some parsley leaves; chopped for serving

Instructions:
1. In a bowl; mix Sriracha sauce with ghee, chives, a pinch of sea salt, pepper and lime juice and whisk well.
2. Cut lobster tails halfway through in the center, open with your fingers, fill them with half of the Sriracha mix, arrange on preheated grill over medium high heat, cook for 4 minutes, flip and cook for 3 minutes more.
3. Divide lobster tails on plates, drizzle the rest of the Sriracha sauce, sprinkle parsley on top and serve.

Nutrition Facts Per Serving: Calories: 240; Fat: 16g; Carbs: 2g; Fiber: 0.5g; Protein: 19g

Shrimp Dish

(Prep + Cook Time: 15 minutes | **Servings**: 4)

Ingredients:
- 1 lb. big shrimp; peeled and deveined
- 1/2 cup olive oil
- 1/4 cup onion; chopped
- 1 cup cilantro; chopped
- 1 cup parsley; chopped
- Juice from 2 limes
- A pinch of sea salt
- 2 tsp. olive oil
- 1/2 tsp. smoked paprika
- 2 garlic cloves; minced

Instructions:
1. Heat up a pan with 2 tsp. olive oil over medium heat, add shrimp, cook them for 5 minutes and reduce heat to low.
2. In your food processor, mix 1/2 cup oil with onion, sea salt, paprika, garlic, lime juice, parsley and cilantro and pulse really well. Divide shrimp on plates, top with the chimichurri and serve.

Nutrition Facts Per Serving: Calories: 120; Fat: 2g; Fiber: 1g; Carbs: 3g; Protein: 8g

Steamed Clams

(Prep + Cook Time: 20 minutes | **Servings**: 2)

Ingredients:
- 1½ lbs. shell clams; scrubbed
- 1/4 cup white wine
- 1/2 cup chicken stock
- 3 garlic cloves; finely chopped
- A pinch of sea salt
- Black pepper to the taste
- 3 tbsp. ghee
- 2 tbsp. parsley; chopped
- Lemon wedges

Instructions:
1. Heat up a pot with the ghee over medium heat, add garlic, stir and cook for 1 minute.
2. Add wine, bring to a boil and simmer for a few minutes.
3. Add stock and clams, cover pot and cook for 4-5 minutes.
4. Divide clams on plates, sprinkle parsley on top, a pinch of sea salt and pepper and serve with lemon wedges on the side.

Nutrition Facts Per Serving: Calories: 79; Fat: 23g; Carbs: 9g; Fiber: 0.4g; Protein: 22g

Paleo Scallops

(Prep + Cook Time: 23 minutes | **Servings**: 3)

Ingredients:
- 1 lb. scallops
- 1 romanesco head; cut in halves
- 1 shallot; minced
- 3 garlic cloves; minced
- 3 tbsp. olive oil
- 1½ cups chicken stock
- 1/4 cup walnuts; toasted and chopped
- 1½ cups grapes; halved
- 2 cups spinach
- 1 tbsp. avocado oil
- A pinch of sea salt
- Black pepper to the taste

Instructions:
1. Put half of the romanesco in a food processor, blend well and put into a bowl.
2. Put the other half of the romanesco in your food processor, blend well again and add to the bowl.
3. Heat up a pan with 2 tbsp. oil over medium high heat, add garlic and shallot, stir and cook for 1 minute.
4. Add romanesco rice, stir and cook for 3 minutes. Add 1 cup stock, some salt and pepper, spinach and 1 cup grapes, stir and blend using an immersion blender.
5. Add the rest of the stock, blend again, cook for 5 minutes, take off heat and divide between plates.
6. Heat up another pan with the rest of the oil over medium high heat, add scallops, season them with a pinch of sea salt and black pepper, cook for 2 minutes, flip, cook for 1 minute more and add next to romanesco rice.
7. Top with walnuts and the rest of the grapes and serve.

Nutrition Facts Per Serving: Calories: 200; Fat: 3g; Fiber: 3g; Carbs: 7g; Protein: 15g

Glazed Salmon

(Prep + Cook Time: 50 minutes | **Servings**: 2)

Ingredients:
- 1 big salmon fillet; cut in halves
- 2 tbsp. mustard
- 1 tbsp. maple syrup
- A pinch of sea salt
- Black pepper to the taste
- 2 sweet potatoes; peeled and chopped
- 2 tsp. coconut oil
- 1/4 cup coconut milk
- 3 garlic cloves; minced

Instructions:
1. In a bowl; mix maple syrup with mustard and whisk well.
2. Season salmon halves with a pinch of sea salt and black pepper to the taste and brush them with half of the maple mix.
3. Heat up a pan with 1 tsp. coconut oil over medium high heat, add salmon, skin side down and cook for 4 minutes.
4. Transfer salmon to a baking dish, brush with the rest of the maple syrup mix, place in the oven at 425 °F and roast for 10 minutes.
5. Put sweet potatoes in a pot, add water to cover, bring to a boil over medium heat, cover and cook for 20 minutes.
6. Heat up a pan with the rest of the oil over medium heat, add garlic, stir and cook for 1 minute.
7. Add sweet potatoes, stir well and then mash everything with a potato masher.
8. Add coconut milk, a pinch of salt and black pepper to the taste and blend using an immersion blender. Divide this mash between plates, add salmon on the side and serve.

Nutrition Facts Per Serving: Calories: 200; Fat: 3g; Fiber: 3g; Carbs: 6g; Protein: 20g

Roasted Cod

(Prep + Cook Time: 30 minutes | **Servings**: 4)

Ingredients:
- 1/4 cup ghee
- 4 medium cod fillets; skinless
- 2 garlic cloves; minced
- 1 tbsp. parsley leaves; finely chopped
- 1 tsp. mustard
- 1 shallot; finely chopped
- 3 tbsp. prosciutto; chopped
- 2 tbsp. lemon juice
- 2 tbsp. coconut oil
- A pinch of sea salt
- Black pepper to the taste
- Lemon wedges for serving

Instructions:
1. In a bowl; mix parsley with ghee, mustard, garlic, shallot, prosciutto, a pinch of sea salt, pepper and lemon juice and whisk very well.
2. Heat up an oven proof pan with the coconut oil over medium high heat, add fish, season with black pepper to the taste and cook for 4 minutes on each side.
3. Spread ghee mix over fish, introduce in the oven at 425 °F and bake for 10 minutes. Divide between plates and serve with lemon wedges on the side.

Nutrition Facts Per Serving: Calories: 138; Fat: 4g; Carbs: 1g; Fiber: 0g; Protein: 23g

Glazed Salmon

(Prep + Cook Time: 25 minutes | **Servings**: 4)

Ingredients:
- 4 salmon fillets; skin on
- White pepper to the taste
- 2 tsp. Dijon mustard
- 2 tbsp. pure maple syrup
- Juice and zest from 1 orange
- 2 garlic cloves; finely chopped
- A pinch of sea salt

Instructions:
1. In a bowl; mix maple syrup with orange zest, juice, mustard, a pinch of sea salt, pepper and garlic and whisk well.
2. Arrange salmon in a baking dish, brush with the maple syrup and orange mix, introduce in the oven at 400 °F and bake for 15 minutes. Divide between plates and serve right away.

Nutrition Facts Per Serving: Calories: 190; Fat: 10g; Carbs: 12g; Fiber: 0.6; Sugar: 13g; Protein: 26g

Salmon and Chives

(Prep + Cook Time: 22 minutes | **Servings**: 4)

Ingredients:
- 4 salmon fillets
- 2 tbsp. chives; chopped
- 1/3 cup maple syrup
- Bacon fat
- 3 tbsp. balsamic vinegar
- A pinch of sea salt
- 2 tbsp. dill; chopped
- Black pepper to the taste
- Lime wedges for serving

Instructions:
1. Heat up a pan with bacon fat over medium high heat, add fish fillets, season them with a pinch of sea salt and black pepper, cook for 3 minutes, cover pan and cook for 6 minutes more.
2. Add balsamic vinegar and maple syrup and cook for 3 minutes basting fish with this mix. Add dill and chives, cook for 1 minute, divide fillets between plates and serve with lime wedges on the side.

Nutrition Facts Per Serving: Calories: 140; Fat: 3g; Fiber: 2g; Carbs: 5g; Protein: 10g

Shrimp and Zucchini Noodles

(Prep + Cook Time: 25 minutes | **Servings**: 2)

Ingredients:
- 1 lb. shrimp; peeled and deveined
- 2 zucchinis; sliced in thin noodles
- 4 garlic cloves; minced
- A pinch of sea salt
- Black pepper to the taste
- 1/4 cup white wine
- 2 tbsp. chives; chopped
- 2 tbsp. lemon juice
- 2 tbsp. coconut oil

Instructions:
1. Heat up a pan with the coconut oil over medium high heat, add garlic, stir and cook for 3 minutes.
2. Add shrimp, stir and cook for 3 minutes and transfer them to a plate.
3. Pour lemon juice and wine into the pan, bring to a boil over medium heat and simmer for a few minutes.
4. Add zucchini noodles, the shrimp, a pinch of sea salt and pepper to the taste stir gently and divide among plates. Sprinkle chives on top and serve.

Nutrition Facts Per Serving: Calories: 140; Fat: 12g; Carbs: 6g; Fiber: 3g; Protein: 18g

Scallops with Delicious Puree

(Prep + Cook Time: 35 minutes | **Servings**: 4)

Ingredients:
- 12 sea scallops
- 3 garlic cloves; minced
- 2 cups cauliflower florets; chopped
- 2 cups sweet potatoes; chopped
- 2 rosemary springs
- A pinch of sea salt
- Black pepper to the taste
- 1/4 cup pine nuts; toasted
- 2 cups veggie stock
- 2 tbsp. extra virgin olive oil
- A handful chives; chopped

Instructions:
1. Put cauliflower, potatoes and stock in a pot, bring to a boil over medium high heat, reduce temperature and simmer until veggies are soft.
2. Drain veggies, transfer them to your blender, add a pinch of sea salt and pepper to the taste and pulse until you obtain a puree.
3. Heat up a pan with the oil over medium high heat, add rosemary and garlic, stir and cook for 1 minute.
4. Add scallops, cook them for 2 minutes, often stirring, season them with pepper to the taste and take them off heat. Divide puree on small plates, arrange scallops on top, sprinkle chives and pine nuts at the end and serve.

Nutrition Facts Per Serving: Calories: 170; Fat: 10g; Fiber: 0g; Carbs: 2g; Protein: 22g

Smoked salmon and veggies

(Prep + Cook Time: 10 minutes | **Servings**: 2)

Ingredients:
- 8 oz. smoked salmon; thinly sliced
- 1 cucumber; thinly chopped
- 2 cups cherry tomatoes; cut in halves
- 1 red onion; thinly sliced
- 6 tbsp. extra virgin olive oil
- 1/2 tsp. garlic; minced
- 2 tbsp. lemon juice
- Black pepper to the taste
- 1 tsp. balsamic vinegar
- Some dill; finely chopped
- 1/2 tsp. oregano; dried

Instructions:
1. In a bowl; mix oil with garlic, balsamic vinegar, oregano and garlic and whisk well.
2. Add black pepper to the taste and stir well again.
3. In a bowl; mix cucumber with tomatoes and onion.

4. Drizzle the dressing over veggies and toss to coat.
5. Roll salmon pieces and divide them among plates. Add mixed veggies on the side, sprinkle dill all over and serve.

Nutrition Facts Per Serving: Calories: 159; Fat: 23g; Carbs: 2g; Fiber: 3g; Protein: 14g

Salmon Dish

(Prep + Cook Time: 40 minutes | **Servings**: 6)

Ingredients:
- 4 salmon fillets; skin on and bone in
- 3 cups apple cider
- 1/2 tsp. fennel seeds
- 1 tsp. mustard seeds
- 1 fennel bulb; chopped
- 1 apple; cored, peeled and chopped
- 2 tbsp. ghee
- A pinch of sea salt
- Black pepper to the taste

Instructions:
1. Put cider in a pot and heat up over medium heat.
2. Add mustard seeds, a pinch of salt, black pepper and fennel seeds, stir and boil for 25 minutes.
3. Strain this into a bowl; add half of the ghee, stir well and leave aside for now.
4. Heat up a pan with the rest of the ghee over medium heat, add fennel and apple pieces, stir and cook for 6 minutes.
5. Brush salmon pieces with some of the cider mix, season with a pinch of salt and black pepper, place on a lined baking sheet.
6. Add fennel and apple pieces as well, introduce everything in the oven at 350 °F and bake for 25 minutes. Divide salmon between plates and serve with the rest of the cider sauce on top.

Nutrition Facts Per Serving: Calories: 150; Fat: 3g; Fiber: 2g; Carbs: 4g; Protein: 10g

Salmon Pie

(Prep + Cook Time: 1 hour 15 minutes | **Servings**: 4)

Ingredients:
- 8 sweet potatoes; thinly sliced
- 4 cups salmon; already cooked and shredded
- 1 red onion; chopped
- 2 carrots; chopped
- 1 celery stalk; chopped
- A pinch of sea salt
- Black pepper to the taste
- 2 tbsp. chives; chopped
- 2 cups coconut milk
- 1 tbsp. tapioca starch
- 2 garlic cloves; minced
- 3 tbsp. ghee

Instructions:
1. Heat up a pan with the ghee over medium heat, add garlic and tapioca, stir and cook for 1 minute.
2. Add coconut milk, stir and cook for 3 minutes.
3. Add a pinch of sea salt and pepper and stir again.
4. In a bowl; mix carrots with salmon, celery, chives, onion and pepper to the taste and stir well.
5. Arrange a layer of potatoes in a baking dish, add some of the coconut sauce, add half of the salmon mix, the rest of the potatoes and top with the remaining sauce.
6. Introduce in the oven at 375 °F and bake for 1 hour. Divide between plates and serve hot.

Nutrition Facts Per Serving: Calories: 260; Fat: 11g; Carbs: 20g; Fiber: 12g; Protein: 14g

Tuna and Chimichurri Sauce

(Prep + Cook Time: 15 minutes | **Servings**: 4)

Ingredients:
- 1 lb. sushi grade tuna
- 2 avocados; pitted, peeled and chopped
- 6 oz. arugula
- 1 small red onion; chopped
- 1/2 cup cilantro; chopped
- 1/3 cup olive oil
- 2 tbsp. olive oil
- 1 jalapeno pepper; chopped
- 2 tbsp. basil; chopped
- 3 tbsp. vinegar
- 3 garlic cloves; minced
- 1 tsp. red pepper flakes
- 1 tsp. thyme; chopped
- A pinch of sea salt
- Black pepper to the taste

Instructions:
1. In a bowl; mix 1/3 cup oil with onion, jalapeno, cilantro, basil, vinegar, garlic, parsley, pepper flakes, thyme, a pinch of salt and black pepper and whisk well.
2. Heat up a pan with 2 tbsp. oil over medium high heat, add tuna, season with a pinch of sea salt and black pepper, cook for 2 minutes on each side, transfer to a cutting board, leave aside to cool down and slice.
3. In a bowl; mix arugula with half of the chimichurri sauce you've made earlier, toss to coat well and divide between plates. Divide tuna slices, avocado pieces and drizzle the rest of the sauce on top.

Nutrition Facts Per Serving: Calories: 140; Fat: 1g; Fiber: 1g; Carbs: 2g; Protein: 6g

Paleo Salmon

(Prep + Cook Time: 30 minutes | **Servings**: 4)

Ingredients:
- 6 cabbage leaves; sliced in half
- 4 medium salmon steaks; skinless
- 2 red bell peppers; chopped
- Some coconut oil
- 1 yellow onion; chopped
- A pinch of sea salt
- Black pepper to the taste

Instructions:
1. Put water in a pot, bring to a boil over medium high heat, add cabbage leaves, blanch them for 2 minutes, transfer to a bowl filled with cold water and pat dry them.
2. Season salmon steaks with a pinch of sea salt and black pepper to the taste and wrap each in 3 cabbage leaf halves.
3. Heat up a pan with some coconut oil over medium high heat, add onion and bell pepper, stir and cook for 4 minutes.
4. Add wrapped salmon, introduce pan in the oven at 350 °F and bake for 12 minutes. Divide salmon and veggies between plates and serve.

Nutrition Facts Per Serving: Calories: 140; Fat: 3g; Fiber: 1g; Carbs: 2g; Protein: 15g

Fish Dish

(Prep + Cook Time: 20 minutes | **Servings**: 4)

Ingredients:
- 4 halibut fish fillets
- 1/4 cup ghee; melted
- 4 garlic cloves; minced
- 2 tbsp. parsley; chopped
- Zest and juice from 1 lemon
- 1 lemon; sliced
- A pinch of sea salt
- Black pepper to the taste

Instructions:
1. In a bowl; mix garlic with ghee, lemon zest, juice, parsley, a pinch of sea salt and pepper and stir well.
2. Arrange fish in a baking dish, season with pepper to the taste, drizzle the mix you've made, top with lemon slices, introduce in the oven at 425 °F and bake for 15 minutes. Divide between plates and serve warm.

Nutrition Facts Per Serving: Calories: 150; Fat: 19g; Carbs: 5g; Fiber: 0.4g; Protein: 31

Thai Shrimp Delight

(Prep + Cook Time: 60 minutes | **Servings**: 4)

Ingredients:
- 1 lb. shrimp; peeled and deveined
- 2 eggs; whisked
- 1 cup carrots; chopped
- 1/4 cup nuts; roasted and chopped
- 1/4 cup cilantro; chopped
- 4 green onions; chopped
- 2 shallots; chopped
- 1 spaghetti squash; cut in halves and seedless
- Juice from 1 lime
- 2 tbsp. coconut aminos
- 1 tbsp. chili sauce
- 1 tsp. ginger; grated
- 3 garlic cloves; minced
- 3 cups mung beans sprouts
- 3 tbsp. coconut oil
- 2 tbsp. almond butter
- A pinch of sea salt
- Black pepper to the taste

Instructions:
1. Brush squash halves with 1 tbsp. coconut oil, arrange pieces on a lined baking sheet, place in the oven at 400 °F and bake for 40 minutes.
2. Leave squash to cool down and make squash noodles using a fork.
3. Heat up a pan over medium heat, add coconut aminos, lime juice, almond butter and chili sauce and stir well until everything combines.
4. Heat up another pan with the rest of the oil over medium high heat, add shrimp, cook for 4 minutes and transfer to a plate.
5. Heat up the pan again over medium high heat, add ginger, shallots and garlic, stir and cook for 2 minutes.
6. Add carrots and sprouts, stir and cook for 1 minute. Add eggs and stir everything.
7. Add almond butter sauce you've made earlier, squash noodles, cilantro, green onions, nuts, shrimp, a pinch of salt and black pepper, stir well, divide between plates and serve right away.

Nutrition Facts Per Serving: Calories: 150; Fat: 3g; Fiber: 2g; Carbs: 3g; Protein: 14g

Salmon Skewers

(Prep + Cook Time: 25 minutes | **Servings**: 4)

Ingredients:
- 1 lb. wild salmon; skinless, boneless and cubed
- 2 Meyer lemons; sliced
- 1/4 cup balsamic vinegar
- 1/4 cup orange juice
- 1/3 cup Paleo orange marmalade
- A pinch of pink salt
- Black pepper to the taste

Instructions:
1. Heat up a small pot with the vinegar over medium heat, add marmalade and orange juice, stir; bring to a simmer for 1 minute and take off heat.
2. Skewer salmon cubes and lemon slices, season with a pinch of salt and black pepper, brush them with half of the vinegar mix, place on preheated grill over medium heat, cook for 4 minutes on each side.
3. Brush skewers with the rest of the vinegar mix, grill for 1 minute more, divide between plates and serve.

Nutrition Facts Per Serving: Calories: 150; Fat: 1g; Fiber: 2g; Carbs: 4g; Protein: 10g

Shrimp Dish

(Prep + Cook Time: 20 minutes | **Servings**: 4)

Ingredients:
- 20 shrimp; peeled and deveined
- 1 small red bell pepper; chopped
- 1 small yellow onion; chopped
- 1 garlic clove; finely chopped
- 5 dried red chilies
- 1-inch ginger; minced
- 1/4 cup coconut aminos
- A pinch of sea salt
- Black pepper to the taste
- 2 tbsp. coconut oil
- 2 tbsp. water
- 1 tbsp. lime juice
- 1 tsp. apple cider vinegar
- 1 tsp. raw honey
- A handful cilantro; finely chopped for serving

Instructions:
1. In a bowl; mix aminos with vinegar, honey, water and lime juice and whisk well.
2. Heat up a pan with the coconut oil over medium heat, add garlic and ginger, stir and cook for 2 minutes.
3. Add red chilies, onion, bell pepper, stir and cook for 4 minutes.
4. Add shrimp, a pinch of salt and pepper to the taste and the vinegar mix you've made, stir and cook for 5 minutes. Divide between plates and serve with cilantro sprinkled on top.

Nutrition Facts Per Serving: Calories: 157; Fat: 7g; Carbs: 11g; Fiber: 0g; Protein: 5g

Salmon Tartar Delight

(Prep + Cook Time: 15 minutes | **Servings**: 4)

Ingredients:
- 7 oz. smoked salmon; minced
- 14 oz. salmon fillet; cut into very small cubes
- 3 tbsp. red onion; minced
- 2 tbsp. pickled cucumber; minced
- Zest and juice from 1 lemon
- 1 garlic clove; finely minced
- 2 tbsp. basil; minced
- 2 tsp. oregano; dried
- Black pepper to the taste
- 2 tbsp. mint leaves; minced
- 2 tbsp. Dijon mustard
- 5 tbsp. extra virgin olive oil
- Lime wedges for serving

Instructions:
1. In a bowl; mix onion with cucumber, garlic, lemon zest and juice, basil, mint, oregano, mustard, oil and pepper and stir well.
2. Add smoked and fresh salmon and stir well again. Divide tartar between plates and serve with lime wedges on the side.

Nutrition Facts Per Serving: Calories: 230; Fat: 16g; Carbs: 2.3g; Fiber: 0.4g; Protein: 17g

Salmon and Chili Sauce

(Prep + Cook Time: 25 minutes | **Servings**: 12)

Ingredients:
- 1 lb. salmon; cut into medium cubes
- 1/3 cup coconut flour
- 1¼ cups coconut; shredded
- 1 egg
- 4 red chilies; chopped
- 3 garlic cloves; minced
- 1/4 cup balsamic vinegar
- 1/2 cup honey
- ¼ cup water
- 2 tbsp. coconut oil
- 1/4 tsp. agar agar
- A pinch of sea salt
- Black pepper to the taste

Instructions:
1. In a bowl; mix coconut flour with a pinch of salt and stir.
2. In another bowl; whisk the egg with black pepper.

3. Put coconut in a third bowl.
4. Dip salmon cubes in flour, egg and coconut and place them all on a working surface.
5. Heat up a pan with the oil over medium high heat, add salmon cubes, fry them for 3 minutes on each side, transfer them to paper towels, drain grease and divide them between plates.
6. Heat up a pan with the water over medium high heat.
7. Add chilies, cloves, vinegar, honey and agar agar, stir very well, bring to a gentle boil and simmer until all ingredients combine. Drizzle this over salmon cubes and serve.

Nutrition Facts Per Serving: Calories: 140; Fat: 1g; Fiber: 2g; Carbs: 4g; Protein: 15g

Salmon with Avocado Sauce

(Prep + Cook Time: 30 minutes | **Servings**: 5)

Ingredients:
- 2 lbs. salmon filets; cut into 4 pieces
- 1 tsp. cumin
- 1 tsp. sweet paprika
- 1 tsp. chili powder
- 1 tsp. onion powder
- 1/2 tsp. garlic powder
- A pinch of sea salt
- Black pepper to the taste

For the avocado sauce:
- 2 avocados; pitted, peeled and chopped
- 1 garlic clove; minced
- Juice from 1 lime
- 1 red onion; chopped
- 1 tbsp. extra virgin olive oil
- Black pepper to the taste
- 1 tbsp. cilantro; finely chopped

Instructions:
1. In a bowl; mix paprika with cumin, onion powder, garlic powder, chili powder, a pinch of sea salt and pepper to the taste.
2. Add salmon pieces, toss to coat and keep in the fridge for 20 minutes.
3. Put avocado in a bowl and mash well with a fork.
4. Add red onion, garlic clove, lime juice, olive oil, chopped cilantro and pepper to the taste and stir very well.
5. Take salmon out of the fridge, place it on preheated grill over medium high heat and cook it for 3 minutes.
6. Flip salmon, cook for 3 more minutes and divide on serving plates. Top each salmon piece with avocado sauce and serve.

Nutrition Facts Per Serving: Calories: 150; Fat: 12g; Carbs: 9g; Fiber: 6g; Protein: 24g

Roasted Trout

(Prep + Cook Time: 30 minutes | **Servings**: 4)

Ingredients:
- 3 trout; cleaned and gutted
- 1 bunch dill
- 2 lemons; sliced
- 1 bunch rosemary
- 2 fennel bulbs; sliced
- A pinch of sea salt
- Black pepper to the taste
- 2 tbsp. extra virgin olive oil

Instructions:
1. Grease a baking dish with some oil, spread fennel slices on the bottom and add trout after you've seasoned them with a pinch of sea salt and pepper.
2. Fill each fish with lemon slices, dill and rosemary springs.
3. Top fish with the rest of the herbs and lemon slices, drizzle the rest of the oil, introduce everything in the oven at 500 °F and bake for 10 minutes.
4. Reduce heat to 425 °F and bake for 12 more minutes. Leave fish to cool down, divide between plates and serve.

Nutrition Facts Per Serving: Calories: 143; Fat: 2.3g; Carbs: 1g; Fiber: 0g; Protein: 6g

Fish Tacos

(Prep + Cook Time: 25 minutes | **Servings**: 4)

Ingredients:
- 4 tilapia fillets; cut into medium pieces
- 1/4 cup coconut flour
- 2 eggs
- 3/4 cup tapioca starch
- 1/2 cup tapioca starch
- 1/4 cup sparkling water
- 2 cups cabbage; shredded
- 2 cups coconut oil
- A pinch of sea salt
- Black pepper to the taste
- Lime wedges for serving
- Cauliflower tortillas

For the Pico de Gallo:
- 2 tomatoes; chopped
- 2 tbsp. jalapeno; finely chopped
- 6 tbsp. yellow onion; finely chopped
- 2 tbsp. lime juice
- 1 tbsp. cilantro; finely chopped

For the mayo:
- 1/4 cup homemade mayonnaise
- 1 tbsp. Sriracha sauce
- 2 tsp. lime juice

Instructions:
1. In a bowl; mix tomatoes with tomatoes with onion, jalapeno, cilantro, 2 tbsp. lime juice and stir well, cover and keep in the fridge for now.
2. In another bowl; mix mayo with Sriracha and 2 tsp. lime juice, stir well, cover and also keep in the fridge.
3. In a bowl; mix 3/4 cup tapioca starch with coconut flour, sparkling water, a pinch of sea salt, pepper and eggs and whisk very well.
4. Put the rest of the tapioca starch in a separate bowl.
5. Pat dry tapioca pieces, coat with tapioca starch and dip each piece in eggs mix.
6. Heat up a pan with the coconut oil over medium high heat, transfer fish fillets to pan, cook for 1 minute, flip them, cook for 1 more minute, transfer to paper towels and drain excess fat.
7. Arrange tortillas on a working surface, divide cabbage on them, add a piece of fish on each, add some of the Pico de Gallo and top with mayo. Serve with lime wedges.

Nutrition Facts Per Serving: Calories: 230; Fat: 10g; Carbs: 12g; Fiber: 4g; Protein: 13g

Lobster and Sauce

(Prep + Cook Time: 18 minutes | **Servings**: 4)

Ingredients:
- 4 lobster tails; cut halfway through the center
- 1/4 cup ghee; melted
- 2 tbsp. sriracha sauce
- 1 tbsp. chives; chopped
- 1 tbsp. parsley; chopped
- 1 tbsp. lime juice
- A pinch of sea salt
- Black pepper to the taste

Instructions:
1. In a bowl; mix ghee with a pinch of salt, black pepper, lime juice, chives and sriracha sauce and whisk well.
2. Fill lobster tails with half of this mix, place them on heated grill over medium high heat, cook for 5 minutes, flip, grill them for 3 minutes more and divide between plates.
3. Top lobster tails with the rest of the Sriracha sauce and parsley.

Nutrition Facts Per Serving: Calories: 223; Fat: 12g; Fiber: 0g; Carbs: 2g; Protein: 6g

Tuna Dish

(Prep + Cook Time: 25 minutes | **Servings**: 4)

Ingredients:
- 4 medium tuna steaks
- 1 tsp. fennel seeds
- 1 tsp. mustard seeds
- 1/4 tsp. black peppercorns
- A pinch of sea salt
- Black pepper to the taste
- 4 tbsp. sesame seeds
- 3 tbsp. coconut oil

Instructions:
1. In your grinder, mix peppercorns with fennel and mustard seeds and grind well.
2. Add sesame seeds, a pinch of sea salt and pepper to the taste and grind again well.
3. Spread this mix on a plate, add tuna steaks and toss to coat.
4. Heat up a pan with the oil over medium high heat, add tuna steaks and cook for 3 minutes on each side. Divide between plates and serve with a side salad.

Nutrition Facts Per Serving: Calories: 240; Fat: 2g; Carbs: 0g; Fiber: 0g; Protein: 53

Salmon and Lemon Relish

(Prep + Cook Time: 1 hour 10 minutes | **Servings**: 2)

Ingredients:
- A drizzle of olive oil
- 1 big salmon fillet; cut in halves
- Black pepper to the taste
- A pinch of sea salt

For the relish:
- 1 shallot; chopped
- 1 Meyer lemon; cut in wedges and then thinly sliced
- 1 tbsp. lemon juice
- 2 tbsp. parsley; chopped
- 1/4 cup olive oil
- Black pepper to the taste

Instructions:
1. Put some water in a dish and place it in the oven.
2. Put the salmon on a lined baking dish, drizzle some olive oil, season with a pinch of sea salt and black pepper, rub well, place in the oven at 370 °F and bake for 1 hour.
3. Meanwhile; in a bowl, mix shallot with the lemon juice, a pinch of salt and black pepper, stir and leave aside for 10 minutes.
4. In another bowl; mix marinated shallot with lemon slices, some salt, pepper, parsley and 1/4 cup oil and whisk well. Cut salmon in chunks, divide on plates and top with lemon relish.

Nutrition Facts Per Serving: Calories: 200; Fat: 3g; Fiber: 3g; Carbs: 6g; Protein: 20g

Salmon and Spicy Slaw

(Prep + Cook Time: 16 minutes | **Servings**: 4)

Ingredients:
- 3 cups cold water
- 3 scallions; chopped
- 2 cups cabbage; chopped
- 4 cups baby arugula
- 2 cups radish; julienne cut
- 1/4 cup pepitas; toasted
- 2 tsp. sriracha sauce
- 4 tsp. honey
- 3 tsp. avocado oil
- 4 tsp. cider vinegar
- 2 tsp. flax seed oil
- 4 medium salmon fillets; skinless and boneless
- A pinch of sea salt
- 1½ tsp. jerk seasoning

Instructions:
1. Put scallions in a bowl; add cold water to them and leave aside.
2. In a bowl; mix Sriracha with honey and stir well.

3. In another bowl; combine 2 tsp. of the honey mix with 2 tsp. avocado oil, vinegar, a pinch of sea salt and black pepper and stir well.
4. Sprinkle salmon fillets with a pinch of sea salt, black pepper and jerk seasoning and rub well.
5. Heat up a pan with the rest of the avocado oil over medium high heat, add salmon, cook for 6 minutes, flip, take off heat, cover pan and leave aside for a few more minutes.
6. In a salad bowl; mix cabbage with arugula, radish, pepitas, a pinch of salt, black pepper, the honey and vinegar salad dressing and flax seed oil and toss to coat well.
7. Divide salmon on plates, drizzle the rest of the Sriracha sauce, add cabbage salad next to them and top with drained scallions.

Nutrition Facts Per Serving: Calories: 180; Fat: 3g; Fiber: 3g; Carbs: 4g; Protein: 8g

Grilled Salmon with Peaches

(Prep + Cook Time: 25 minutes | **Servings**: 4)

Ingredients:
- 2 red onions; cut into wedges
- 3 peaches; cut in wedges
- 4 salmon steaks
- 1 tsp. thyme; chopped
- 1 tbsp. ginger; grated
- A pinch of sea salt
- Black pepper to the taste
- 1 tbsp. white wine vinegar
- 3 tbsp. extra virgin olive oil

Instructions:
1. In a bowl; mix wine with ginger, vinegar, thyme, a pinch of sea salt, pepper and olive oil and whisk very well.
2. In a bowl; mix peaches with onion, salt and pepper and toss to coat.
3. Heat up your kitchen grill over medium high heat, add salmon steaks after you've seasoned them with pepper to the taste, grill for 6 minutes on each side and divide between plates.
4. Add peaches and onions to grill, cook for 4 minutes on each side and transfer next to salmon on plates. Drizzle the vinaigrette you've made all over salmon, onions and peaches and serve right away.

Nutrition Facts Per Serving: Calories: 448; Fat: 26g; Carbs: 13g; Fiber: 2; Sugar: 8g; Protein: 40

Stuffed Salmon Fillets

(Prep + Cook Time: 30 minutes | **Servings**: 2)

Ingredients:
- 2 medium salmon fillets; boneless
- 5 oz. tiger shrimp; peeled, deveined and chopped
- 6 mushrooms; chopped
- 3 green onions; chopped
- 2 cups spinach; chopped
- 1/4 cup macadamia nuts; toasted and chopped
- A pinch of sea salt
- Black pepper to the taste
- A pinch of nutmeg; ground
- 1/4 cup Paleo mayonnaise
- Bacon fat for cooking

Instructions:
1. Heat up a pan with some bacon fat over medium heat, add onions and mushrooms, a pinch of salt and black pepper, stir and cook for 4 minutes.
2. Add nuts, stir and cook for 2 minutes more.
3. Add spinach, stir and cook for 1 minute.
4. Add shrimp, stir and cook for another minute.
5. Take this mix off heat, leave it aside to cool down a bit, add Paleo mayo and nutmeg and stir everything.
6. Make an incision lengthwise in each salmon fillet, season with some black pepper and stuff with the shrimp mix.
7. Heat up a pan with some bacon fat over high heat, add salmon fillets and cook skin side down for 1 minute.
8. Cover the pan, reduce temperature to medium-low and cook for 8 minutes more.

9. Introduce pan in preheated broiler and broil for 2 minutes. Divide stuffed salmon fillets on plates and serve.

Nutrition Facts Per Serving: Calories: 450; Fat: 6g; Fiber: 4g; Carbs: 7g; Protein: 40

Shrimp Burgers

(**Prep + Cook Time**: 30 minutes | **Servings**: 4)

Ingredients:
- 1½ lbs. shrimp; peeled and deveined
- 1/4 cup celery; minced
- 1/4 cup almond meal
- 1 egg; whisked
- 2 tbsp. chives; chopped
- 2 tbsp. cilantro; chopped
- Black pepper to the taste
- 1 garlic clove; minced
- 1/4 cup radishes; minced
- 1 tsp. lemon zest
- 1 tbsp. lemon juice

For the salsa:
- 1 avocado; pitted, peeled and chopped
- 1 cup pineapple; chopped
- 2 tbsp. red onion; chopped
- 1/4 cup bell peppers; chopped
- 1 tbsp. lime juice
- 1 tbsp. cilantro; finely chopped
- A pinch of sea salt
- Black pepper to the taste

Instructions:
1. In a bowl; mix pineapple with avocado, bell peppers, 2 tbsp. red onion, 1 tbsp. lime juice, pepper to the taste and 1 tbsp. cilantro, stir well and keep in the fridge for now.
2. In your food processor, mix shrimp with 2 tbsp. cilantro, chives and garlic and blend well.
3. Transfer to a bowl and mix with radishes, celery, lemon zest, lemon juice, egg, almond meal, a pinch of sea salt and pepper to the taste and stir well.
4. Shape 4 burgers, place them on preheated grill over medium high heat and cook for 5 minutes on each side. Divide shrimp burgers between plates and serve with the salsa you've made earlier on the side.

Nutrition Facts Per Serving: Calories: 238; Fat: 12g; Carbs: 13.2g; Fiber: 3g; Protein: 15.4

Salmon Delight

(**Prep + Cook Time**: 37 minutes | **Servings**: 4)

Ingredients:
- 10 oz. spinach; chopped
- 5 sun-dried tomatoes; chopped
- 1/4 tsp. red pepper flakes
- 4 medium salmon fillets
- A pinch of sea salt
- Black pepper to the taste
- 1 tbsp. coconut oil
- 1/4 cup shallots; chopped
- 4 garlic cloves

Instructions:
1. Heat up a pan with the oil over medium high heat, add shallots, stir and cook for 3 minutes.
2. Add garlic, stir and cook for 1 minute. Add tomatoes, pepper flakes and spinach, stir and cook for 3 minutes.
3. Season with a pinch of salt and black pepper to the taste, stir; take off heat and leave aside for now.
4. Arrange salmon fillets on a lined baking sheet, season with a pinch of salt and some black pepper, top with the spinach mix, place in the oven at 350 °F and bake for 20 minutes.
5. Divide between plates and serve right away.

Nutrition Facts Per Serving: Calories: 140; Fat: 2g; Fiber: 2g; Carbs: 3g; Protein: 10g

Scallops Tartar

(Prep + Cook Time: 15 minutes | **Servings**: 2)

Ingredients:
- 6 scallops; diced
- A pinch of sea salt
- Black pepper to the taste
- 3 strawberries; chopped
- 1 tbsp. extra virgin olive oil
- 1 tbsp. green onions; minced
- Juice from 1/2 lemon
- 1/2 tbsp. basil leaves; finely chopped

Instructions:
1. In a bowl; mix strawberries with scallops, basil and onions and stir well.
2. Add olive oil, a pinch of salt, pepper to the taste and lemon juice and stir well again. Keep in the fridge until you serve.

Nutrition Facts Per Serving: Calories: 180; Fat: 27g; Carbs: 3g; Fiber: 0g; Protein: 24g

Shrimp Skewers

(Prep + Cook Time: 20 minutes | **Servings**: 4)

Ingredients:
- 1/2 lb. sausages; chopped and already cooked
- 1/2 lb. shrimp; peeled and deveined
- 2 tbsp. extra virgin olive oil
- 2 zucchinis; cubed
- A pinch of sea salt
- Black pepper to the taste

For the Creole seasoning:
- 1/2 tbsp. garlic powder
- 2 tbsp. paprika
- 1/2 tbsp. onion powder
- 1/4 tbsp. oregano; dried
- 1/2 tbsp. chili powder
- 1/4 tbsp. thyme; dried

Instructions:
1. In a bowl; mix paprika with garlic powder, onion one, chili powder, oregano and thyme and stir well.
2. In another bowl; mix shrimp with sausage, zucchini and oil and toss to coat.
3. Pour paprika mix over shrimp mix and stir well.
4. Arrange sausage, shrimp and zucchini on skewers alternating pieces, season with a pinch of sea salt and black pepper, place them on preheated grill over medium high heat and cook for 8 minutes, flipping skewers from time to time. Arrange on a platter and serve.

Nutrition Facts Per Serving: Calories: 360; Fat: 32g; Carbs: 4.3g; Fiber: 0.8; Sugar: 1g; Protein: 18.1

Infused Clams

(Prep + Cook Time: 22 minutes | **Servings**: 2)

Ingredients:
- 2 lb. little clams; scrubbed
- 1 shallot; minced
- 2 garlic cloves; minced
- 1 tbsp. olive oil
- 3 oz. pancetta
- 3 tbsp. ghee
- 1 bottle infused cider
- 1 apple; cored and chopped
- Juice of 1/2 lemon

Instructions:
1. Heat up a pan with the oil over medium high heat, add pancetta and brown for 3 minutes.
2. Add ghee, shallot and garlic, stir and cook for 3 minutes.
3. Add cider, stir well and cook for 1 minute.
4. Add clams and thyme, cover and simmer for 5 minutes. Add apple and lemon juice, stir; divide everything into bowls and serve.

Nutrition Facts Per Serving: Calories: 120; Fat: 1g; Fiber: 2g; Carbs: 4g; Protein: 10g

Halibut and Tasty Salsa

(Prep + Cook Time: 25 minutes | **Servings**: 4)

Ingredients:
- 4 medium halibut fillets
- 2 tsp. olive oil
- 4 tsp. lemon juice
- 1 garlic clove; minced

For the salsa:
- 1/4 cup green onions; chopped
- 1 cup red bell pepper; chopped
- 4 tsp. oregano; chopped
- 1 tsp. sweet paprika
- A pinch of sea salt
- Black pepper to the taste
- 1 small habanero pepper; chopped
- 1 garlic clove; minced
- 1/4 cup lemon juice

Instructions:
1. In a bowl; mix red bell pepper with habanero, green onion, 1/4 cup lemon juice, 1 garlic clove, oregano, a pinch of sea salt and black pepper, stir well and keep in the fridge for now.
2. In a large bowl; mix paprika, olive oil, 1 garlic clove and 4 tsp. lemon juice and stir well.
3. Add fish, rub well, cover bowl and leave aside for 10 minutes.
4. Place marinated fish on preheated grill over medium high heat, season with a pinch of sea salt and black pepper, cook for 4 minutes on each side and divide between plates. Top fish with the salsa you've made earlier and serve.

Nutrition Facts Per Serving: Calories: 150; Fat: 3g; Fiber: 2g; Carbs: 3g; Protein: 12g

Shrimp with Mango and Avocado Mix

(Prep + Cook Time: 15 minutes | **Servings**: 2)

Ingredients:
- 1 lb. shrimp; peeled and deveined
- 1 avocado; pitted, peeled and chopped
- 1 tomato; chopped
- 1 mango; peeled and chopped
- 1 jalapeno; chopped
- 1 tbsp. lime juice
- Bacon fat
- 1/4 cup green onions; chopped
- 4 garlic cloves; minced
- A pinch of sea salt
- Black pepper to the taste

Instructions:
1. In a bowl; mix lime juice with jalapeno, mango, tomato, avocado and green onions, stir well and leave aside.
2. Heat up a pan with some bacon fat over medium high heat, add garlic, stir and cook for 2 minutes.
3. Add shrimp, a pinch of sea salt and black pepper, stir and cook for 5 minutes. Divide shrimp on plates, add mango and avocado mix on the side.

Nutrition Facts Per Serving: Calories: 140; Fat: 2g; Fiber: 3g; Carbs: 3g; Protein: 8g

Grilled Oysters

(Prep + Cook Time: 17 minutes | **Servings**: 7)

Ingredients:
- 1/4 cup red onion; chopped
- 2 tomatoes; chopped
- A handful cilantro; chopped
- 1 jalapeno; chopped
- A pinch of sea salt
- Black pepper to the taste
- Juice from 1 lime
- 2 limes; cut into wedges
- 24 oysters; scrubbed

Instructions:
1. In a bowl; tomatoes with onion, cilantro, jalapeno, a pinch of salt, black pepper and juice from 1 lime, stir well and leave aside.
2. Heat up your grill over medium high heat, add oysters, grill them for 7 minutes.

3. Open them completely and divide oysters between plates. Top with the tomatoes mix and serve with lime wedges on the side.

Nutrition Facts Per Serving: Calories: 140; Fat: 2g; Fiber: 2g; Carbs: 4g; Protein: 8g

Stuffed Calamari

(**Prep + Cook Time**: 1 hour 5 minutes | **Servings**: 4)

Ingredients:
- 4 big calamari; tentacles separated and chopped
- 2 tbsp. parsley; chopped
- 5 oz. kale; chopped
- 2 garlic cloves; minced
- 1 red bell pepper; chopped
- 1 tsp. oregano; dried
- 14 oz. canned tomato puree
- Some bacon fat
- 1 onion; chopped
- A pinch of sea salt
- Black pepper to the taste

Instructions:
1. Heat up a pan with some bacon fat over medium heat, add onion and garlic, stir and cook for 2 minutes.
2. Add bell pepper, stir and cook for 3 minutes.
3. Add calamari tentacles, stir and cook for 6 minutes more.
4. Add kale, a pinch of sea salt and black pepper, stir; cook for a couple more minutes and take off heat.
5. Stuff calamari tubes with this mix and secure with toothpicks.
6. Heat up a pan with some bacon fat over medium high heat, add calamari, brown them for 2 minutes on each side and then mix with tomato puree.
7. Also add parsley, oregano and some black pepper to the pan, stir gently, cover, reduce heat to medium-low and simmer for 40 minutes. Divide stuffed calamari on plates and serve.

Nutrition Facts Per Serving: Calories: 222; Fat: 10g; Fiber: 1g; Carbs: 7g; Protein: 15g

Shrimp Cocktail

(**Prep + Cook Time**: 36 minutes | **Servings**: 4)

Ingredients:
- 20 jumbo shrimp; deveined but shelled
- 2 cups ice
- A pinch of sea salt
- A drizzle of olive oil
- 1 cup water

For the cocktail sauce:
- 1 cup tomato sauce
- 1/4 tsp. Worcestershire sauce
- Juice of 1 lemon
- Zest from 1 lemon
- 1 tbsp. prepared horseradish
- Chili sauce to the taste

Instructions:
1. In a bowl; mix water with ice, a pinch of sea salt and shrimp, stir; cover and keep in the fridge for 30 minutes.
2. Discard water from shrimp, rinse them, pat dry them, drizzle olive oil over them and rub well.
3. Arrange shrimp on a lined baking sheet, place in preheated broiler and broil them for 3 minutes.
4. Flip, broil for 2 minutes more and leave aside.
5. In a bowl; mix tomato sauce with Worcestershire sauce, lemon juice, lemon zest, chili sauce to the taste and horseradish and whisk well. Arrange shrimp on a platter and serve with the cocktail sauce on the side.

Nutrition Facts Per Serving: Calories: 160; Fat: 3g; Fiber: 2g; Carbs: 3g; Protein: 14g

Grilled Calamari

(Prep + Cook Time: 15 minutes | **Servings**: 4)

Ingredients:
- 2 lbs. calamari tentacles and tubes cut into rings
- 2 tbsp. parsley; minced
- 1 lemon; sliced
- 1 lime; sliced
- 2 garlic cloves; minced
- 3 tbsp. lemon juice
- 1/4 cup olive oil
- A pinch of sea salt
- Black pepper to the taste

Instructions:
1. In a bowl; mix calamari with parsley, lime slices, lemon slices, garlic, lemon juice, a pinch of salt, black pepper and olive oil and stir well.
2. Place calamari rings on preheated grill over medium high heat, cook for 5 minutes and divide between plates. Serve with the lemon and lime slices and some of the marinade drizzled on top.

Nutrition Facts Per Serving: Calories: 130; Fat: 4g; Fiber: 1g; Carbs: 3g; Protein: 12g

Grilled Salmon and Avocado Sauce

(Prep + Cook Time: 25 minutes | **Servings**: 4)

Ingredients:
- 1 avocado; pitted, peeled and chopped
- 4 salmon fillets
- 1/4 cup cilantro; chopped
- 1/3 cup coconut milk
- 1 tbsp. lime juice
- 1 tbsp. lime zest
- 1 tsp. onion powder
- 1 tsp. garlic powder
- A pinch of sea salt
- Black pepper to the taste

Instructions:
1. Season salmon fillets with a pinch of salt, black pepper and lime zest, rub well, place on heated grill over medium heat, cook for 15 minutes flipping once and divide between plates.
2. In your food processor, mix avocado with cilantro, garlic powder, onion powder, lime juice and coconut milk and blend well.
3. Add a pinch of sea salt and some black pepper, blend again and drizzle this over salmon fillets. Serve right away.

Nutrition Facts Per Serving: Calories: 170; Fat: 7g; Fiber: 2g; Carbs: 3g; Protein: 20g

Crusted Salmon

(Prep + Cook Time: 30 minutes | **Servings**: 4)

Ingredients:
- 1 cup pistachios; chopped
- 4 salmon fillets
- 1/4 cup lemon juice
- 2 tbsp. honey
- 1 tsp. dill; chopped
- A pinch of sea salt
- Black pepper to the taste
- 1 tbsp. mustard

Instructions:
1. In a bowl; mix pistachios with mustard, honey, lemon juice, a pinch of salt, black pepper and dill and stir well.
2. Spread this over salmon fillets, press well, place them on a lined baking sheet, place in the oven at 375 °F and bake for 20 minutes. Divide salmon between plates and serve with a side salad.

Nutrition Facts Per Serving: Calories: 150; Fat: 3g; Fiber: 2g; Carbs: 5g; Protein: 12g

Salmon Tartar

(Prep + Cook Time: 30 minutes | **Servings**: 4)

Ingredients:
- 1 lb. salmon fillet; skinless, boneless and cut into small cubes
- 1 small red onion; chopped
- 1 tbsp. basil; chopped
- Juice from lemon
- 2 tbsp. capers
- 1 tbsp. chives; minced
- 1/4 cup olive oil
- 1 tsp. mustard
- 2 green onions; chopped
- A pinch of sea salt
- Black pepper to the taste

Instructions:
1. In a big bowl mix chives with onion, basil, capers, salmon and green onions and stir.
2. In another bowl; mix lemon juice with mustard, oil, a pinch of salt and black pepper the taste and stir well. Add this dressing over salad, toss to coat well, divide between plates and serve.

Nutrition Facts Per Serving: Calories: 130; Fat: 1g; Fiber: 2g; Carbs: 2g; Protein: 7g

Tuna and Salsa

(Prep + Cook Time: 2 hours 18 minutes | **Servings**: 4)

Ingredients:
- 4 tuna pieces
- 3 cherry tomatoes; cut in quarters
- 1 red onion; chopped
- 1 jalapeno; chopped
- 2 avocados; pitted, peeled and chopped
- 1/2 tsp. coriander
- 2 tbsp. cilantro; chopped
- 2 tbsp. lime juice
- A pinch of sea salt
- Black pepper to the taste

Instructions:
1. In a bowl; mix cherry tomatoes with avocados, cilantro, lime juice, jalapeno, a pinch of sea salt and black pepper, stir well and keep in the fridge for 2 hours.
2. Season tuna with a pinch of sea salt, black pepper and coriander and rub well.
3. Place tune on preheated grill over medium high heat, cook for 3 minutes on each side and divide between plates. Serve with the avocado salsa on the side.

Nutrition Facts Per Serving: Calories: 150; Fat: 2g; Fiber: 1g; Carbs: 2g; Protein: 14g

Crab Cakes and Red Pepper Sauce

(Prep + Cook Time: 17 minutes | **Servings**: 8)

Ingredients:
- 1 cup crab meat
- 2 tbsp. parsley; chopped
- 2 tbsp. old bay seasoning
- 2 tsp. Dijon mustard
- 1 egg; whisked
- 1 tbsp. lemon juice
- 2 tbsp. coconut oil
- 1½ tbsp. coconut flour

For the sauce:
- 1/4 cup roasted red peppers
- 1/4 cup avocado; peeled and chopped
- 1 tbsp. olive oil
- 1 tbsp. lemon juice

Instructions:
1. In a bowl; mix crabmeat with old bay seasoning, parsley, mustard, egg, 1 tbsp. lemon juice and coconut flour and stir everything very well.
2. Shape 8 patties from this mix and place them on a plate.
3. Heat up a pan with 2 tbsp. coconut oil over medium high heat, add crab patties, cook for 3 minutes on each side and divide between plates.
4. In your food processor, mix olive oil with red peppers, avocado and 1 tbsp. lemon juice and blend really well. Spread this on your crab patties and serve.

Nutrition Facts Per Serving: Calories: 100; Fat: 4g; Fiber: 3g; Carbs: 5g; Protein: 7g

Tilapia Surprise

(**Prep + Cook Time**: 35 minutes | **Servings**: 4)

Ingredients:
- 28 oz. canned coconut milk
- 2 red bell peppers; seedless and cut in halves
- 4 tilapia fillets
- 2 green onions; chopped
- 4 tbsp. Thai red curry paste
- A drizzle of olive oil
- 1/2 cup water
- 2 tbsp. coconut aminos
- 8 lime wedges
- 1 cup basil; chopped
- A pinch of sea salt
- Black pepper to the taste

Instructions:
1. In your food processor, mix half of the coconut milk with basil, curry paste and blend well.
2. Heat up a pan over medium heat, add curry mix and cook for 3 minutes.
3. Add the rest of the coconut milk, water and coconut aminos, stir and cook for 10 minutes.
4. In a bowl; mix fish with bell pepper, a drizzle of oil, a pinch of salt and black pepper to the taste.
5. Heat up a grill over medium high heat, add peppers, grill them for 5 minutes and transfer to a plate.
6. Place fish on the grill, cook for 6 minutes and divide between plates. Add bell peppers on the side, sprinkle green onions, drizzle curry sauce and serve with lime wedges on the side.

Nutrition Facts Per Serving: Calories: 160; Fat: 3g; Fiber: 1g; Carbs: 2g; Protein: 12g

Shrimp and Zucchini Noodles

(**Prep + Cook Time**: 25 minutes | **Servings**: 2)

Ingredients:
- 1 lb. shrimp; peeled and deveined
- 2 zucchinis; cut with a spiralizer
- 4 garlic cloves; minced
- 2 tbsp. bacon fat
- 2 tbsp. lemon juice
- 2 tbsp. chives; minced
- A pinch of sea salt
- Black pepper to the taste

Instructions:
1. Heat up a pan with the bacon fat over medium heat, add garlic, stir and cook for 3 minutes.
2. Add shrimp, stir; cook for 4 minutes more and transfer to a plate.
3. Heat up the pan again, add lemon juice and zucchini noodles, stir and cook for 4 minutes.
4. Return shrimp to pan, season with a pinch of salt, black pepper and chives, stir; cook for a couple more minutes and divide between plates. Serve right away.

Nutrition Facts Per Serving: Calories: 140; Fat: 3g; Fiber: 3g; Carbs: 4g; Protein: 8g

Squid and Guacamole

(**Prep + Cook Time**: 15 minutes | **Servings**: 2)

Ingredients:
- 2 medium squid; cleaned, tentacles and tubes separated
- A pinch of sea salt
- Black pepper to the taste
- 1 tbsp. olive oil
- Juice of 1/2 lime

For the guacamole:
- 2 red chilies; chopped
- 2 avocados; pitted, peeled and chopped
- 1 tomato; chopped
- 1 red onion; chopped
- 1 tbsp. coriander; chopped
- Juice from 2 limes

Instructions:
1. In a bowl; mix chilies with avocados, coriander, tomato, red onion and juice from 2 limes and stir well.
2. Heat up your grill over medium high heat, add squid pieces after you've rubbed it with 1 tbsp. olive oil, season with salt and pepper to the taste, grill for 3 minutes, flip and cook for 2 minutes on the other side.

3. Transfer squid to a cutting board, slice, drizzle juice from 1/2 lime toss to coat and divide between plates. Serve with the guacamole on the side.

Nutrition Facts Per Serving: Calories: 360; Fat: 7g; Fiber: 5g; Carbs: 8g; Protein: 17g

Swordfish

(**Prep + Cook Time**: 16 minutes | **Servings**: 2)

Ingredients:
- 2 medium wild swordfish fillets
- 1 tbsp. cilantro; chopped
- 1 avocado; pitted, peeled and chopped
- 1 mango; peeled and chopped
- 2 tsp. avocado oil
- 1 tsp. cumin powder
- 1 tsp. onion powder
- 1 tsp. garlic powder
- A pinch of sea salt
- Black pepper to the taste
- 1/2 cup balsamic vinegar
- Juice of 1/2 lime

Instructions:
1. Season fish fillets with a pinch of sea salt, black pepper, onion powder, garlic powder and cumin powder and rub well.
2. Heat up a pan with half of the oil over medium high heat, add fish and vinegar, cook for 3 minutes on each side and transfer to plates.
3. In a bowl; mix avocado with mango, lime juice, cilantro and the rest of the oil and stir well. Divide this salsa next to fish fillets and serve.

Nutrition Facts Per Serving: Calories: 120; Fat: 2g; Fiber: 2g; Carbs: 4g; Protein: 16g

Spicy Shrimp

(**Prep + Cook Time**: 14 minutes | **Servings**: 2)

Ingredients:
- 12 jumbo shrimp; peeled and deveined
- 2 garlic cloves; minced
- 2 tbsp. olive oil
- 1/4 tsp. red pepper flakes
- 1 tsp. steak seasoning
- 1 tsp. lemon zest
- 1 tbsp. parsley; chopped
- 2 tsp. lemon juice
- A pinch of sea salt
- Black pepper to the taste

Instructions:
1. Heat up a pan with the oil over medium high heat, add pepper flakes, garlic and shrimp, stir and cook for 4 minutes.
2. Season with a pinch of sea salt, black pepper, parsley, lemon juice and lemon zest, stir well, divide between plates and serve.

Nutrition Facts Per Serving: Calories: 152; Fat: 12g; Fiber: 1g; Carbs: 2g; Protein: 6g

Scallops Tartar

(**Prep + Cook Time**: 10 minutes | **Servings**: 2)

Ingredients:
- 6 scallops; chopped
- 3 strawberries; chopped
- Juice of 1/2 lemon
- 1 tbsp. green onions; chopped
- 1 tbsp. olive oil
- 1/2 tbsp. basil; chopped
- A pinch of sea salt
- Black pepper to the taste

Instructions:
1. In a bowl; mix green onions with lemon juice, olive oil, scallops, strawberries, basil, a pinch of sea salt and black pepper to the taste, stir well, divide into small bowls and serve cold.

Nutrition Facts Per Serving: Calories: 140; Fat: 2g; Fiber: 2g; Carbs: 3g; Protein: 9g

Salmon and Tomato Pesto

(Prep + Cook Time: 25 minutes | **Servings**: 4)

Ingredients:
- 4 salmon fillets; skin on
- 1 shallot; chopped
- 1/2 cup cherry tomatoes; cut in quarters
- 2 garlic cloves; minced
- 1/2 cup sun-dried tomatoes; chopped
- 1 tbsp. red bell pepper; chopped
- 2 tbsp. basil; chopped
- 3 tbsp. olive oil
- A pinch of sea salt
- Black pepper to the taste

Instructions:
1. In your food processor, mix sun-dried tomatoes with garlic, oil, basil, shallots, a pinch of sea salt and black pepper and blend really well.
2. Rub salmon with some of this mix, place on preheated grill over medium high heat, cook for 12 minutes flipping once and divide between plates. Add the rest of the tomato pesto on top and serve with cherry tomatoes and bell pepper pieces on the side.

Nutrition Facts Per Serving: Calories: 140; Fat: 2g; Fiber: 2g; Carbs: 3g; Protein: 9g

Crusted Snapper

(Prep + Cook Time: 18 minutes | **Servings**: 1)

Ingredients:
- 1 red snapper fillet; skinless
- 1 tbsp. sesame seeds
- 1 tsp. coconut oil
- A pinch of sea salt
- Black pepper to the taste

Instructions:
1. Season red snapper with a pinch of sea salt and black pepper to the taste and spread sesame seeds on one side.
2. Press seeds down, flip fish and spread the remaining sesame seeds on this side.
3. Heat up a pan with the oil over medium high heat, add crusted red snapper, cook for 3 minutes on each side and transfer to a plate. Serve with a side salad.

Nutrition Facts Per Serving: Calories: 120; Fat: 1g; Fiber: 1g; Carbs: 2g; Protein: 10g

Cod and Herb Sauce

(Prep + Cook Time: 25 minutes | **Servings**: 4)

Ingredients:
- Grated zest from 1/2 lemon
- 4 medium cod fillets
- 1 shallot; chopped
- 3/4 cup coconut milk
- 1 tbsp. chives; chopped
- 1 tbsp. thyme; chopped
- 1 tbsp. parsley; chopped
- 6 tbsp. ghee
- 2 garlic cloves
- A pinch of sea salt
- Black pepper to the taste

Instructions:
1. In a bowl; mix garlic with ghee, shallots, chives, parsley and thyme and stir well.
2. Season cod with a pinch of salt and black pepper to the taste.
3. Heat up a pan over medium heat, add herbed ghee and fish, toss to coat and cook for 2 minutes on each side.
4. Transfer fish to a lined baking sheet, place in the oven at 400 °F and bake for 7 minutes.
5. Heat up the pan with the herbed ghee over medium heat, add lemon zest and coconut milk, stir and bring to a simmer over medium heat. Divide fish on plates, drizzle the herbed sauce on top and serve.

Nutrition Facts Per Serving: Calories: 160; Fat: 3g; Fiber: 2g; Carbs: 3g; Protein: 14g

Mussels Mix

(Prep + Cook Time: 25 minutes | **Servings**: 6)

Ingredients:
- 2 lbs. mussels; scrubbed
- 28 oz. canned tomatoes; chopped
- 2 cups chicken stock
- 29 oz. canned crushed tomatoes
- 3 garlic cloves; minced
- 1 yellow onion; chopped
- 1 tbsp. olive oil
- 1 handful parsley; chopped
- 1/2 cup white wine
- 1 tsp. red pepper flakes

Instructions:
1. Heat up a pot with the oil over medium heat, add onions, garlic, parsley and pepper flakes, stir and cook for 2 minutes.
2. Add wine, crushed and chopped tomatoes, black pepper and stock, stir; cover and bring to a boil.
3. Add mussels, stir; cover and cook until they open. Ladle this into bowls and serve.

Nutrition Facts Per Serving: Calories: 150; Fat: 3g; Fiber: 2g; Carbs: 6g; Protein: 12g

Mahi Mahi Dish

(Prep + Cook Time: 20 minutes | **Servings**: 4)

Ingredients:
- 4 mahi-mahi fillets
- 1/2 tbsp. sweet paprika
- 1/2 tsp. garlic powder
- 1/2 tsp. oregano; dried
- 1 tbsp. chili powder
- 2 tbsp. olive oil
- 2 tbsp. coconut oil
- 1/2 tsp. onion powder
- A handful cilantro; chopped
- Lime wedges

For the cilantro butter:
- Juice of 1 lemon
- 1 garlic clove; minced
- 1/4 cup ghee; melted
- 2 tbsp. cilantro; chopped

Instructions:
1. In a bowl; mix 1/4 cup ghee with 1 garlic clove, juice from 1 lemon and 2 tbsp. cilantro, whisk very well and leave aside for now.
2. In another bowl; mix garlic powder with onion powder, chili powder, oregano and paprika and stir well.
3. Season mahi-mahi with this mix, drizzle the olive oil over them and rub well.
4. Heat up a pan with the coconut oil over medium high heat, add fish fillets, cook for 4 minutes on each side and divide them between plates. Add cilantro butter over fish and serve.

Nutrition Facts Per Serving: Calories: 160; Fat: 4g; Fiber: 3g; Carbs: 6g; Protein: 15g

Roasted Cod

(Prep + Cook Time: 30 minutes | **Servings**: 4)

Ingredients:
- 4 medium cod filets
- 1/4 cup ghee
- 2 garlic cloves; minced
- 1 shallot; chopped
- 2 tbsp. bacon fat
- 2 tbsp. lemon juice
- 1 tbsp. parsley; chopped
- 3 tbsp. prosciutto; chopped
- 1 tsp. Dijon mustard
- A pinch of sea salt
- Black pepper to the taste
- Lemon wedges

Instructions:
1. In a bowl; mix mustard with ghee, garlic, parsley, shallot, lemon juice, prosciutto, salt and pepper and whisk well.
2. Heat up a pan with the bacon fat over medium high heat, add fish fillets, season them with some black pepper and cook for 4 minutes on each side.
3. Spread mustard and ghee mix over fish, transfer everything to a lined baking sheet, place in the oven at 425 °F and bake for 10 minutes. Divide fish between plates and serve with lemon wedges on the side.

Nutrition Facts Per Serving: Calories: 150; Fat: 4g; Fiber: 1g; Carbs: 3g; Protein: 20g

Meat Recipes

Beef Dish

(Prep + Cook Time: 45 minutes | **Servings**: 4)

Ingredients:
- 1 lb. beef; ground
- 1 lb. sweet potatoes; cubed
- 1 tsp. cumin seeds
- 3 tbsp. ghee
- 2 onions; chopped
- 1 small ginger pieces; grated
- 1 Serrano pepper; chopped
- 2 tsp. coriander powder
- 2 tsp. garam masala
- Black pepper to the taste
- 1 cup green peas
- A handful cilantro; chopped

Instructions:
1. Heat up a pan with 2 tbsp. ghee over medium heat, add sweet potato cubes, stir; cook them for 20 minutes and transfer them to a bowl.
2. Heat up the same pan over medium heat, add cumin, stir and brown them for 1 minute. Add Serrano pepper and onion, stir and cook for 4 minutes.
3. Add beef, ginger, coriander, garam masala, cayenne and black pepper, stir and cook for 5 minutes more.
4. Add green peas and sweet potatoes, stir; cook for 5 minutes more, divide between plates and serve with cilantro on top.

Nutrition Facts Per Serving: Calories: 160; Fat: 3g; Fiber: 1g; Carbs: 5g; Protein: 12g

Turkey Casserole

(Prep + Cook Time: 1 hour 10 minutes | **Servings**: 6)

Ingredients:
- 1 lb. turkey meat; ground
- 1 sweet potato; chopped
- 1 eggplant; thinly sliced
- 1 yellow onion; finely chopped
- 1 tbsp. garlic; finely minced
- A pinch of sea salt
- Black pepper to the taste
- 1/4 tsp. chili powder
- 1/4 tsp. cumin
- 15 oz. canned tomatoes; chopped and drained
- 8 oz. tomato paste
- A drizzle of olive oil
- 1/2 tsp. tarragon flakes
- 1/8 tsp. cardamom; ground
- 1/8 tsp. oregano

For the sauce:
- 1 cup almond milk
- 1 tbsp. almond flour
- 1½ tbsp. extra virgin olive oil
- 1 tbsp. coconut flour

Instructions:
1. Heat up a pan over medium-high heat, add turkey meat, onion and garlic, stir and cook until the meat turns brown.
2. Add tomatoes, tomato paste and sweet potatoes, stir and cook for 5 minutes.
3. Add a pinch of sea salt, pepper to the taste, chili powder, cumin, oregano, tarragon flakes and cardamom, stir well and cook for 2 minutes.
4. Grease a baking dish with a drizzle of olive oil, arrange eggplant slices on the bottom and add turkey mix on top.
5. Spread turkey mix evenly, introduce dish in the oven at 350 °F and bake for 15 minutes.
6. Meanwhile; heat up a pot over medium-high heat, add the rest of the olive oil, almond flour and coconut one, stir well 1 minute, reduce heat, add almond milk and stir well.
7. Cook this for 10 minutes.
8. Take the baking dish out of the oven and pour this almond milk mix over it.
9. Introduce in the oven again and bake for 45 minutes. Take casserole out of the oven, leave aside a few minutes to cool down, slice and divide between plates and serve.

Nutrition Facts Per Serving: Calories: 278; Fat: 2.6g; Carbs: 29g; Fiber: 6.7; Sugar: 13g; Protein: 28.5

Beef Lasagna

(**Prep + Cook Time**: 6 hours 10 minutes | **Servings**: 6)

Ingredients:
- 1 lb. beef; ground
- 1 red bell pepper; chopped
- 1 eggplant; sliced lengthwise
- 2 zucchinis; sliced lengthwise
- 2 cups tomatoes; chopped
- 2 tsp. oregano; dried
- 4 cups tomato sauce
- 1/4 cup basil; chopped
- 2 garlic cloves; minced
- 1 yellow onion; chopped
- 2 tbsp. tomato paste
- 1 tbsp. parsley; chopped
- 2 tbsp. olive oil
- A pinch of sea salt
- Black pepper to the taste

Instructions:
1. Heat up a pan with the oil over medium high heat, add onion and garlic, stir and cook for 2 minutes.
2. Add beef, stir and brown for 5 minutes more.
3. Add bell pepper, tomatoes, oregano, basil, tomato paste and parsley, stir and cook for 4 minutes more.
4. Add tomato sauce, black pepper to the taste and a pinch of salt and stir well again.
5. Arrange layers of eggplant and zucchini slices with the sauce you've made in your slow cooker.
6. Cover and cook on Low for 4 hours and 45 minutes. Divide your lasagna between plates and serve.

Nutrition Facts Per Serving: Calories: 240; Fat: 10g; Fiber: 5g; Carbs: 7g; Protein: 12g

Beef and Bok Choy

(**Prep + Cook Time**: 30 minutes | **Servings**: 4)

Ingredients:
- 2 lb. beef sirloin; cut into strips
- 1 onion; sliced
- 12 baby bok choy heads; halved
- 2 garlic cloves; minced
- 3 tbsp. coconut oil
- 5 red chilies; dried and chopped
- A pinch of sea salt
- Black pepper to the taste
- 1 ginger piece; grated

Instructions:
1. Heat up a pan with the oil over high heat, add chilies, garlic and ginger, stir and cook for 1 minute.
2. Add beef, stir; cook for 3 minutes and transfer to a bowl.
3. Heat up the pan again over medium high heat, add onion, stir and cook for 2 minutes.
4. Add bok choy, stir and cook for 4 minutes more. Return beef mix to the pan, stir; cook for 1 minute more, divide between plates and serve hot.

Nutrition Facts Per Serving: Calories: 140; Fat: 3g; Fiber: 5g; Carbs: 9g; Protein: 20g

Grilled Steaks

(**Prep + Cook Time**: 20 minutes | **Servings**: 4)

Ingredients:
- 4 rib eye steaks
- 1½ tbsp. coffee; ground
- 1/2 tbsp. sweet paprika
- 2 tbsp. chili powder
- 2 tsp. garlic powder
- 2 tsp. onion powder
- 1/4 tsp. ginger; ground
- 1/4 teaspoon; coriander, ground
- A pinch of cayenne pepper
- Black pepper to the taste

Instructions:
1. In a bowl; mix coffee with paprika, chili powder, garlic powder, onion powder, ginger, coriander, cayenne and black pepper and stir well.
2. Rub steaks with the coffee mix, place them on your preheated grill over medium high heat, cook them for 5 minutes on each side and divide between plates. Leave steaks to cool down for 5 minutes before serving them with a side salad!

Nutrition Facts Per Serving: Calories: 160; Fat: 10g; Fiber: 1g; Carbs: 4g; Protein: 8g

Pulled Pork

(Prep + Cook Time: 20 hours 30 minutes | **Servings**: 4)

Ingredients:
- 3 lbs. organic pork shoulder
- 1/2 cup salsa
- 1/2 cup beef stock
- 1/2 cup enchilada sauce
- 2 green chilies; chopped
- 1 tbsp. garlic powder
- 1 tbsp. chili powder
- 1 tsp. onion powder
- 1 tsp. cumin
- 1 tsp. paprika
- Black pepper to the taste

Instructions:
1. In a bowl; mix chili powder with onion and garlic one.
2. Add cumin, paprika and pepper to the taste and stir everything.
3. Add pork, rub well and keep in the fridge for 12 hours.
4. Transfer pork to your slow cooker, add enchilada sauce, stock, salsa and green chilies, stir; cover and cook on Low for 8 hours.
5. Transfer pork to a plate, leave aside to cool down and shred.
6. Strain sauce from slow cooker into a pan, bring to a boil over medium heat and simmer for 8 minutes stirring all the time.
7. Add shredded pork to the sauce, stir; reduce heat to medium and cook for 20 more minutes. Divide between plates and serve hot.

Nutrition Facts Per Serving: Calories: 250; Fat: 35g; Carbs: 5g; Fiber: 2g; Protein: 50

Beef Casserole

(Prep + Cook Time: 8 hours 10 minutes | **Servings**: 4)

Ingredients:
- 3½ lbs. grass fed beef meat; cubed
- 2 cups pearl onions
- 4 garlic cloves; minced
- 2 sweet potatoes; chopped
- 2 celery stalks; chopped
- A pinch of sea salt
- Black pepper to the taste
- 2 tbsp. tomato paste
- 2 bay leaves
- 2 cups carrot; chopped
- 2 cups broth
- 1 tsp. thyme; dried
- 1 tbsp. coconut oil

Instructions:
1. Heat up a pan with the oil over medium-high heat, add beef, stir and brown for 2 minutes on each side and transfer to your slow cooker.
2. Add pearl onions, potatoes, celery, garlic, carrots, tomato paste, stock, bay leaves, thyme, a pinch of salt and pepper to the taste, stir; cover and cook on Low for 8 hours. Uncover cooker, leave stew aside for 10 minutes, divide between plates and serve.

Nutrition Facts Per Serving: Calories: 210g; Carbs: 14; Fat: 20g; Fiber: 4g; Protein: 38

Grilled Lamb Chops

(Prep + Cook Time: 20 minutes | **Servings**: 6)

Ingredients:
- 8 lamb chops
- 2 garlic cloves; minced
- 3 tbsp. coconut amino
- 4 tbsp. extra virgin olive oil
- A pinch of sea salt
- Black pepper to the taste
- 2 tbsp. ginger; minced
- 1 tbsp. parsley leaves; chopped

Instructions:
1. In a bowl; mix olive oil with coconut amino, garlic, ginger and parsley and stir well.
2. Season lamb chops with a pinch of sea salt and pepper to the taste, place them on preheated grill over medium-high heat and cook for 4 minutes on each side, basting all the time with the marinade you've made.
3. Divide lamb chops on plates, leave aside to cool down for 4 minutes and serve.

Nutrition Facts Per Serving: Calories: 214; Fat: 33g; Carbs: 2g; Protein: 28g; Fiber: 0.2

Pork Dish with Delicious Blueberry Sauce

(**Prep + Cook Time**: 40 minutes | **Servings**: 4)

Ingredients:
- 1 cup blueberries
- 1/2 tsp. thyme; dried
- 2 lbs. pork loin
- 1 tbsp. balsamic vinegar
- 1/2 tsp. red chili flakes
- 1 tsp. ginger powder
- A pinch of sea salt
- Black pepper to the taste
- 2 tbsp. water

Instructions:
1. Put pork loin in a baking dish and season with a pinch of sea salt and pepper to the taste.
2. Heat up a pan over medium heat, add blueberries and mix with vinegar, water, thyme, chili flakes and ginger.
3. Stir well, cook for 5 minutes and pour over pork loin. Introduce in the oven at 375 °F and bake for 25 minutes.
4. Take pork out of the oven, leave aside for 5 minutes, slice, divide between plates and serve with blueberries sauce.

Nutrition Facts Per Serving: Calories: 325; Fat: 23g; Carbs: 6g; Fiber: 1g; Protein: 64

Stuffed Quail

(**Prep + Cook Time**: 1 hour 15 minutes | **Servings**: 4)

Ingredients:
- 1 lb. grapes
- 8 bacon slices
- 4 quails
- 1 apple; chopped
- 1 tbsp. rosemary; chopped
- 1/2 cup cranberries; chopped
- 2 tbsp. extra virgin olive oil
- 2 garlic cloves; chopped
- 4 rosemary springs
- 1/2 cup chicken stock
- A pinch of sea salt
- Black pepper to the taste

Instructions:
1. Pat dry quail, season with a pinch of sea salt and pepper and leave aside for now.
2. In a bowl; mix cranberries with chopped rosemary, apple, olive oil, garlic, salt and pepper to the taste and stir well.
3. Fill quail with this mix, wrap each with 2 bacon slices and tie with cooking twine.
4. Spread half of the grapes in a baking dish, mash gently with a fork, arrange quail on top, spread the rest of the grapes and pour chicken stock at the end.
5. Introduce everything in the oven at 425 °F and bake for 1 hour. Divide between plates and serve with baked grapes on the side.

Nutrition Facts Per Serving: Calories: 260; Fat: 18g; Carbs: 22g; Fiber: 3g; Protein: 29g

Beef in Tomato Marinade

(Prep + Cook Time: 2 hours 15 minutes | **Servings**: 4)

Ingredients:
- 1 jalapeno pepper; chopped
- 2 tsp. chili powder
- 1 cup tomatoes; crushed
- 4 beef medallions
- 2 tsp. onion powder
- 2 tbsp. coconut aminos
- A pinch of sea salt
- Black pepper to the taste
- 1 tbsp. hot pepper
- 2 tbsp. lime juice

Instructions:
1. In a bowl; mix tomatoes with hot pepper, aminos, chili powder, onion powder, a pinch of salt, black pepper and lime juice and whisk well.
2. Arrange beef medallions in a baking dish, pour the sauce over them and leave them aside for 2 hours.
3. Discard tomato marinade, place beef on preheated grill over medium high heat, cook them for 5 minutes one each side basting them with the marinade.
4. Divide beef medallions on plates, sprinkle jalapeno on top and serve.

Nutrition Facts Per Serving: Calories: 230; Fat: 4g; Fiber: 1g; Carbs: 3g; Protein: 14g

Lamb Chops and Mint Sauce

(Prep + Cook Time: 30 minutes | **Servings**: 4)

Ingredients:
- 8 lamb chops
- 2 garlic cloves; minced
- 1 tbsp. lemon zest
- 1 tbsp. oregano; chopped
- 2/3 cup olive oil
- 1/3 cup mint; chopped
- 2 tbsp. balsamic vinegar
- A pinch of sea salt
- Black pepper to the taste
- 3 tbsp. Dijon mustard

Instructions:
1. In a bowl; mix oil with oregano, garlic and lemon zest and whisk well.
2. Brush lamb chops with this mix, season them with a pinch of salt and black pepper to the taste, place them on preheated grill over medium high heat and cook for 5 minutes on each side.
3. In a bowl; mix mustard with a pinch of salt, mint, vinegar and black pepper and whisk well. Divide lamb chops on plates, drizzle mint sauce over them and serve.

Nutrition Facts Per Serving: Calories: 17; Fat: 11g; Fiber: 1g; Carbs: 6g; Protein: 14g

Lamb Casserole

(Prep + Cook Time: 3 hours | **Servings**: 4)

Ingredients:
- 3 lbs. lamb shoulder; chopped
- 1 butternut squash; cubed
- 4 shallots; chopped
- 4 carrots; chopped
- 4 tomatoes; chopped
- 2 Thai chilies; chopped
- 2 tbsp. tomato paste
- 1 cinnamon stick
- 2½ cups warm beef broth
- 2-star anise
- 2 tbsp. tapioca starch
- 1 lemongrass stalk; finely chopped
- 1 tsp. Chinese five spice powder
- 1 tbsp. ginger; minced
- 2 tbsp. coconut amino
- 1½ tbsp. coconut oil
- 3 garlic cloves; chopped
- Black pepper to the taste

Instructions:
1. In a bowl; mix lamb with coconut amino, tapioca starch, ginger, lemongrass, garlic and pepper, stir well, cover and keep in the fridge for 2 hours.
2. Heat up a pot with the oil over medium-high heat, add marinated lamb, stir and brown for 3 minutes.
3. Add tomato paste and tomatoes, stir and cook for 2 more minutes.

4. Add squash, shallots, Thai chilies, carrots, cinnamon stick, star anise, beef stock and five spices, stir well, introduce in the oven at 325 °F and bake for 1 hour. Divide between plates and serve hot.

Nutrition Facts Per Serving: Calories: 456; Fat: 31g; Carbs: 5g; Fiber: 3g; Protein: 22g

Paleo Steak

(**Prep + Cook Time**: 40 minutes | **Servings**: 4)

Ingredients:
- 2 sweet potatoes; chopped
- 4 sirloin steaks
- 1 red onion; chopped
- 1 broccoli head; florets separated
- 8 cherry tomatoes; halved
- 4 thyme springs
- 4 garlic cloves; minced
- A pinch of sea salt
- Black pepper to the taste
- 4 tbsp. olive oil
- 1/2 tbsp. sweet paprika

Instructions:
1. In a bowl; mix oil with a pinch of salt, black pepper, garlic and paprika and stir well.
2. Spread broccoli and sweet potatoes on a lined baking sheet, place in the oven at 425 degrees f and bake for 10 minutes.
3. Heat up a pan over medium high heat, add steaks, season them with a pinch of sea salt and black pepper, cook for 2 minutes on each side and add to the baking sheet.
4. Also add onions and tomatoes, drizzle the oil and garlic mix, toss to coat, top with thyme and bake in the oven for 15 minutes more. Divide everything between plates and serve.

Nutrition Facts Per Serving: Calories: 170; Fat: 2g; Fiber: 2g; Carbs: 4g; Protein: 10g

Lamb Chops with Mint Sauce

(**Prep + Cook Time**: 35 minutes | **Servings**: 4)

Ingredients:
- 8 lamb chops
- 2 garlic cloves; finely minced
- 2/3 cup extra virgin olive oil
- 1 tbsp. oregano; finely chopped
- 3 tbsp. Dijon mustard
- 1 tbsp. lemon zest
- 2 tbsp. white wine vinegar
- 1/3 cup mint; chopped
- Black pepper to the taste

Instructions:
1. In a bowl; mix olive oil with oregano, garlic and lemon zest and stir well.
2. Season lamb with black pepper to the taste and brush with the mix you've just made.
3. Heat up your grill over medium high heat, add lamb chops, cook for 5 minutes on each side and transfer to plates.
4. In a bowl; mix mustard with vinegar, pepper and mint and whisk well. Serve lamb chops with vinegar mix drizzled on top.

Nutrition Facts Per Serving: Calories: 160; Fat: 5.6g; Carbs: 1g; Fiber: 0.2g; Protein: 23.2

Beef Kabobs

(Prep + Cook Time: 22 minutes | **Servings**: 4)

Ingredients:
- 2 lbs. sirloin steak; cut into medium pieces
- 2 red bell peppers; chopped
- 1 red onion; chopped
- 1 zucchini; sliced
- Juice from 1 lime
- 2 tbsp. chili powder
- 2 tbsp. hot sauce
- 1/2 tbsp. cumin powder
- 1/4 cup olive oil
- 1/4 cup Paleo Salsa
- A pinch of sea salt and black pepper to the taste

Instructions:
1. In a bowl; mix salsa with lime juice, oil, hot sauce, chili powder, cumin, salt and black pepper and whisk well.
2. Layer steaks pieces, bell peppers, zucchini and onion on skewers.
3. Brush kabobs with the salsa mix you made earlier, place them on preheated grill over medium high heat and cook them for 5 minutes on each side. Divide kabobs between plates and serve.

Nutrition Facts Per Serving: Calories: 170; Fat: 5g; Fiber: 2g; Carbs: 3g; Protein: 8g

Pork Chops

(Prep + Cook Time: 40 minutes | **Servings**: 4)

Ingredients:
- 4 pork chops; bone-in
- 8 sage springs
- 4 tbsp. ghee
- 4 garlic cloves; crushed
- 1 tbsp. coconut oil
- A pinch of sea salt
- Black pepper to the taste

Instructions:
1. Season pork chops with a pinch of sea salt and pepper to the taste.
2. Heat up a pan with the oil over medium high heat, add pork chops and cook for 10 minutes turning them often.
3. Take pork chops off heat, add ghee, sage and garlic and toss to coat. Return to heat, cook for 4 minutes often stirring, divide between plates and serve.

Nutrition Facts Per Serving: Calories: 250; Fat: 41g; Carbs: 1g; Fiber: 1; Sugar: 0.1g; Protein: 18.3

Chicken Thighs with Tasty Squash

(Prep + Cook Time: 40 minutes | **Servings**: 6)

Ingredients:
- 1/2 lb. bacon; chopped
- 6 chicken thighs; boneless and skinless
- 2 tbsp. coconut oil
- A pinch of sea salt
- A handful sage; chopped
- Black pepper to the taste
- 3 cups butternut squash; cubed

Instructions:
1. Heat up a pan over medium heat, add bacon, cook until it's crispy, drain on paper towels, transfer to a plate, crumble and leave aside for now.
2. Heat up the same pan over medium heat, add butternut squash, a pinch of salt and black pepper to the taste, stir; cook until it's soft, transfer to a plate and also leave aside.
3. Heat up the pan again with the coconut oil over medium-high heat, add chicken, salt and pepper and cook for 10 minutes, turning often.
4. Take the pan off the heat, add squash, introduce in the oven at 425 °F and bake for 15 minutes. Divide chicken and butternut on plates, top with sage and bacon and serve.

Nutrition Facts Per Serving: Calories: 241; Fat: 11g; Carbs: 17g; Fiber: 2.5; Sugar: 3g; Protein: 16g

Sausage Casserole

(Prep + Cook Time: 60 minutes | Servings: 6)

Ingredients:
- 6 sausage
- 2 green bell peppers; chopped
- 3 sweet potatoes; chopped
- 1-pint grape tomatoes; chopped
- A pinch of sea salt
- Black pepper to the taste
- 2 garlic cloves; minced
- 1 red onion; chopped
- A few thyme springs

Instructions:
1. In a baking dish, mix potatoes with tomatoes, onion, bell pepper, garlic, a pinch of sea salt and pepper and stir gently.
2. Heat up a pan over high heat, add sausages, brown them for 2 minutes on each side and transfer on top of veggies in the baking dish.
3. Add thyme, introduce in the oven at 400 °F and bake for 45 minutes. Divide between plates and serve hot.

Nutrition Facts Per Serving: Calories: 355; Fat: 10g; Carbs: 25g; Fiber: 2g; Protein: 16g

Mexican Steaks

(Prep + Cook Time: 25 minutes | Servings: 4)

Ingredients:
- 4 medium sirloin steaks
- 2 tbsp. chili powder
- 1 tsp. cumin; ground
- 1/2 tbsp. sweet paprika

For the Pico de gallo:
- 1 small red onion; chopped
- 2 garlic cloves; minced
- 2 tomatoes; chopped
- 2 tbsp. lime juice
- 1 small green bell pepper; chopped
- 1 tsp. onion powder
- 1 tsp. garlic powder
- A pinch of sea salt and black pepper to the taste
- 1 jalapeno; chopped
- 1/4 cup cilantro; chopped
- 1/4 tsp. cumin; ground
- Black pepper to the taste

Instructions:
1. In a bowl; mix chili powder with a pinch of salt, black pepper, onion powder, garlic powder, paprika and 1 tsp. cumin and stir well.
2. Season steaks with this mix, rub well and place them on preheated grill over medium high heat.
3. Cook steaks for 5 minutes on each side and divide them between plates.
4. In a bowl; mix red onion with tomatoes, garlic, lime juice, bell pepper, jalapeno, cilantro, black pepper to the taste and 1/4 tsp. cumin and stir well. Top steaks with this mix and serve.

Nutrition Facts Per Serving: Calories: 200; Fat: 12g; Fiber: 4g; Carbs: 5g; Protein: 12g

Beef Tenderloin with Special Sauce

(Prep + Cook Time: 50 minutes | Servings: 4)

Ingredients:
- 3 lbs. beef tenderloin
- 3 tbsp. Dijon mustard
- A pinch of sea salt

For the sauce:
- 1/2 cup parsley leaves; chopped
- 3 tbsp. basil leaves; chopped
- Zest from 1 lemon
- 2 garlic cloves; finely chopped
- Black pepper to the taste
- 1 tbsp. coconut oil
- 3 tbsp. balsamic vinegar
- A pinch of sea salt
- Black pepper to the taste
- 1/4 cup extra virgin olive oil

Instructions:
1. In a bowl; mix mustard with vinegar, stir very well and leave aside.
2. Season beef with a pinch of sea salt and pepper to the taste put in a pan heated with the coconut oil over medium-high heat and cook for 2 minutes on each side.
3. Transfer beef to a baking pan, cover with the mustard mix, introduce in the oven at 475 °F and bake for 25 minutes.
4. Meanwhile; in a bowl, mix parsley with basil, lemon zest, garlic, olive oil, a pinch of sea salt and pepper to the taste and whisk very well.
5. Take beef tenderloin out if the oven, leave aside for a few minutes to cool down, slice and divide between plates. Serve with herbs sauce on the side.

Nutrition Facts Per Serving: Calories: 180; Fat: 13g; Carbs: 2g; Fiber: 2g; Protein: 7g

Roasted Duck Dish

(Prep + Cook Time: 2 hours 10 minutes | **Servings**: 4)

Ingredients:
- 4 duck legs
- 4 thyme springs
- 1 lemon; sliced
- 1 orange; sliced
- 1 cup chicken broth
- 2 tsp. allspice; ground
- A pinch of sea salt
- Black pepper to the taste
- 1/2 cup orange juice

Instructions:
1. Heat up a pan over medium high heat, add duck legs, season with a pinch of salt and pepper to the taste and brown them for 3 minutes on each side.
2. Arrange half of lemon and orange slices on the bottom of a baking dish, place duck legs, top with the rest of the orange and lemon slices and thyme springs.
3. Add chicken stock, orange juice, sprinkle allspice, introduce in the oven at 350 °F and bake for 2 hours. Divide between plates and serve hot.

Nutrition Facts Per Serving: 255; Fat: 17g; Carbs: 6g; Protein: 33g; Fiber: 1

Steaks and Scallops

(Prep + Cook Time: 30 minutes | **Servings**: 2)

Ingredients:
- 10 sea scallops
- 4 garlic cloves; minced
- 2 beef steaks
- 1 shallot; chopped
- 2 tbsp. lemon juice
- 2 tbsp. parsley; chopped
- 2 tbsp. basil; chopped
- 1 tsp. lemon zest
- 1/4 cup ghee
- 1/4 cup veggie stock
- Some bacon fat
- A pinch of sea salt
- Black pepper to the taste

Instructions:
1. Heat up a pan with some bacon fat over medium high heat, add steaks, season them with a pinch of salt and black pepper to the taste and cook for 4 minutes on each side.
2. Add shallot and garlic, stir and cook for 2 minutes more.
3. Add ghee and stir everything.
4. Add stock, basil, lemon juice, parsley and lemon zest and stir.
5. Add scallops, season them with some black pepper as well and cook for a couple more minutes. Divide steaks and scallops between plates and serve with pan juices.

Nutrition Facts Per Serving: Calories: 150; Fat: 2g; Fiber: 2g; Carbs: 4g; Protein: 14g

Beef Stir Fry

(Prep + Cook Time: 30 minutes | **Servings:** 4)

Ingredients:
- 1½ lbs. beef steak; thinly sliced
- 10 oz. mushrooms; sliced
- 10 oz. asparagus; sliced
- 2 tbsp. honey
- 1/3 cup coconut amino
- 2 tsp. apple cider vinegar
- 1/2 tsp. ginger; minced
- 6 garlic cloves; minced
- 1 chili; sliced
- 1 tbsp. coconut oil
- Black pepper to the taste

Instructions:
1. In a bowl; mix garlic with coconut amino, honey, ginger and vinegar and whisk well.
2. Put some water in a pan, heat up over medium high heat, add asparagus and black pepper, cook for 3 minutes, transfer to a bowl filled with ice water, drain and leave aside.
3. Heat up a pan with the oil over medium-high heat, add mushrooms, cook for 2 minutes on each side, transfer to a bowl and also leave aside.
4. Heat up the same pan over high heat, add meat, brown for a few minutes and mix with chili pepper.
5. Cook for 2 more minutes and mix with asparagus, mushrooms and vinegar sauce you've made at the beginning. Stir well, cook for 3 minutes, take off heat, divide between plates and serve.

Nutrition Facts Per Serving: Calories: 165; Fat: 7.2g; Carbs: 6.33g; Fiber: 1.3; Sugar: 3g; Protein: 18.4

Pork with Pear Salsa

(Prep + Cook Time: 55 minutes | **Servings:** 4)

Ingredients:
- 1 yellow onion; chopped
- 1 organic pork tenderloin
- 2 pears; chopped
- 2 garlic cloves; minced
- 1 tbsp. chives; chopped
- 1/4 cup walnuts; chopped
- 3 tbsp. balsamic vinegar
- Black pepper to the taste
- 1/2 cup chicken stock
- 1 tbsp. coconut oil
- 1 tbsp. lemon juice

Instructions:
1. In a bowl; mix walnuts with pear, chives, pepper and lemon juice and stir well.
2. Heat up a pan with the oil over medium high heat, add tenderloin and brown for 3 minutes on each side.
3. Reduce heat, add onion and garlic, stir and cook for 2 minutes. Add balsamic vinegar, stock, pear mix, stir; introduce in the oven at 400 °F and bake for 20 minutes.
4. Take pork out of the oven, leave aside for 4 minutes, slice, divide between plates and serve with pear salsa on top.

Nutrition Facts Per Serving: Calories: 170; Fat: 3g; Carbs: 19g; Fiber: 4.4; Sugar: 10g; Protein: 12g

Pork Tenderloin with Carrot Puree

(Prep + Cook Time: 55 minutes | **Servings:** 4)

Ingredients:
- 2 sausages; casings removed
- A handful arugula
- Black pepper to the taste
- 1 grass fed pork tenderloin
- 1 tbsp. coconut oil

For the puree:
- 1 sweet potato; chopped
- 3 carrots; chopped
- A pinch of sea salt
- Black pepper to the taste
- 1 tbsp. curry paste

For the sauce:
- 2 shallots; finely chopped
- 2 tbsp. balsamic vinegar
- 1 tsp. mustard
- Black pepper to the taste
- 4 tbsp. extra virgin olive oil

Instructions:
1. Slice pork tenderloin in half horizontally but not all the way and open it up.
2. Use a meat tenderizer to even it up.
3. Place sausage in the middle, roll pork around it, tie with twine, season pepper to the taste and leave aside.
4. Heat up an oven proof pan with the coconut oil over medium high heat, add pork roll, cook for 3 minutes on each side, introduce in the oven at 350 °F and bake for 25 minutes.
5. Meanwhile; put potatoes and carrots in a pot, add water to cover, bring to a boil over medium high heat, cook for 20 minutes, drain and transfer to your food processor.
6. Pulse a few times until you obtain a puree, add a pinch of sea salt and pepper to the taste, blend again, transfer to a bowl and leave aside.
7. Take pork roll out of the oven, slice and divide between plates.
8. Heat up a pan with the olive oil over medium high heat, add shallots, stir and cook for 10 minutes.
9. Add balsamic vinegar, mustard, pepper, stir well and take off heat. Divide carrots puree next to pork slices, drizzle vinegar sauce on to and serve with arugula on the side.

Nutrition Facts Per Serving: Calories: 250; Fat: 34g; Carbs: 19g; Fiber: 2g; Protein: 53

Pork with Strawberry Sauce

(Prep + Cook Time: 45 minutes | **Servings**: 4)

Ingredients:
- 4 lbs. pork tenderloin
- 1 cup strawberries; sliced
- 10 bacon slices
- A pinch of sea salt
- Black pepper to the taste
- 4 garlic cloves; minced
- 1/2 cup balsamic vinegar
- 2 tbsp. extra virgin olive oil

Instructions:
1. Wrap bacon slices around tenderloin, secure with toothpicks and season with salt and pepper.
2. Heat up your grill over indirect medium high heat, put tenderloin on it and cook for 30 minutes.
3. Heat up a pan with the oil over medium high heat, add garlic, stir and cook for 2 minutes.
4. Add vinegar and half of the strawberries, stir and bring to a boil.
5. Reduce heat to medium and simmer for 10 minutes.
6. Add black pepper to the taste and the rest of the strawberries and stir.
7. Baste pork with some of the sauce and continue cooking over indirect heat until bacon is crispy enough.
8. Transfer pork to a cutting board, leave aside for a few minutes to cool down, slice and divide between plates. Serve with the strawberry sauce right away.

Nutrition Facts Per Serving: Calories: 279; Fat: 30g; Carbs: 8g; Fiber: 22g; Protein: 125

Beef and Veggies

(Prep + Cook Time: 3 hours 10 minutes | **Servings**: 4)

Ingredients:
- 3 lbs. beef; cut into cubes
- 1 yellow onion; sliced
- 3 garlic cloves; minced
- 1 cup beef stock
- 2 tbsp. coconut oil
- A pinch of sea salt
- Black pepper to the taste
- 8 oz. carrots; sliced
- 8 oz. mushrooms; sliced
- 1 tsp. thyme; chopped

Instructions:

1. Heat up a Dutch oven with 1 tbsp. oil over medium high heat, add beef cubes, season with a pinch of sea salt and black pepper, brown for 2 minutes on each side and transfer to a bowl.
2. Heat up the same Dutch oven over medium heat, add garlic, stir and cook for 2 minutes.
3. Add stock, stir well and heat it up.
4. Return meat to the pot, stir; place in the oven at 250 °F and roast for 3 hours.
5. In a bowl; mix carrots with mushrooms, 1 tbsp. oil, a pinch of sea salt, black pepper to the taste and thyme and stir well.
6. Spread these into a pan, place in the oven at 250 °F and roast them for 15 minutes. Divide beef and juices between plates and serve with roasted veggies on the side.

Nutrition Facts Per Serving: Calories: 200; Fat: 3g; Fiber: 4g; Carbs: 7g; Protein: 20g

Chicken Meatballs

(**Prep + Cook Time**: 30 minutes | **Servings**: 4)

Ingredients:
- 2 lbs. chicken meat; ground
- 1 pineapple; diced
- 1 egg
- 1 tsp. sweet paprika
- A pinch of sea salt
- Black pepper to the taste
- 1 tsp. garlic powder
- 1 tsp. onion powder

For the sauce:
- 1/4 cup coconut amino
- 4 tbsp. ketchup
- 1 tbsp. ginger; grated
- 1/2 cup pineapple juice
- 2 tsp. raw honey
- 1/2 tsp. red pepper flakes
- 1 tbsp. garlic; minced
- Salt and black pepper to the taste

Instructions:
1. In a pot, mix amino with ketchup, ginger, pineapple sauce, garlic, pepper flakes, honey, a pinch of sea salt and pepper to the taste, stir well, bring to a boil over medium heat, simmer for 8 minutes and take off heat.
2. In a bowl; mix chicken meat with paprika, egg, onion powder, garlic powder, salt and black pepper to the taste and stir well.
3. Shape meatballs, arrange them on a lined baking sheet, introduce them in the oven at 475 °F and bake for 15 minutes.
4. Heat up a pan over medium heat, add pineapple pieces, stir and cook for 2 minutes.
5. Add baked meatballs, pour sauce you've made at the beginnings, stir gently, cook for 5 minutes, divide between plates and serve.

Nutrition Facts Per Serving: Calories: 264; Fat: 20g; Carbs: 47g; Fiber: 2g; Protein: 47

Chicken and Veggies Stir Fry

(**Prep + Cook Time**: 35 minutes | **Servings**: 4)

Ingredients:
- 1 red bell pepper; chopped
- 1 zucchini; chopped
- 1 yellow onion; finely chopped
- 1 broccoli head; florets separated
- 4 chicken breasts; skinless, boneless and chopped
- A pinch of sea salt
- Black pepper to the taste
- 1 tbsp. coconut oil

For the sauce:
- 1/4 cup chicken broth
- 2 garlic cloves; finely chopped
- 3 tbsp. coconut amino
- 1/2 cup orange juice
- 1 tbsp. orange zest
- 1 tsp. Sriracha sauce
- 1/4 tsp. ginger; grated
- A pinch of red pepper flakes

Instructions:
1. In a bowl; mix broth with orange juice, zest, amino, ginger, garlic, pepper flakes and Sriracha sauce and stir well.
2. Heat up a pan with the oil over medium heat, add chicken, cook for 8 minutes and transfer to a plate.
3. Heat up the same pan over medium heat, add bell pepper, broccoli florets, onion and zucchini, stir and cook for 4-5 minutes.
4. Add a pinch of sea salt, pepper, orange sauce you've made, stir; bring to a boil, add chicken, reduce heat and simmer for 8 minutes. Divide between plates and serve hot.

Nutrition Facts Per Serving: Calories: 320; Fat: 13g; Carbs: 17g; Protein: 45g; Fiber: 3.7; Sugar: 4

Beef and Brussels Sprouts

(Prep + Cook Time: 22 minutes | **Servings**: 4)

Ingredients:
- 1 lb. beef; ground
- 1 apple; cored, peeled and chopped
- 1 yellow onion; chopped
- 3 cups Brussels sprouts; shredded
- A pinch of sea salt
- Black pepper to the taste
- 3 tbsp. ghee

Instructions:
1. Heat up a pan with the ghee over medium high heat, add beef, stir and brown for 2 minutes.
2. Add Brussels sprouts, stir and cook for 3 minutes more.
3. Add onion and apple, stir and cook for 5 minutes more.
4. Add a pinch of sea salt and black pepper to the taste, stir; cook for 1 minute more, divide among plates and serve.

Nutrition Facts Per Serving: Calories: 150; Fat: 1g; Fiber: 2g; Carbs: 3g; Protein: 9g

Steaks and Apricots

(Prep + Cook Time: 35 minutes | **Servings**: 2)

Ingredients:
- 2 medium skirt steaks
- 2 tbsp. Cajun spice
- 1/4 cup coconut oil
- 1/3 cup lemon juice
- 1/4 cup apricot preserves
- 1/4 cup coconut aminos

Instructions:
1. In a bowl; mix half of the Cajun spice with lemon juice, aminos, oil and apricot preserves and stir well.
2. Pour this into a pan, bring to a boil over medium high heat and simmer for 8 minutes.
3. Blend this using an immersion blender and leave aside for now.
4. Season steaks with the rest of the Cajun spice, brush them with half of the apricots mix, place them on preheated grill over medium high heat and cook them for 6-minute son each side. Divide steaks on plates and top with the rest of the apricots mix.

Nutrition Facts Per Serving: Calories: 160; Fat: 6g; Fiber: 0.1g; Carbs: 1g; Protein: 22g

Beef and Wonderful Gravy

(Prep + Cook Time: 30 minutes | **Servings**: 4)

Ingredients:
- 1½ lb. beef; ground
- 1 egg; whisked
- 1 tbsp. mustard
- 1 tbsp. tomato paste
- 1 tsp. garlic powder
- 1 tsp. onion powder
- Some coconut oil for cooking
- A pinch of sea salt and black pepper to the taste

For the gravy:
- 1 small yellow onion; chopped
- 1¼ cups beef stock
- 2 tsp. parsley; chopped
- 2 tbsp. ghee
- 1 tsp. tapioca
- Black pepper to the taste

Instructions:
1. In a bowl; mix beef with tomato paste, egg, mustard, onion powder, garlic powder, a pinch of salt and black pepper to the taste and stir well.
2. Heat up a pan with the ghee over medium heat, add onion, stir and cook for 2 minutes.
3. Add stock, some black pepper, tapioca mixed with water, stir; cook until it thickens and take off heat.
4. Shape 4 patties from the beef mix. Heat up a pan with the coconut oil over medium high heat, add beef patties and cook for 5 minutes on each side.
5. Pour the gravy over beef patties, sprinkle parsley on top, cook for a couple more minutes, divide between plates and serve.

Nutrition Facts Per Serving: Calories: 200; Fat: 4g; Fiber: 2g; Carbs: 4g; Protein: 20g

Sheppard's Pie

(**Prep + Cook Time**: 60 minutes | **Servings**: 6)

Ingredients:
- 2 lbs. sweet potatoes; chopped
- 1½ lbs. beef; ground
- 2 cups beef stock
- 1 onion; chopped
- 2 carrots; chopped
- 2 thyme springs
- 2 bay leaves
- 2 garlic cloves; minced
- 2 celery stalks; chopped
- 1/4 cup ghee
- Bacon fat
- A handful parsley; chopped
- 2 tbsp. tomato paste
- A pinch of sea salt
- Black pepper to the taste

Instructions:
1. Put sweet potatoes in a pot, add water to cover, bring to a boil over medium high heat, cook for 20 minutes, drain, leave them to cool down and transfer to a bowl.
2. Add ghee, a pinch of salt and pepper and mash potatoes well.
3. Heat up a pan with the bacon fat over medium high heat, add beef, stir and cook for a couple of minutes.
4. Add carrots, garlic, onions, celery, stock, tomato paste, bay leaves, thyme springs, some black pepper and another pinch of salt, stir and cook for 10 minutes.
5. Discard bay leaves and thyme and spread beef mix on the bottom of a baking dish.
6. Top with mashed potatoes, spread well, place in the oven at 375 °F and bake for 25 minutes. Leave pie to cool down a bit before slicing and serving it.

Nutrition Facts Per Serving: Calories: 254; Fat: 7g; Fiber: 4g; Carbs: 7g; Protein: 14g

Barbeque Ribs

(**Prep + Cook Time**: 3 hour 2 minutes | **Servings**: 4)

Ingredients:
- 4 lbs. baby ribs
- 1 tbsp. smoked paprika
- 1/2 tbsp. onion powder
- 1/2 tbsp. garlic powder
- 1/2 tsp. cayenne pepper
- 1 cup paleo BBQ sauce
- 2 tbsp. raw honey
- 4 tsp. Sriracha
- 1/4 cup cilantro; chopped
- 1/4 cup chives; chopped
- 1/4 cup parsley; chopped
- Black pepper to the taste

Instructions:
1. In a bowl; mix paprika with onion powder, garlic powder, pepper and cayenne and stir well.
2. Add ribs, toss to coat and arrange them on a lined baking sheet.
3. Introduce in the oven at 325 °F and bake them for 2 hours and 30 minutes.

4. In a bowl; mix BBQ sauce with honey and Sriracha and stir well.
5. Take ribs out of the oven, mix them with BBQ sauce, place them on preheated grill over medium-high heat and cook for 7 minutes on each side. Divide ribs on plates, sprinkle chives, cilantro and parsley on top and serve.

Nutrition Facts Per Serving: Calories: 120; Fat: 6.4g; Carbs: 2g; Fiber: 03; Sugar: 0.3g; Protein: 6.2

Souvlaki

(Prep + Cook Time: 30 minutes | **Servings**: 4)

Ingredients:
- 3 sweet potatoes; cubed
- 4 medium round steaks
- 1/4 cup olive oil
- 1 lemon; sliced
- 1/4 cup kalamata olives; pitted and chopped
- 4 dill springs
- 2 garlic cloves; minced
- Some bacon fat
- 1 yellow onion; chopped
- 12 mini bell peppers; chopped
- 1/2 cup sun dried tomatoes; chopped
- 1 tbsp. sweet paprika
- 2 tbsp. balsamic vinegar
- 1 tbsp. oregano; dried
- A pinch of sea salt and black pepper
- Juice of 1 lemon

Instructions:
1. Heat up a pan with some bacon fat over medium high heat, add steaks, season them with a pinch of sea salt and some black pepper, brown them for 2 minutes on each side and transfer to a baking dish.
2. Heat up the pan again over medium high heat, add sweet potatoes, cook them for 4 minutes and add them to the baking dish.
3. Also add bell peppers, tomatoes, onion, olives and lemon slices.
4. Meanwhile; in a bowl, mix lemon juice with olive oil, vinegar, garlic, paprika and oregano and whisk well.
5. Pour this over steak and veggies, add dill springs on top, toss to coat, place in the oven at 425 °F and bake for 12 minutes. Divide steak and veggies between plates and serve.

Nutrition Facts Per Serving: Calories: 180; Fat: 11g; Fiber: 0g; Carbs: 0g; Protein: 21g

Turkey Casserole

(Prep + Cook Time: 1 hour 10 minutes | **Servings**: 6)

Ingredients:
- 1 lb. turkey meat; ground
- 1/4 cup onion; chopped
- 1 sweet potato; cut with a spiralizer
- 1 eggplant; chopped
- 1 tbsp. garlic; minced
- 8 oz. tomato paste
- 15 oz. canned tomatoes; chopped
- A pinch of sea salt
- Black pepper to the taste
- A pinch of oregano; dried
- 1/4 tsp. chili powder
- 1/4 tsp. cumin; ground
- Cooking spray
- A pinch of cardamom; ground
- 1/2 tsp. tarragon flakes

For the sauce:
- 1 cup almond milk
- 1 tbsp. coconut flour
- 1 tbsp. almond flour
- 1½ tbsp. olive oil

Instructions:
1. Heat up a pan over medium heat, add onion, turkey and garlic, stir and brown for a few minutes.
2. Add tomatoes, tomato paste and sweet potatoes, stir and cook for a few minutes more.
3. In a bowl; mix eggplant pieces with a pinch of sea salt, black pepper, chili powder, cumin, oregano, cardamom and tarragon flakes and stir well.
4. Spread eggplant into a baking dish after you sprayed it with some cooking spray and top with the turkey mix.

5. Place in the oven at 350 °F and bake for 15 minutes.
6. Meanwhile; heat up a pan with the oil over medium heat, add coconut and almond flour and stir for 1 minute.
7. Add almond milk and cook for 10 minutes stirring often.
8. Top turkey casserole with this sauce, place in the oven again and bake for 40 minutes more. Slice and serve hot.

Nutrition Facts Per Serving: Calories: 278; Fat: 3g; Fiber: 7g; Carbs: 9g; Protein: 18g

Moroccan Lamb

(Prep + Cook Time: 17 minutes | **Servings:** 4)

Ingredients:
- 8 lamb chops
- 2 tbsp. ras el hanout
- 1 tsp. olive oil

For the sauce:
- 1/4 cup parsley; chopped
- 2 tbsp. mint; chopped
- 3 garlic cloves; minced
- 2 tbsp. lemon zest
- 1/4 cup olive oil
- 1/2 tsp. smoked paprika
- 1 tsp. red pepper flakes
- 2 tbsp. lemon juice
- A pinch of sea salt
- Black pepper to the taste

Instructions:
1. Rub lamb chops with ras el hanout and 1 tsp. oil, place them on preheated grill over medium high heat, cook them for 2 minutes on each side and divide them between plates.
2. In your food processor, mix parsley with mint, garlic, lemon zest, 1/4 cup oil, paprika, pepper flakes, lemon juice, a pinch of salt and black pepper and pulse really well. Drizzle this over lamb chops and serve.

Nutrition Facts Per Serving: Calories: 400; Fat: 23g; Fiber: 1g; Carbs: 3g; Protein: 32

Carne Asada

(Prep + Cook Time: 55 minutes | **Servings:** 2)

Ingredients:
- 1/4 cup olive oil
- 1/2 tsp. oregano; dried
- 2 garlic cloves; minced
- Juice from 1 lime
- 2 skirt steaks
- 1/4 tsp. cumin; ground
- 1 Serrano chili pepper; minced
- 1/4 cup cilantro; chopped
- A pinch of sea salt
- Black pepper to the taste

For the veggie mix:
- 2 red bell peppers; chopped
- 3 Portobello mushrooms; sliced
- 1 yellow onion; chopped
- 1 tbsp. olive oil
- 1 tbsp. lime juice
- 1 tbsp. taco seasoning

Instructions:
1. In a bowl; mix 1/4 cup oil with oregano, garlic, lime juice, cumin, cilantro, chili pepper, a pinch of salt and black pepper and whisk very well.
2. Add steaks, toss to coat and keep in the fridge for 30 minutes.
3. Place steaks on preheated grill over medium high heat, cook them for 4 minutes on each side and transfer to a plate.
4. Heat up a pan with 1 tbsp. oil over medium high heat, add bell pepper and onion, stir and cook for 3 minutes,
5. Add mushrooms, taco seasoning and lime juice, stir and cook for 6 minutes more. Divide steaks between plates and serve with mixed veggies on the side.

Nutrition Facts Per Serving: Calories: 190; Fat: 2g; Fiber: 1g; Carbs: 4g; Protein: 20g

Steak and Blueberry Sauce

(**Prep + Cook Time**: 30 minutes | **Servings**: 4)

Ingredients:
- 1 cup beef stock
- 2 garlic cloves; minced
- 1 cup blueberries
- 4 medium flank steaks
- 2 tbsp. shallots; chopped
- 2 tbsp. ghee
- 1 tsp. thyme; chopped
- A pinch of sea salt
- Black pepper to the taste

Instructions:
1. Heat up a pan with the ghee over medium heat, add shallot and garlic, stir and cook for 4 minutes.
2. Add thyme, stock, a pinch of salt and black pepper, stir; bring to a simmer and cook for 10 minutes.
3. Add blueberries, stir and cook for 2 minutes more
4. Place steaks on preheated grill over medium high heat, cook for 4 minutes son each side and transfer to plates. Drizzle the blueberry sauce on top and serve them.

Nutrition Facts Per Serving: Calories: 170; Fat: 4g; Fiber: 3g; Carbs: 7g; Protein: 15g

Filet Mignon and Special Sauce

(**Prep + Cook Time**: 35 minutes | **Servings**: 4)

Ingredients:
- 12 mushrooms; sliced
- 4 fillet mignons
- 1 shallot; chopped
- 2 garlic cloves; minced
- 2 tbsp. olive oil
- 1/4 cup Dijon mustard
- 1/4 cup wine
- 1¼ cup coconut cream
- 2 tbsp. parsley; chopped
- Black pepper to the taste
- A pinch of sea salt

Instructions:
1. Heat up a pan with the oil over medium high heat, add garlic and shallots, stir and cook for 3 minutes.
2. Add mushrooms, stir and cook for 4 minutes more.
3. Add wine, stir and cook until it evaporates.
4. Add coconut cream, mustard, parsley, a pinch of salt and black pepper to the taste, stir and cook for 6 minutes more.
5. Heat up another pan over high heat, add fillets, season them with a pinch of salt and some black pepper and cook them for 4 minutes on each side. Divide fillets between plates and serve with the mushroom sauce on top.

Nutrition Facts Per Serving: Calories: 300; Fat: 12g; Fiber: 1g; Carbs: 4g; Protein: 23g

Veal Rolls

(**Prep + Cook Time**: 30 minutes | **Servings**: 4)

Ingredients:
- 2 zucchinis; cut in quarters
- 1/4 cup balsamic vinegar
- 8 veal scallops
- 2 tbsp. olive oil
- 2 tsp. garlic powder
- A pinch of sea salt
- Black pepper to the taste

Instructions:
1. Flatten veal scallops with a meat tenderizer, season them with a pinch of sea salt and black pepper to the taste and leave aside.
2. Season zucchini with a pinch of sea salt, black pepper and garlic powder, place on preheated grill over medium high heat, cook for 2 minutes on each side and transfer to a working surface.
3. Roll veal around each zucchini piece.
4. In a bowl; mix oil with balsamic vinegar and whisk well.

5. Brush veal rolls with this mix, place them on your grill and cook for 3 minutes on each side. Serve right away.

Nutrition Facts Per Serving: Calories: 160; Fat: 3g; Fiber: 2g; Carbs: 5g; Protein: 14g

Roasted Lamb

(Prep + Cook Time: 2 hours 40 minutes | **Servings:** 4)

Ingredients:
- 6 lamb shanks
- 15 garlic cloves; peeled
- 2 tsp. onion powder
- 2 tsp. cumin powder
- 1 cup water
- 3 tsp. oregano; dried
- 1/2 cup olive oil
- A pinch of sea salt
- Black pepper to the taste
- 1/2 cup lemon juice

Instructions:
1. Place garlic cloves in a roasting pan.
2. Add lamb on top, drizzle half of the oil and season with a pinch of salt and black pepper.
3. Also add onion powder and cumin and rub well.
4. Introduce this in the oven at 450 °F and roast for 35 minutes.
5. In a bowl mix the rest of the oil with the water, lemon juice and oregano and whisk very well.
6. Take lamb shanks out of the oven, drizzle this mix, toss to coat well and roast in the oven at 350 °F for 2 hours and 30 minutes. Divide lamb pieces between plates and serve.

Nutrition Facts Per Serving: Calories: 170; Fat: 2g; Fiber: 2g; Carbs: 4g; Protein: 12g

Beef Curry

(Prep + Cook Time: 45 minutes | **Servings:** 4)

Ingredients:
- 1 lb. beef; ground
- 2 curry leaves
- 1 Serrano pepper; chopped
- 1 onion; chopped
- 3 carrot; chopped
- 10 oz. canned coconut milk
- 1/4 cup water
- 1 tsp. mustard seeds
- 2 tbsp. coconut oil
- 1 tbsp. garlic; minced
- 2 tsp. garam masala
- 1 small ginger piece; grated
- 1/4 tsp. chili powder
- 1/2 tsp. turmeric powder
- 1 tsp. coriander powder
- A pinch of sea salt
- Black pepper to the taste

Instructions:
1. Heat up a pan with the oil over medium high heat, add mustard seeds, stir and toast them for 1 minute.
2. Add Serrano pepper, onion and curry leaves, stir and cook for 5 minutes.
3. Add ginger and garlic, stir and cook for 1 minute.
4. Add beef, a pinch of salt, black pepper, coriander powder, turmeric, chili and garam masala, stir and cook for 10 minutes.
5. Add carrot and 1/4 cup water, stir and cook for 5 minutes more.
6. Add coconut milk, stir well and cook for 15 minutes. Divide curry into bowls and serve.

Nutrition Facts Per Serving: Calories: 260; Fat: 4g; Fiber: 5g; Carbs: 9g; Protein: 14g

Beef Teriyaki

(**Prep + Cook Time**: 30 minutes | **Servings**: 4)

Ingredients:
- 1½ lbs. steaks; sliced
- 2 green onions; chopped
- 1/4 cup honey
- 1/2 cup coconut aminos
- 1 tbsp. ginger; minced
- 1 tbsp. tapioca flour
- 1 tbsp. water
- 2 garlic cloves; minced
- 1/4 cup pear juice
- Some bacon fat
- 4 tbsp. white wine

Instructions:
1. Heat up a pan with the bacon fat over medium heat, add ginger and garlic, stir and cook for 2 minutes.
2. Add wine, stir and cook until it evaporates.
3. Add honey, aminos, pear juice, stir; bring to a simmer and cook for 12 minutes.
4. Add tapioca mixed with the water, stir and cook until it thickens.
5. Heat up a pan with some bacon fat over medium high heat, add steak slices and brown them for 2 minutes on each side.
6. Add green onions and half of the sauce you've just made, stir gently and cook for 3 minutes more. Divide steaks between plates and serve with the rest of the sauce on top.

Nutrition Facts Per Serving: Calories: 170; Fat: 3g; Fiber: 2g; Carbs: 2g; Protein: 8g

Beef Skillet

(**Prep + Cook Time**: 50 minutes | **Servings**: 4)

Ingredients:
- 1 lb. beef; ground
- 1 tbsp. parsley flakes
- 2 big tomatoes
- 2 yellow squash; chopped
- 2 green bell peppers; chopped
- 1 yellow onion; chopped
- A pinch of sea salt
- Black pepper to the taste

Instructions:
1. Place tomatoes on a lined baking sheet, place in preheated broiler for 5 minutes, leave them to cool down, peel and roughly chop them.
2. Heat up a pan over medium high heat, add onion and beef, stir and cook for 10 minutes.
3. Add tomatoes, stir and cook for a couple more minutes.
4. Add parsley flakes, black pepper and a pinch of sea salt, stir and cook for 10 minutes more.
5. Add bell pepper pieces and squash ones, stir and cook for 10 minutes. Divide between plates and serve.

Nutrition Facts Per Serving: Calories: 190; Fat: 3g; Fiber: 4g; Carbs: 6g; Protein: 20g

Thai Curry

(**Prep + Cook Time**: 40 minutes | **Servings**: 4)

Ingredients:
- 1 lb. beef; ground
- 1 yellow onion; chopped
- 3 Thai chilies; chopped
- 2 tbsp. avocado oil
- 1 small ginger pieces; grated
- 3 garlic cloves; minced
- 1/2 tsp. cumin
- 1/2 tsp. turmeric
- A pinch of sea salt
- Black pepper to the taste
- A pinch of cayenne pepper
- 1 tbsp. red curry paste
- 1 cup tomato sauce
- 1 broccoli head; florets separated
- 1 handful basil; chopped
- 2 tsp. lime juice
- 2 tbsp. coconut aminos

Instructions:
1. Heat up a pan with the oil over medium heat, add chilies and onion, stir and cook for 5 minutes.
2. Add a pinch of salt, ginger, garlic, cumin, turmeric, black pepper, cayenne and beef, stir and cook for 10 minutes.
3. Add broccoli and curry paste, stir and cook for 1 minute more.
4. Add basil, tomato paste and coconut aminos, stir; bring to a simmer, cover, reduce heat to medium-low and cook for 15 minutes. Add lime juice, stir; divide into bowls and serve.

Nutrition Facts Per Serving: Calories: 200; Fat: 3g; Fiber: 5g; Carbs: 7g; Protein: 24g

Hamburger Salad

(Prep + Cook Time: 18 minutes | **Servings:** 4)

Ingredients:
- 1 lb. beef; ground
- 2 garlic cloves; minced
- 1 sweet onion; chopped
- 1 tbsp. coconut oil
- 1 cup cherry tomatoes; chopped

For the dressing:
- 2 tbsp. water
- 4 tbsp. mayonnaise
- 2 tbsp. Paleo ketchup
- 1 dill pickle; chopped
- 1 lettuce head; leaves separated and chopped
- A pinch of sea salt
- Black pepper to the taste
- 1 tbsp. yellow onion; chopped
- 1 tsp. balsamic vinegar
- 1 tbsp. pickle; minced

Instructions:
1. Heat up a pan with the oil over medium heat, add garlic and onion, stir and cook for 2 minutes.
2. Add beef, a pinch of sea salt and black pepper, stir; cook for 8 minutes more and take off heat.
3. In a salad bowl; combine beef mix and with lettuce leaves, 1 dill pickle and cherry tomatoes.
4. In another bowl; mix water with mayo, ketchup, yellow onion, vinegar and 1 tbsp. pickle and whisk well. Drizzle this over salad, toss to coat and serve.

Nutrition Facts Per Serving: Calories: 170; Fat: 3g; Fiber: 2g; Carbs: 5g; Protein: 12g

Lamb Chops

(Prep + Cook Time: 20 minutes | **Servings:** 6)

Ingredients:
- 8 lamb chops
- 2 garlic cloves; minced
- 3 tbsp. coconut aminos
- 4 tbsp. olive oil
- 2 tbsp. ginger; grated
- 1 tbsp. parsley; chopped
- A pinch of sea salt
- Black pepper to the taste

Instructions:
1. In a bowl; mix oil with aminos, parsley, ginger and garlic and stir well.
2. Place lamb chops on a preheated grill over medium high heat, season them with a pinch of salt and black pepper to the taste and grill them for 4 minutes on each side basting them with the oil and ginger mix you've made. Leave lamb chops to cool down for a couple of minutes and then serve.

Nutrition Facts Per Serving: Calories: 160; Fat: 5g; Fiber: 0g; Carbs: 1g; Protein: 20g

Beef and Cabbage Delight

(Prep + Cook Time: 20 minutes | **Servings**: 4)

Ingredients:
- 1 lb. beef; ground
- 1 onion; chopped
- 1 napa cabbage head; shredded
- 1 carrot; grated
- A pinch of sea salt
- Black pepper to the taste
- 2 tbsp. coconut oil

Instructions:
1. Heat up a pan with the oil over medium high heat, add onion and beef, stir and brown them for 5 minutes.
2. Add carrots, cabbage, a pinch of salt and black pepper to the taste, stir and cook for 5 minutes more. Divide between plates and serve.

Nutrition Facts Per Serving: Calories: 150; Fat: 1g; Fiber: 2g; Carbs: 5g; Protein: 9g

Slow Cooked Lamb Shanks

(Prep + Cook Time: 4 hours 10 minutes | **Servings**: 4)

Ingredients:
- 2 big lamb shanks
- A pinch of sea salt
- 1 garlic head; cloves peeled
- 4 tbsp. olive oil
- Juice of 1/2 lemon
- Zest from 1/2 lemon; grated
- 1/2 tsp. oregano; dried

Instructions:
1. Put lamb shanks in your slow cooker, sprinkle a pinch of sea salt, add garlic cloves, cover and cook on High for 4 hours.
2. In a bowl; mix olive oil with lemon juice, lemon zest and oregano and whisk well.
3. Transfer lamb shanks to a cutting board, discard bones, shred meat and divide between plates. Drizzle the lemon dressing on top and serve with a Paleo side salad.

Nutrition Facts Per Serving: Calories: 180; Fat: 2g; Fiber: 2g; Carbs: 4g; Protein: 9g

Rosemary Lamb Chops

(Prep + Cook Time: 20 minutes | **Servings**: 4)

Ingredients:
- 4 lamb chops
- 12 rosemary springs
- 4 garlic cloves; halved
- 1/2 tsp. black peppercorns
- 3 tbsp. avocado oil
- A pinch of sea salt

Instructions:
1. In a bowl; mix lamb chops with a pinch of salt, black peppercorns and oil and massage well.
2. Spread lamb chops on a lined baking sheet and add garlic next to them. Rub rosemary into your palms and add over lamb chops.
3. Introduce everything in preheated broiler over medium high heat for 10 minutes, divide between plates and serve.

Nutrition Facts Per Serving: Calories: 160; Fat: 3g; Fiber: 1g; Carbs: 2g; Protein: 20g

Slow-Cooked Beef

(Prep + Cook Time: 8 hours 50 minutes | **Servings**: 4)

Ingredients:
- 2 cups beef stock
- 1/4 cup honey
- 1 cup tomato paste
- 1 cup balsamic vinegar
- 4 lbs. beef chuck
- 1 tbsp. mustard
- 1 tbsp. sweet paprika
- 1 tsp. onion powder
- 2 tbsp. chili powder
- 2 garlic cloves; minced
- Black pepper to the taste

Instructions:
1. In a bowl; mix beef chuck with chili powder, paprika, onion powder, garlic and black pepper and rub well.
2. Transfer beef roast to your slow cooker, add stock over it, cover and cook on Low for 8 hours.
3. Meanwhile; heat up a pan over medium heat, add tomato paste, vinegar, mustard, honey and black pepper, stir; bring to a boil and cook for 12 minutes.
4. Transfer beef roast to a cutting board, leave it to cool down a bit, shred with a fork and return to your crock pot.
5. Add the sauce you've made in the pan, cover and cook everything on High for 30 minutes more. Divide this whole mix between plates and serve.

Nutrition Facts Per Serving: Calories: 340; Fat: 5g; Fiber: 2g; Carbs: 5g; Protein: 24g

Lamb and Eggplant Puree

(Prep + Cook Time: 3 hours 25 minutes | **Servings**: 4)

Ingredients:
- 4 lamb shoulder chops
- 1 cup yellow onion; chopped
- 7 oz. tomato paste
- 2 garlic cloves; minced
- 3 cups water
- 8 oz. white mushrooms; halved
- 1 tbsp. ghee
- A pinch of sea salt
- Black pepper to the taste

For the eggplant puree:
- 2 eggplants
- Juice of 1 lemon
- 1/4 tsp. white pepper
- 4 tbsp. ghee
- A pinch of sea salt

Instructions:
1. Place eggplants on your preheated grill, cookfor 30 minutes, flipping them from time to time, leave them to cool down and peel.
2. In your food processor, mix eggplant flesh with a pinch of salt, white pepper, lemon juice and 4 tbsp. ghee and pulse really well.
3. Spoon eggplant puree on plates and leave aside for now.
4. Heat up a pot with 1 tbsp. ghee, add lamb chops, season with a pinch of salt and black pepper to the taste, stir; brown them for a few minutes on each side and transfer to a plate.
5. Heat up the pot again over medium high heat, add onion, stir and cook for a couple of minutes.
6. Add garlic, stir and cook for 1 minute more.
7. Add mushrooms and tomato paste, stir and cook for 3 minutes more.
8. Add water, return lamb chops, stir; bring to a simmer, cover pot, reduce heat to medium-low heat and cook everything for 2 hours and 20 minutes. Divide lamb chops on eggplant puree and serve.

Nutrition Facts Per Serving: Calories: 200; Fat: 3g; Fiber: 3g; Carbs: 5g; Protein: 10g

Beef and Spinach

(**Prep + Cook Time**: 22 minutes | **Servings**: 2)

Ingredients:
- 1 big oyster mushroom; chopped
- 2 tbsp. almonds; chopped
- 2 tbsp. ghee
- 4 oz. beef; ground
- 1/2 tsp. chili flakes
- A pinch of sea salt
- White pepper to the taste
- 1 tbsp. capers
- 1/4 cup kalamata olives; pitted
- 1 tbsp. roasted almond butter
- 3 oz. spinach leaves; torn

Instructions:
1. Heat up a pan with the ghee over medium high heat, add mushroom, stir and cook for 3 minutes.
2. Add almonds, stir and cook for 1 minute. Add beef, chili flakes, a pinch of salt and white pepper, stir and cook for 6 minutes.
3. Add almond butter, capers, olives and spinach, stir; cook for a couple more minutes, divide into 2 bowls and serve.

Nutrition Facts Per Serving: Calories: 320; Fat: 2g; Fiber: 5g; Carbs: 9g; Protein: 23g

Lavender Lamb Chops

(**Prep + Cook Time**: 2 hours 10 minutes | **Servings**: 4)

Ingredients:
- 4 lamb chops
- 2 garlic cloves; minced
- 1 tbsp. lavender; chopped
- 2 tbsp. rosemary; chopped
- A pinch of sea salt
- Black pepper to the taste
- 1 tbsp. ghee
- 3 small orange peel; grated

Instructions:
1. In a bowl; mix lamb chops with garlic, lavender, rosemary, orange peel, a pinch of salt and black pepper, rub well and keep in the fridge for 2 hours.
2. Heat up your grill over medium high heat, grease it with the ghee, place lamb chops on it, grill for 5 minutes on each side, divide between plates and serve with a side salad on the side.

Nutrition Facts Per Serving: Calories: 160; Fat: 2g; Fiber: 1g; Carbs: 4g; Protein: 10g

Beef Patties

(**Prep + Cook Time**: 35 minutes | **Servings**: 4)

Ingredients:
- 1 lb. beef; ground
- 2 sweet potatoes; boiled and grated
- 1 cup red onion; chopped
- 2 Serrano peppers; chopped
- 1 small ginger piece; grated
- A handful cilantro; chopped
- 4 garlic cloves; minced
- 1/2 tsp. meat masala
- A pinch of cayenne pepper
- 1/4 tsp. turmeric powder
- Black pepper to the taste
- 1 egg; whisked
- 4 tbsp. almond meal
- 1 cup water
- 5 tbsp. ghee

Instructions:
1. Heat up a pan over medium high heat, add beef, masala, turmeric, black pepper to the taste and cayenne pepper, stir and brown for a few minutes.
2. Add water, stir; cook for 10 minutes more and take off heat.
3. Heat up a pan with 2 tbsp. ghee over medium heat, add Serrano peppers and onion, stir and cook for 2 minutes.
4. Add garlic and ginger, stir and cook for 1 minute more.
5. Add cilantro and the meat mixture, stir well and take off heat.

6. Add grated sweet potatoes, stir well, cool everything down and shape patties from this mix.
7. Put the egg in a bowl and almond meal in another.
8. Dip patties in egg and then in almond meal.
9. Heat up a pan with the rest of the ghee over medium heat, add beef patties, cook them well on one side, flip, cook on the other as well and transfer them to paper towels. Serve them with a side salad.

Nutrition Facts Per Serving: Calories: 180; Fat: 3g; Fiber: 3g; Carbs: 6g; Protein: 15g

Thai Lamb Chops

(**Prep + Cook Time**: 1 hour 15 minutes | **Servings**: 4)

Ingredients:
- 2 lbs. lamb chops
- 1/3 cup basil; chopped
- 2 garlic cloves; chopped
- 2 tbsp. Thai green curry paste
- 2 tbsp. avocado oil
- 1 tbsp. gluten free tamari sauce
- 1 small ginger piece; grated
- 1 tbsp. coconut oil
- 1 tbsp. coconut aminos

Instructions:
1. In your food processor, mix basil with garlic, curry paste, avocado oil, tamari sauce, aminos and ginger and blend really well.
2. Put lamb chops in a bowl; add basil mix over them, toss well and keep in the fridge for 1 hour.
3. Heat up a pan with the coconut oil over medium high heat, add lamb chops, cook for 2 minutes on each side, introduce pan in the oven and roast lamb at 400 °F for 10 minutes. Serve lamb chops with a side salad.

Nutrition Facts Per Serving: Calories: 170; Fat: 3g; Fiber: 2g; Carbs: 5g; Protein: 14g

Greek Beef Bowls

(**Prep + Cook Time**: 35 minutes | **Servings**: 4)

Ingredients:
- 1 lb. beef; ground
- 3 oz. kale; chopped
- 3 oz. endives; chopped
- 1/4 cup kalamata olives; pitted and sliced
- 1/4 cup green olives; pitted and sliced
- 1 tbsp. coconut oil
- 2 garlic cloves; minced
- 1 yellow onion; chopped
- A pinch of sea salt
- Black pepper to the taste
- 1 tbsp. savory; dried
- 1 tbsp. parsley; dried
- 2 tbsp. oregano; dried

Instructions:
1. Heat up a pan with the coconut oil over medium high heat, add garlic, onion, a pinch of salt and black pepper, stir and cook for 3 minutes.
2. Add beef, stir and cook for 10 minutes.
3. Add endives, kale, savory, oregano and parsley, stir and cook for 5 minutes more.
4. Add green and kalamata olives, stir; place in preheated broiler and broil for 4 minutes. Divide into bowls and serve.

Nutrition Facts Per Serving: Calories: 367; Fat: 7g; Fiber: 4g; Carbs: 9g; Protein: 30g

Beef and Basil

(**Prep + Cook Time**: 26 minutes | **Servings**: 4)

Ingredients:

- 1½ lbs. beef; ground
- 6 garlic cloves; minced
- 3 cups basil; chopped
- 1/2 cup chicken stock
- 2 cups carrot; grated
- 2 red chilies; chopped
- 1 tbsp. coconut oil
- 1 yellow onion; chopped
- A pinch of sea salt
- Black pepper to the taste
- 4 tbsp. lime juice
- 2 tbsp. coconut aminos
- 1 tbsp. olive oil
- 1/2 tbsp. honey
- Cauliflower rice for serving

Instructions:

1. Heat up a pan with the coconut oil over medium heat, add onions and a pinch of salt, stir and cook for 4 minutes.
2. Add garlic and chili peppers, stir and cook for 1 minute more.
3. Add beef and black pepper, stir and brown everything for 8 minutes. Add stock and half of the basil, stir and cook for 2 minutes more.
4. In a bowl; mix carrots with 1 tbsp. lime juice, the rest of the basil and the olive oil and stir well.
5. In another bowl; mix coconut aminos with the rest of the lime juice and honey and also stir very well.
6. Divide cauliflower rice on plates, add beef and carrot mix on top and drizzle the honey sauce you've made at the end.

Nutrition Facts Per Serving: Calories: 200; Fat: 3g; Fiber: 5g; Carbs: 7g; Protein: 17g

Salad Recipes

Pear Salad with Tasty Dressing

(Prep + Cook Time: 10 minutes | **Servings**: 4)

Ingredients:
- 1 pear; sliced
- 5 cups lettuce leaves; torn
- 1 small cucumber; chopped
- 1/2 cup cherry tomatoes; cut in halves
- 1/2 cup red grapes; cut in halves
- A pinch of sea salt
- Black pepper to the taste
- 3 tbsp. orange juice
- 1/4 cup extra virgin olive oil
- 1 tbsp. orange zest
- 2 tsp. raw honey
- 1 tbsp. parsley; minced

Instructions:
1. In a bowl; mix orange juice with olive oil, orange zest, honey, a pinch of sea salt, pepper to the taste and parsley and whisk very well.
2. In a salad bowl; mix pear with lettuce, cucumber, tomatoes and grapes. Add salad dressing, toss to coat and serve right away.

Nutrition Facts Per Serving: Calories: 100; Fat: 14g; Carbs: 15g; Fiber: 1g; Protein: 3g

Carrot and Cucumber Salad

(Prep + Cook Time: 15 minutes | **Servings**: 4)

Ingredients:
- 3 carrots; thinly sliced with a spiralizer
- 2 cucumbers; thinly sliced with a spiralizer
- 1 green onion; sliced
- 1 tbsp. sesame seeds
- 2 tbsp. lime juice
- A pinch of sea salt
- 2 tbsp. white wine vinegar
- Black pepper to the taste
- 2 tbsp. extra virgin olive oil

Instructions:
1. In a salad bowl; mix cucumbers with green onion and carrots.
2. In a small bowl; mix vinegar with olive oil, lime juice, a pinch of sea salt and pepper to the taste and stir well. Pour this over salad, toss to coat and keep in the fridge until you serve it.

Nutrition Facts Per Serving: Calories: 60; Fat: 1.7g; Carbs: 12g; Fiber: 2.5g; Protein: 1.3

Broccoli Salad

(Prep + Cook Time: 12 minutes | **Servings**: 4)

Ingredients:
- 2 bacon slices
- 4 cups broccoli florets; roughly chopped
- 1/4 cup walnuts; chopped
- 1/4 cup cranberries
- 1 tsp. lemon juice
- 1/4 cup olive oil

Instructions:
1. Heat up a pan over medium high heat, add bacon, cook for 2 minutes, leave aside to cool down and chop.
2. In a salad bowl; mix broccoli with bacon, cranberries, walnuts, lemon juice and olive oil, toss to coat and serve.

Nutrition Facts Per Serving: Calories: 120; Fat: 2g; Fiber: 1g; Carbs: 5g; Protein: 8g

Cabbage and Salmon Slaw

(Prep + Cook Time: 18 minutes | **Servings**: 4)

Ingredients:
- 2 salmon fillets; skin on
- 1 fennel bulb; sliced
- 1 small red cabbage head; sliced
- 1½ tsp. coconut aminos
- 1/2 cup mayonnaise
- 1 tsp. lime juice
- 1 tsp. honey
- A bunch of coriander; chopped
- A pinch of sea salt
- Black pepper to the taste

Instructions:
1. Put water in a pot and bring to a simmer over medium high heat.
2. Place salmon fillets in a vacuum bag, place in water, cook for 8 minutes, leave aside to cool down and cut into medium pieces.
3. Put salmon cubes in a salad bowl; add fennel, cabbage and coriander and toss gently.
4. In another bowl; mix coconut aminos with mayo, lime, honey, salt and pepper and whisk well. Add this to salad, toss to coat well and serve.

Nutrition Facts Per Serving: Calories: 160; Fat: 3g; Fiber: 2g; Carbs: 5g; Protein: 17g

Beef Salad

(Prep + Cook Time: 20 minutes | **Servings**: 4)

Ingredients:
- 1 lb. organic beef steak; cut into strips
- 3 cups broccoli; florets separated
- 8 cups baby salad greens
- 1 red onion; sliced
- 1 red bell pepper; sliced

For the vinaigrette:
- 1/2 cup extra virgin olive oil
- 1 tbsp. ginger; minced
- 2 tbsp. lime juice
- 1 tbsp. rice wine vinegar
- 2 tbsp. shallots; finely chopped
- A pinch of sea salt
- Black pepper to the taste

Instructions:
1. In a bowl; mix ginger with oil, lime juice, vinegar, shallots, a pinch of sea salt and pepper to the taste and stir well.
2. Heat up a pan over medium high heat, add 2 tbsp. of vinaigrette, warm up, add broccoli and cook for 3 minutes.
3. Add beef, stir and cook for 4 more minutes and take off heat.
4. In a salad bowl; mix salad greens with onion, bell pepper, broccoli and beef. Add some black pepper, drizzle the rest of the vinaigrette, toss to coat and serve.

Nutrition Facts Per Serving: Calories: 260; Fat: 12g; Carbs: 11g; Fiber: 4.3g; Protein: 32

Lobster Salad

(Prep + Cook Time: 10 minutes | **Servings**: 2)

Ingredients:
- 1 grapefruit; peeled and chopped
- 1 lb. lobster meat; cooked and chopped
- 1 avocado; pitted, peeled and chopped
- 1 shallot; chopped
- 3 cups mixed greens
- 2 tbsp. grapefruit juice
- 1 tbsp. chives; chopped
- A pinch of sea salt
- Black pepper to the taste
- 4 tbsp. extra virgin olive oil
- 2 tbsp. white wine vinegar
- Some dill; finely chopped for serving

Instructions:
1. In a bowl; mix grapefruit juice with oil, vinegar, chives, shallot, a pinch of sea salt and pepper to the taste and stir very well.

2. Add lobster meat and toss to coat.
3. In a large bowl; mix avocado with greens and grapefruit. Add lobster meat and dressing on top, sprinkle dill all over and serve.

Nutrition Facts Per Serving: Calories: 180; Fat: 10g; Carbs: 6.5g; Fiber: 1.4; Sugar: 3.4g; Protein: 11.1

Summer Salad

(Prep + Cook Time: 10 minutes | **Servings**: 6)

Ingredients:
- 8 oz. prosciutto
- 1 cup blackberries; halved
- 2 cups honeydew; sliced
- 3 tbsp. chives; chopped
- Juice of 1 lemon
- Zest from 1 lemon
- 1 shallot; chopped
- 2 cup cantaloupe; sliced
- A pinch of sea salt
- Black pepper to the taste

Instructions:
1. In a large salad bowl; mix blackberries with prosciutto, honeydew, cantaloupe, chives, lemon juice and zest, shallot, a pinch of sea salt and black pepper to the taste, toss to coat and serve cold.

Nutrition Facts Per Serving: Calories: 80; Fat: 0.5g; Fiber: 1g; Carbs: 1g; Protein: 3g

Special Salad

(Prep + Cook Time: 30 minutes | **Servings**: 4)

Ingredients:
- 4 parsnips; cut into medium wedges
- 2 red onions; cut into medium wedges
- 1 garlic clove; minced
- 1 butternut squash; cut into medium wedges
- 6 cups spinach
- Black pepper to the taste
- 2 tbsp. white wine vinegar
- 1/3 cup nuts; roasted
- 1 tsp. Dijon mustard
- 1/2 tbsp. oregano; dried
- 6 tbsp. extra virgin olive oil

Instructions:
1. Spread squash, onions and parsnips in a baking dish.
2. Drizzle half of the oil, sprinkle oregano and pepper to the taste, toss to coat, introduce in the oven at 400 °F and bake for 10 minutes.
3. Take veggies out of the oven, turn them and bake for another 10 minutes.
4. In a bowl; mix vinegar with the rest of the oil, garlic, mustard and pepper to the taste and stir very well.
5. Put spinach in a salad bowl; add roasted veggies, pour salad dressing, sprinkle nuts, toss to coat and serve warm.

Nutrition Facts Per Serving: Calories: 131; Fat: 5.5g; Carbs: 14g; Fiber: 4.7; Sugar: 5g; Protein: 5.2

Summer Salad

(Prep + Cook Time: 15 minutes | **Servings**: 4)

Ingredients:
- 1 cucumber; chopped
- 4 medium tomatoes; chopped
- 1 red onion; sliced
- 1 green bell pepper; chopped
- 3/4 cup kalamata olives; pitted and chopped
- 1 tbsp. lemon juice
- 1/4 cup extra virgin olive oil
- 1/2 tsp. oregano; dried
- 2 tbsp. red wine vinegar
- Black pepper to the taste

Instructions:
1. In a small bowl; mix lemon juice with oil, oregano, vinegar and pepper to the taste and whisk very well.

2. In a salad bowl; mix tomatoes with bell pepper, onion and cucumber. Add salad dressing, toss to coat and serve with olives on top.

Nutrition Facts Per Serving: Calories: 140; Fat: 9g; Carbs: 3g; Fiber: 5g; Protein: 7g

Shrimp Salad

(Prep + Cook Time: 30 minutes | Servings: 2)

Ingredients:
- 1 lb. shrimp; peeled and deveined
- 1 small red onion; thinly sliced
- 5 cups mixed greens
- 1/2 cup cherry tomatoes; cut in halves
- 1 avocado; pitted, peeled and chopped
- Black pepper to the taste
- 1/2 tbsp. sweet paprika
- 1/2 tsp. cumin
- 1 tbsp. chili powder
- 1/3 cup cilantro; finely chopped
- 1/2 cup lime juice
- 1/4 cup extra virgin olive oil

Instructions:
1. In a bowl; mix chili powder with cumin, paprika, 1/4 cup lime juice and shrimp, toss to coat and leave aside for 20 minutes.
2. Place shrimps on preheated grill over medium high heat, cook for 4 minutes on each side and transfer to a bowl.
3. In a small bowl; mix cilantro with oil, the rest of the lime juice and pepper to the taste and whisk very well.
4. In a large salad bowl; mix greens with tomatoes, onion, avocado and shrimp. Add salad dressing, toss to coat and serve right away.

Nutrition Facts Per Serving: Calories: 190; Fat: 40g; Carbs: 19g; Fiber: 3g; Protein: 50

Egg Salad

(Prep + Cook Time: 20 minutes | Servings: 4)

Ingredients:
- 1 avocado; pitted, peeled and chopped
- 1 small red onion; chopped
- 4 eggs
- 1 small red bell pepper; chopped
- 1/4 cup homemade mayonnaise
- A pinch of sea salt
- Black pepper to the taste
- 1 tbsp. lemon juice

Instructions:
1. Put eggs in a pot, add water to cover, place on stove over medium high heat, bring to a boil, reduce heat to low and cook for 10 minutes.
2. Drain eggs, leave them in cold water to cool down, peel, chop them and put in a salad bowl.
3. Add a pinch of sea salt and pepper to the taste, onion, bell pepper, avocado, lemon juice and mayo, toss to coat and serve right away.

Nutrition Facts Per Serving: Calories: 109; Fat: 4.6g; Carbs: 7.5g; Fiber: 3.3g; Protein: 9g

Chicken Salad

(Prep + Cook Time: 10 minutes | Servings: 2)

Ingredients:
- 1 smoked chicken breast; sliced
- 1 avocado; pitted, peeled and cubed
- 2 eggs; hard-boiled and halved
- 2 handfuls lettuce leaves; torn
- A handful walnuts; chopped
- 2 tbsp. flaxseed oil

Instructions:
1. In a salad bowl; mix lettuce with avocado, walnuts and chicken slices and toss.
2. Add eggs and oil, toss gently and serve.

Nutrition Facts Per Serving: Calories: 110; Fat: 0.9g; Fiber: 1g; Carbs: 4g; Protein: 12g

Chicken Salad

(Prep + Cook Time: 60 minutes | **Servings**: 4)

Ingredients:
- 2 chicken breasts; skinless and boneless
- 1 pineapple; sliced
- 6 cups mixed salad greens
- 1 red onion; thinly sliced
- 1/4 cup pineapple sauce

For the sauce:
- 1 yellow onion; minced
- 1 garlic clove; minced
- 6 oz. tomato paste
- 1/2 cup apple cider vinegar
- 1/2 cup water
- 1/2 cup cherry tomatoes; cut in halves
- A pinch of sea salt
- Black pepper to the taste
- 1/4 cup extra virgin olive oil
- 2 tbsp. apple cider vinegar
- 1/4 cup ketchup
- 3 tbsp. mustard
- 1 pinch cloves; ground
- A pinch of cinnamon
- A pinch of smoked paprika

Instructions:
1. Heat up a pan over medium high heat, add 1 yellow onion, stir and brown for 3 minutes.
2. Add garlic and cook 1 more minute.
3. Add tomato paste, 1/2 cup vinegar, water, ketchup, mustard, cloves, cinnamon and a pinch of smoked paprika, stir everything well, bring to a boil, reduce heat to medium-low and simmer for 30 minutes.
4. Take sauce off heat, reserve 1 cup and keep the rest in the fridge for another occasion.
5. Season chicken breast with a pinch of sea salt and pepper to the taste, place them on preheated grill over medium high heat, cook for 8 minutes on each side.
6. Brush chicken with 1 cup of the sauce you've just made and cook for 4 more minutes on each side.
7. Transfer chicken to a cutting board, leave aside to cool down, slice and put in a salad bowl.
8. Grill pineapple on medium high heat, transfer to a cutting board as well, cut into small cubes and add to chicken.
9. Also add greens, red onion, grape tomatoes and pepper to the taste.
10. In a small bowl; mix pineapple juice with 2 tbsp. vinegar, 1/4 cup olive oil, a pinch of sea salt and pepper to the taste and stir well. Pour this over chicken salad, toss to coat and serve.

Nutrition Facts Per Serving: Calories: 120; Fat: 16g; Carbs: 45g; Fiber: 4g; Protein: 16g

Winter Salad

(Prep + Cook Time: 17 minutes | **Servings**: 2)

Ingredients:
- 1 red onion; chopped
- 12 Brussels sprouts; sliced
- A pinch of sea salt
- Black pepper to the taste
- 1 tbsp. olive oil
- 1/3 cup pecans; chopped
- 1/4 cup raisins
- 2/3 cup hemp seeds
- 1/2 red apple; cored and chopped

Instructions:
1. Heat up a pan with the oil over medium heat, add onion, stir and cook for a few minutes.
2. Add Brussels sprouts, cook for 4 minutes, take off heat and leave aside to cool down. Add apple pieces, hemp seeds, raisins, a pinch of sea salt, black pepper and pecans, stir salad and serve.

Nutrition Facts Per Serving: Calories: 100; Fat: 0.7g; Fiber: 1g; Carbs: 3g; Protein: 9g

Shrimp and Radish Salad

(Prep + Cook Time: 14 minutes | **Servings**: 4)

Ingredients:
- 2 lbs. shrimp; deveined
- A pinch of sea salt
- Black pepper to the taste
- 2 tbsp. olive oil
- 4 oz. watermelon radish; thinly sliced
- 4 oz. radishes; sliced
- 1/2 cup fennel bulb; chopped
- 4 green onions; chopped
- 1 tsp. maple syrup
- 2 tbsp. lemon juice
- 1/4 cup mint; chopped
- 2 tbsp. mayonnaise

Instructions:
1. Heat up a pan with the oil over medium high heat, add shrimp, season with a pinch of salt and some black pepper, cook for 2 minutes on each side and transfer them to a salad bowl.
2. Add watermelon radish, radishes, fennel and onions and stir gently.
3. In a small bowl; mix maple syrup with lemon juice, mint and mayo and whisk well. Add this to salad, toss to coat well and serve.

Nutrition Facts Per Serving: Calories: 170; Fat: 3g; Fiber: 3g; Carbs: 6g; Protein: 10g

Scallops Salad

(Prep + Cook Time: 17 minutes | **Servings**: 4)

Ingredients:
- 1 lb. bay scallops
- 2 tsp. cayenne pepper
- Black pepper to the taste
- 3 tbsp. lemon juice
- 1 tbsp. homemade mayonnaise
- 1 tsp. mustard
- A pinch of cayenne pepper
- 1/2 cup extra virgin olive oil
- 1 garlic clove; minced
- 2 handfuls mixed greens
- 1 avocado; pitted, peeled and cubed
- 1 red bell pepper; cut into thin strips
- 3 tbsp. melted coconut oil

Instructions:
1. In a salad bowl; mix salad greens with avocado and pepper and leave aside for now.
2. In a bowl; mix lemon juice with mustard, garlic, mayo, pepper and a pinch of cayenne, stir well and leave aside.
3. Add olive oil gradually and whisk very well again.
4. Rinse and pat dry scallops, put them in another bowl; add pepper to the taste and 2 tsp. cayenne and toss to coat.
5. Heat up a pan with the coconut oil over medium high heat, add scallops, cook for 2 minutes on each side and transfer them to the bowl with the veggies. Add mustard dressing you've made, toss to coat and serve.

Nutrition Facts Per Serving: Calories: 235; Fat: 4.1g; Carbs: 18g; Fiber: 3.3g; Protein: 30.7

Potato Salad

(Prep + Cook Time: 45 minutes | **Servings**: 4)

Ingredients:
- 8 sweet potatoes; chopped
- 4 bacon slices; already cooked and crumbled
- 1 tbsp. coriander seeds
- 1 tsp. cumin seeds
- 1 red onion; sliced
- 1/2 tbsp. oregano; dried
- A pinch of sea salt
- Black pepper to the taste
- 1/2 tsp. chili flakes
- 1/4 cup extra virgin olive oil
- 3 tbsp. parsley; chopped
- 1 tbsp. coconut oil
- 2 tbsp. red wine vinegar

Instructions:
1. Put potatoes in a pot, add water to cover, bring to a boil over medium high heat, cook for 20 minutes, drain water and put them in a bowl.
2. Heat up a pan with the coconut oil over medium high heat, add onions, stir; reduce temperature to low, cook for 10 minutes and transfer them to a bowl
3. Return pan to medium high heat, add cumin seeds and coriander seeds, stir; toast for 2 minutes and add them to the bowl with the onions.
4. Also add chili flakes, oregano, bacon, parsley, olive oil, vinegar, a pinch of sea salt and pepper to the taste and stir everything well. Add potatoes, toss to coat and serve cold.

Nutrition Facts Per Serving: Calories: 142; Fat: 24g; Carbs: 47g; Fiber: 2g; Protein: 10g

Taco Salad

(**Prep + Cook Time**: 25 minutes | **Servings**: 4)

Ingredients:
- 1 romaine lettuce head; chopped
- 1 avocado; pitted, peeled and chopped
- 1 small red onion; chopped
- Some black olives; pitted and chopped
- 1 red bell pepper; chopped
- 1/2 cup Pico de gallo
- 1 tbsp. chili powder
- 1 tsp. onion powder
- 1/2 tsp. garlic powder
- 1 tsp. cumin; ground
- 2 tsp. paprika
- 3 tbsp. olive oil
- A pinch of cayenne pepper
- 1 lb. beef; ground
- 3 cups cilantro; chopped
- Juice from 1 lime
- A pinch of sea salt
- Black pepper to the taste

Instructions:
1. In a bowl; mix chili powder with paprika, onion and garlic powder, 1/2 tsp. cumin, cayenne and some black pepper and stir.
2. Heat up a pan with 1 tbsp. oil over medium heat, add beef, stir and cook for 7 minutes.
3. Add spice mix, stir and cook until meat is done.
4. Meanwhile; in your food processor, blend 1 cup cilantro with lime juice, 1/2 tsp. cumin, a pinch of salt, black pepper to the taste and 2 tbsp. oil and pulse really well.
5. In a salad bowl; mix lettuce leaves with avocado, 2 cups cilantro, onion, bell pepper, olives and Pico de gallo and stir. Divide this between plates, top with beef and drizzle the salad dressing on top.

Nutrition Facts Per Serving: Calories: 190; Fat: 3g; Fiber: 2g; Carbs: 5g; Protein: 12g

Chorizo Salad

(**Prep + Cook Time**: 30 minutes | **Servings**: 4)

Ingredients:
- 2 garlic cloves; minced
- 4 sweet potatoes; peeled and cubed
- 4 cups arugula
- 2 green onions; chopped
- 2 chorizo sausages; sliced
- 1 tbsp. rosemary; chopped
- 1 tbsp. bacon fat
- A pinch of sea salt
- Black pepper to the taste

For the salad dressing:
- 2 tsp. mustard
- 2 tbsp. apple vinegar
- 4 tbsp. olive oil
- 1/2 tsp. lemon juice

Instructions:
1. Heat up a pan with the bacon fat over medium heat, add sweet potatoes, stir and cook for 7 minutes.
2. Add a pinch of salt, black pepper, rosemary and garlic, stir and cook for 6 minutes more.
3. Add chorizo slices, stir; cook for 3 minutes, take off heat, cool down and transfer everything to a salad bowl.
4. Add green onions and arugula and stir.

5. In a small bowl; mix olive oil with lemon juice, vinegar, mustard and some black pepper and whisk well. Add this to salad, toss to coat and serve.

Nutrition Facts Per Serving: Calories: 190; Fat: 3g; Fiber: 2g; Carbs: 5g; Protein: 9g

Paleo Salad

(**Prep + Cook Time**: 50 minutes | **Servings**: 4)

Ingredients:
- 2 lettuce heads; leaves, torn
- 4 bacon strips
- 2 cups chicken meat; already cooked and shredded
- 4 cups arugula
- 1 small red onion; finely chopped
- 2 tbsp. ghee
- 1 tbsp. balsamic vinegar
- 1 zucchini; cubed
- 4 eggs
- 1/3 cup cranberries
- A pinch of sea salt
- Black pepper to the taste
- A pinch of garlic powder
- 1/3 cup pecans; chopped
- 2 apples; chopped
- 2 tbsp. maple syrup
- 1 tbsp. apple cider vinegar
- 1 tsp. shallot; minced
- 1 tsp. mustard
- 1 tsp. garlic; minced
- 1/4 cup extra virgin olive oil

Instructions:
1. Spread zucchini cubes on a lined baking sheet, sprinkle with a pinch of sea salt, pepper, garlic powder, drizzle balsamic vinegar and add ghee, toss to coat, introduce in the oven at 400 °F and bake for 25 minutes.
2. Meanwhile; put eggs in a pot, add water to cover, bring to a boil over medium high heat, boil for 15 minutes, drain, place in a bowl filled with ice water, leave aside to cool down, peel them, chop and put in a salad bowl.
3. Heat up a pan over medium high heat, add bacon, brown for a few minutes, take off heat, leave to cool down and add to the same bowl with the eggs.
4. Add lettuce leaves, arugula, chicken, onion, pecans, apple pieces, roasted squash cubes and cranberries.
5. In a small bowl; mix maple syrup with apple cider vinegar, mustard, garlic, shallot, olive oil and pepper and whisk very well. Pour this over salad, toss to coat and serve.

Nutrition Facts Per Serving: Calories: 249; Fat: 10g; Carbs: 35g; Fiber: 6; Sugar: 2.8g; Protein: 5g

Brussels Sprouts Salad

(**Prep + Cook Time**: 20 minutes | **Servings**: 4)

Ingredients:
- 4 cups Brussels sprouts
- 2 cups red cabbage; shredded
- 1/4 cup walnuts; chopped
- 1/4 cup homemade mayonnaise
- Black pepper to the taste
- 1 red apple; sliced
- 2 celery stalks; chopped
- 2 tbsp. lemon juice
- 4 tbsp. apple cider vinegar

Instructions:
1. In a bowl; mix lemon juice with mayo, vinegar and pepper to the taste and stir very well.
2. In a big bowl; mix Brussels sprouts with cabbage, celery, apple and walnuts. Add salad dressing you've just made, toss to coat and keep in the fridge for 10 minutes before you serve it.

Nutrition Facts Per Serving: Calories: 80; Fat: 1g; Carbs: 3g; Fiber: 1; Sugar: 1g; Protein: 2g

Kale and Carrots Salad

(Prep + Cook Time: 10 minutes | **Servings:** 1)

Ingredients:
- 1 carrot; grated
- A handful kale; chopped
- 1 small lettuce head; chopped
- 1 tbsp. tahini paste
- 1 tbsp. olive oil
- A pinch of sea salt
- Black pepper to the taste
- Juice of 1/2 lime
- A pinch of garlic powder

Instructions:
1. In a salad bowl; mix carrots with kale and lettuce leaves.
2. In your blender, mix tahini with a pinch of salt, black pepper, garlic powder, lime juice and oil and pulse well.
3. Pour this over salad, toss to coat well and serve.

Nutrition Facts Per Serving: Calories: 100; Fat: 1g; Fiber: 0g; Carbs: 0g; Protein: 7g

Chicken Salad

(Prep + Cook Time: 25 minutes | **Servings:** 2)

Ingredients:
- 2 chicken breasts; skinless and boneless
- 8 strawberries; sliced
- 1 small red onion; sliced
- 6 cups baby spinach
- 1 avocado; peeled and cut into small chunks
- 1/2 tsp. onion powder
- 1/2 cup lemon juice
- 2 tsp. paprika
- A pinch of sea salt
- Black pepper to the taste
- 2 tsp. parsley; dried
- 1/4 cup extra virgin olive oil
- 1 tbsp. tarragon; chopped
- 2 tbsp. balsamic vinegar

Instructions:
1. Put chicken in a bowl; add lemon juice, parsley, onion powder and paprika and toss to coat.
2. Place chicken on preheated grill over medium high heat, cook for 10 minutes on each side, transfer to a cutting board and slice.
3. In a bowl; mix oil with vinegar, a pinch of sea salt, pepper and tarragon and whisk well.
4. In a salad bowl; mix spinach with onion, avocado and strawberry. Add chicken pieces and the vinaigrette, toss to coat and serve.

Nutrition Facts Per Serving: Calories: 230; Fat: 42g; Carbs: 13g; Fiber: 5g; Protein: 30g

Radish Salad

(Prep + Cook Time: 10 minutes | **Servings:** 4)

Ingredients:
- 8 radishes; sliced
- 1 cucumber; sliced
- 1 apple; chopped
- 1 celery stalk; chopped
- Black pepper to the taste
- 1/4 cup homemade mayonnaise
- 2 tbsp. chives; chopped
- 2 tbsp. apple cider vinegar
- 2 tbsp. lemon juice

Instructions:
1. In a bowl; mix radishes with apple, celery and cucumber.
2. In a small bowl; mix mayo with vinegar, pepper, lemon juice and chives and whisk well. Pour this over salad, toss to coat and keep in the fridge until you serve it.

Nutritional value: Calories: 50; Fat: 7g; Carbs: 3g; Fiber: 1g; Protein: 1g

Salmon Salad

(Prep + Cook Time: 15 minutes | **Servings:** 2)

Ingredients:
- 1 lettuce head; chopped
- 2 salmon fillets
- 1 tbsp. olive oil
- 1 tbsp. coconut aminos
- 1 avocado; pitted, peeled and sliced
- 1 cucumber; sliced
- A pinch of sea salt
- Black pepper to the taste

Instructions:
1. Heat up a pan with the oil over medium high heat, add salmon fillets skin side down, cook for 3 minutes, flip and cook for 2 minutes more.
2. In a salad bowl; mix lettuce with cucumber, avocado, a pinch of salt, black pepper and coconut aminos and stir. Flake salmon using a fork, add to salad, drizzle some of the oil from the pan, toss to coat and serve.

Nutrition Facts Per Serving: Calories: 140; Fat: 3g; Fiber: 2g; Carbs: 6g; Protein: 15g

Summer Salad

(Prep + Cook Time: 10 minutes | **Servings:** 3)

Ingredients:
- 1 lettuce head; chopped
- A handful kale; chopped
- A handful green beans
- A handful walnuts; chopped
- 8 cherry tomatoes; halved
- A handful radishes; chopped
- 1 tbsp. lemon juice
- 8 dates; chopped
- A drizzle of olive oil

Instructions:
1. In a salad bowl; mix lettuce with kale, green beans, walnuts, tomatoes, radishes and dates.
2. In smaller bowl; mix lemon juice with olive oil and whisk well. Add this to salad, toss to coat and serve.

Nutrition Facts Per Serving: Calories: 100; Fat: 0g; Fiber: 1g; Carbs: 1g; Protein: 6g

Sashimi Salad

(Prep + Cook Time: 10 minutes | **Servings:** 2)

Ingredients:
- 1/2 lb. salmon sashimi; sliced
- 1 mango; peeled and roughly chopped
- 2 handfuls kale; chopped
- 1 tsp. balsamic vinegar
- 1/2 tbsp. honey
- 3 tbsp. tamari sauce
- 2 tbsp. olive oil

Instructions:
1. In a bowl; mix tamari with oil, honey and vinegar and whisk well.
2. In a salad bowl; mix kale with mango and sashimi. Add salad dressing, toss to coat and serve.

Nutrition Facts Per Serving: Calories: 140; Fat: 1g; Fiber: 2g; Carbs: 2g; Protein: 16g

Steak Salad

(Prep + Cook Time: 1 hour 15 minutes | **Servings:** 4)

Ingredients:
- 1 lb. steak
- 1 red bell pepper; cut into strips
- 1 cucumber; sliced
- 4 cups lettuce leaves; torn
- 1/4 cup mint leaves; chopped
- 1/4 cup cilantro; chopped
- 1 tbsp. ginger; grated
- 1/4 cup coconut aminos
- 1 Thai red chili pepper; chopped
- 3 garlic cloves; minced
- Juice from 1 lime
- A pinch of sea salt

- Black pepper to the taste
- Silvered almonds for serving

For the salad dressing:
- 1 Thai red chili pepper; chopped
- 3 tbsp. coconut aminos
- 2 tbsp. melted coconut oil
- 1 tsp. fish sauce
- Zest from 1 lime
- Juice from 1 lime

Instructions:
1. In a bowl; mix garlic with ginger, 1 red chili, juice from 1 lime and 1/4 cup coconut aminos and stir.
2. Add steak, toss to coat, cover bowl and keep in the fridge for 1 hour.
3. In another bowl; mix 2 tbsp. coconut oil with 3 tbsp. coconut aminos, 1 lime chili pepper, fish sauce, zest and juice from 1 lime, stir well and leave aside for now.
4. Place steak on preheated grill over medium high heat, cook for 4 minutes on each side, transfer to a cutting board, leave aside for 4 minutes, slice very thinly and put in a salad bowl.
5. Add lettuce, cucumber, bell pepper, a pinch of sea salt and pepper to the taste. Add salad dressing you've made, toss to coat, sprinkle cilantro, mint and almonds and serve.

Nutrition Facts Per Serving: Calories: 300; Fat: 10g; Carbs: 15g; Fiber: 4; Sugar: 4g; Protein: 38

Pomegranate Salad

(Prep + Cook Time: 15 minutes | **Servings**: 4)

Ingredients:
- 1 avocado; pitted, peeled and chopped
- 8 cups mixed salad greens
- 2 tbsp. pine nuts; toasted
- 6 figs; cut into quarters
- 3/4 cup pomegranate seeds
- 4 clementines; peeled and chopped
- 1/4 cup extra virgin olive oil
- 1 tbsp. lemon juice
- 4 tbsp. orange juice
- 2 tbsp. white wine vinegar
- 1 tsp. orange zest
- A pinch of sea salt
- Black pepper to the taste

Instructions:
1. In a salad bowl; mix greens with avocado, figs, clementines, pine nuts and pomegranate seeds.
2. In another bowl; mix orange juice with lemon juice, olive oil, orange zest, vinegar, a pinch of sea salt and pepper to the taste and whisk well. Pour this over salad, toss to coat and serve.

Nutrition Facts Per Serving: Calories: 120; Fat: 6g; Carbs: 12g; Fiber: 2g; Protein: 4.7

Green Apple and Shrimp Salad

(Prep + Cook Time: 10 minutes | **Servings**: 3)

Ingredients:
- 1 green apple; cored and chopped
- 1 small red onion; chopped
- 1/4 cup Dijon mustard
- 4 celery stalks; chopped
- 2 cups shrimp; peeled, deveined, cooked and chopped
- 3 eggs; hard-boiled, peeled and chopped
- 1 tbsp. olive oil
- 2 tbsp. vinegar
- 1/2 tsp. thyme; chopped
- 1/2 tsp. parsley; chopped
- 1/2 tsp. basil; chopped
- A pinch of sea salt
- Black pepper to the taste

Instructions:
1. In a big salad bowl; mix apple pieces with shrimp, eggs, onion and celery and stir.
2. In another bowl; mix mustard with oil, vinegar, thyme, parsley, basil, a pinch of salt and black pepper and whisk well. Add this to your salad, toss well and serve.

Nutritional value: Calories: 110; Fat: 2g; Fiber: 4g; Carbs: 7g; Protein: 15g

Quick Paleo Salad

(Prep + Cook Time: 10 minutes | **Servings**: 4)

Ingredients:
For the salad dressing:
- 1/2 cup avocado mayonnaise
- 1 tbsp. basil; chopped
- 1 tsp. rosemary ; chopped
- 1 garlic clove; minced
- A pinch of sea salt
- Black pepper to the taste
- 1 tsp. lemon juice

For the salad:
- 6 baby lettuce heads; chopped
- 1 cup cherry tomatoes; halved
- 1/2 lb. bacon; cooked and chopped
- 2 green onions; chopped

Instructions:
1. In a bowl; mix basil with rosemary, mayo, garlic, lemon juice, a pinch of salt and black pepper and whisk well.
2. In a salad bowl; mix lettuce with tomatoes, green onions and bacon. Add salad dressing, toss to coat and serve.

Nutrition Facts Per Serving: Calories: 140; Fat: 3g; Fiber: 2g; Carbs: 4g; Protein: 15g

Eggplant and Tomato Salad

(Prep + Cook Time: 18 minutes | **Servings**: 4)

Ingredients:
- 1/2 cup sun-dried tomatoes; sliced
- 1 eggplant; sliced
- 1 green onion; sliced
- Black pepper to the taste
- 4 cups mixed salad greens
- 1 tbsp. mint leaves; finely chopped
- 1 tbsp. oregano; finely chopped
- 1 tbsp. parsley leaves; finely chopped
- 4 tbsp. extra virgin olive oil

For the salad dressing:
- 2 garlic cloves; minced
- 1/4 cup extra virgin olive oil
- 1/2 tbsp. mustard
- 1 tbsp. lemon juice
- 1/2 tsp. smoked paprika
- A pinch of sea salt
- Black pepper to the taste

Instructions:
1. Brush eggplant slices with olive oil, season with black pepper, place them on preheated grill over medium high heat, cook for 3 minutes on each side and transfer them to a salad bowl.
2. Add sun-dried tomatoes, onion, greens, mint, parsley, oregano and pepper to the taste and 4 tbsp. olive oil and toss to coat.
3. In a small bowl; mix 1/4 cup olive oil with garlic, mustard, paprika, lemon juice, salt and pepper to the taste and whisk very well. Pour this over salad, toss to coat gently and serve.

Nutrition Facts Per Serving: Calories: 130; Fat: 27g; Carbs: 14g; Fiber: 2g; Protein: 4g

Salmon and Strawberry Salad

(Prep + Cook Time: 18 minutes | **Servings**: 4)

Ingredients:
- 1 lb. salmon fillet
- 2 tbsp. olive oil
- 1/4 tsp. coriander; ground
- 1/2 tsp. cumin; ground
- 1 tsp. chili powder
- 1/4 tsp. paprika
- A pinch of sea salt
- Black pepper to the taste

For the vinaigrette:
- 1/4 cup balsamic vinegar
- 1/3 cup olive oil
- 1/2 tsp. lemon zest
- 3 strawberries; chopped

- 6 strawberries; chopped
- 1/4 cup red onion; chopped
- 1 jalapeno; chopped
- Juice from 1 lime
- 1 garlic clove; minced
- 5 oz. baby arugula
- 1/2 avocado; pitted, peeled and chopped
- 3 radishes; chopped

- 1 tbsp. lemon juice
- 1½ tbsp. maple syrup
- 1½ tbsp. mustard

Instructions:
1. chili powder, paprika, a pinch of salt and black pepper to the taste and whisk well.
2. Brush salmon with this mix, place on preheated grill over medium high heat, cook for 6 minutes skin side down, flip, cook for 2 minutes more, transfer to a cutting board, leave aside to cool down, cut into medium pieces and transfer to a bowl.
3. Add radishes, avocado, 6 strawberries, garlic, arugula, red onion, jalapeno and lime juice and toss gently.
4. In another bowl; mix 1/3 cup oil with 3 strawberries, vinegar, lemon zest, 1 tbsp. lemon juice, maple syrup and mustard and whisk very well.
5. Add this to salad, toss to coat and serve. In a bowl; mix 2 tbsp. oil with coriander, cumin,

Nutrition Facts Per Serving: Calories: 120; Fat: 2g; Fiber: 2g; Carbs: 4g; Protein: 10g

Cucumber Salad

(Prep + Cook Time: 10 minutes | **Servings**: 4)

Ingredients:
- 1 zucchini; cut with a spiralizer
- 3 big cucumbers; cut with a spiralizer
- 2 garlic cloves; minced
- 1½ tbsp. balsamic vinegar
- 1/4 tsp. ginger; grated

- A pinch of sea salt
- Black pepper to the taste
- 2 tsp. sesame oil
- 1 small red jalapeno pepper; chopped
- 5 mint leaves; chopped

Instructions:
1. In a salad bowl; mix zucchini noodles with cucumber ones, garlic, ginger, salt and pepper and stir.
2. Add vinegar, oil, jalapeno and mint, toss to coat and serve right away.

Nutrition Facts Per Serving: Calories: 90; Fat: 0g; Fiber: 1g; Carbs: 1g; Protein: 5g

Sweet Potato Salad

(Prep + Cook Time: 40 minutes | **Servings**: 4)

Ingredients:
- 1/2 lb. bacon; chopped
- 3 sweet potatoes; cubed
- 2 tbsp. coconut oil
- 4 garlic cloves; minced
- Juice from 1 lime

- A pinch of sea salt
- Black pepper to the taste
- 2 tbsp. balsamic vinegar
- 2 tbsp. olive oil
- A handful dill; chopped

- 2 green onions; chopped
- A pinch of cinnamon; ground
- A pinch of red pepper flakes

Instructions:
1. Arrange bacon and sweet potatoes on a lined bacon sheet, add garlic and coconut oil, toss well, place in the oven at 375 °F and bake for 30 minutes.
2. Meanwhile; in a bowl, mix vinegar with lime juice, olive oil, green onions, pepper flakes, dill, a pinch of sea salt, black pepper and cinnamon and stir well.
3. Transfer bacon and sweet potatoes to a salad bowl; add salad dressing, toss well and serve.

Nutrition Facts Per Serving: Calories: 170; Fat: 3g; Fiber: 2g; Carbs: 5g; Protein: 12g

Swiss Chard Salad

(Prep + Cook Time: 13 minutes | Servings: 4)

Ingredients:
- 1 garlic clove; minced
- 1 shallot; chopped
- 1 bunch Swiss chard; sliced
- 1½ cup walnuts; halved
- 1 tbsp. rosemary; chopped
- A pinch of sea salt
- Black pepper to the taste
- 2 tbsp. avocado oil
- 1 tbsp. vinegar
- 1 tbsp. lemon juice

Instructions:
1. Heat up a pan with the oil over medium high heat, add garlic, rosemary, shallot, a pinch of salt and black pepper, stir and cook for 3 minutes.
2. Add walnuts, stir; reduce heat and cook for a few seconds more. In a salad bowl; mix Swiss chard with vinegar, lemon juice and shallots mix and toss to coat.

Nutrition Facts Per Serving: Calories: 195; Fat: 2g; Fiber: 2g; Carbs: 4g; Protein: 10g

Dinner Salad

(Prep + Cook Time: 10 minutes | Servings: 2)

Ingredients:
- 1/4 cup carrot; grated
- 4 radishes; chopped
- 1/2 cup red cabbage; shredded
- 1/2 cup green cabbage; shredded
- 1½ tbsp. vinegar
- 3 tbsp. olive oil
- 1 tsp. thyme; dried
- 2 tbsp. macadamia nuts; chopped
- A pinch of sea salt
- Black pepper to the taste
- 3/4 cup chicken; cooked and shredded
- 3 tbsp. onion; chopped

Instructions:
1. In a salad bowl; mix chicken with macadamia nuts, carrot, onion, radishes, green and red cabbage.
2. In a bowl; mix vinegar with oil, a pinch of salt, black pepper and thyme and whisk well. Add this to salad, toss to coat and serve.

Nutrition Facts Per Serving: Calories: 120; Fat: 2g; Fiber: 3g; Carbs: 4g; Protein: 12g

Steak Salad

(Prep + Cook Time: 10 minutes | Servings: 4)

Ingredients:
- 3/4 lb. flank steak; cooked and sliced
- 6 cups romaine lettuce; chopped
- 1 red onion; chopped
- 1 yellow bell pepper; chopped
- 1 red bell pepper; chopped
- A pinch of sea salt
- Black pepper to the taste
- 1 cucumber; sliced
- 1/2 cup kalamata olives; pitted and sliced
- 1/4 cup parsley; chopped
- 1 tbsp. olive oil

Instructions:
1. In a salad bowl; mix lettuce with onion, yellow bell pepper, red bell pepper, cucumber, olives, parsley and steak slices and toss well.
2. Add a pinch of salt, black pepper and the oil, toss to coat well and serve.

Nutrition Facts Per Serving: Calories: 150; Fat: 3g; Fiber: 2g; Carbs: 3g; Protein: 10g

Fresh Salad

(Prep + Cook Time: 10 minutes | **Servings:** 4)

Ingredients:
- 2 cup red cabbage; chopped
- 1/4 cup Paleo mayonnaise
- 1 red apple; cored and chopped
- 2 celery sticks; chopped
- 1/4 cup walnuts; chopped
- 4 cups Brussels sprouts; shredded
- 2 tbsp. lemon juice
- 4 tbsp. balsamic vinegar
- A pinch of sea salt
- Black pepper to the taste

Instructions:
1. In a salad bowl; mix cabbage with Brussels sprouts, apple, celery and walnuts.
2. In another bowl; mix lemon juice with vinegar, a pinch of salt, black pepper and mayo and whisk well. Add this to salad, toss to coat and serve.

Nutrition Facts Per Serving: Calories: 90; Fat: 0g; Fiber: 1g; Carbs: 1g; Protein: 7g

Awesome Pork Salad

(Prep + Cook Time: 15 minutes | **Servings:** 4)

Ingredients:
- 2 cups pork; already cooked and shredded
- 2 lettuce heads; torn
- 1 avocado; pitted, peeled and chopped
- 1 cup cherry tomatoes; cut in halves
- 1 green bell pepper; sliced
- 2 green onions; thinly sliced
- A pinch of sea salt
- Black pepper to the taste
- Juice of 1/2 lime
- 1 tbsp. apple cider vinegar
- 1/4 cup BBQ sauce
- 2 tbsp. extra virgin olive oil

Instructions:
1. In a small bowl; mix oil with lime juice, vinegar, black pepper and BBQ sauce and whisk well.
2. Heat up a pan over medium heat, add pork meat and heat it up.
3. Meanwhile; in a salad bowl; mix lettuce leaves with tomatoes, bell pepper, avocado and green onions. Add pork, drizzle the BBQ dressing, toss to coat and serve.

Nutrition Facts Per Serving: Calories: 322; Fat: 45g; Carbs: 23g; Fiber: 4g; Protein: 36

Broccoli and Carrots Salad

(Prep + Cook Time: 10 minutes | **Servings:** 2)

Ingredients:
- 3 carrots; sliced
- 1 cup broccoli; chopped
- 1/3 cup mushrooms; sliced
- 2 tbsp. walnuts; chopped
- 3 tbsp. red onion; chopped
- 3 tbsp. black olives; pitted and chopped
- A pinch of sea salt
- Black pepper to the taste
- 1 tsp. mustard
- 3 tbsp. olive oil
- 1½ tbsp. red vinegar

Instructions:
1. In a salad bowl; mix carrots with olives, onion, walnuts, mushrooms and broccoli.
2. In a small bowl; mix oil with vinegar, mustard, salt and pepper and whisk well. Add this to salad, toss to coat and serve.

Nutrition Facts Per Serving: Calories: 140; Fat: 1g; Fiber: 3g; Carbs: 4g; Protein: 15g

Seafood Salad

(Prep + Cook Time: 3 hours 10 minutes | **Servings**: 6)

Ingredients:
- 8 ounces; baby shrimp, already cooked, peeled, deveined and chopped
- 8 oz. crab meat; already cooked
- 2/3 cup homemade mayonnaise
- 2/3 cup yellow onion; chopped
- 2/3 cup celery; chopped
- 2 tbsp. Dijon mustard
- Black pepper to the taste
- 1/4 tsp. onion powder
- 1/2 tsp. garlic powder
- 1 tbsp. hot sauce

Instructions:
1. In a salad bowl; mix shrimp with crab meat, onion and celery.
2. In another bowl; mix mayo with mustard, pepper, onion powder, garlic powder and hot sauce and stir very well. Pour this over seafood salad, toss to coat and keep in the fridge for 3 hours before you serve it.

Nutrition Facts Per Serving: Calories: 240; Fat: 22g; Carbs: 3.3g; Fiber: 0.6g; Protein: 24g

Red Cabbage Salad

(Prep + Cook Time: 25 minutes | **Servings**: 4)

Ingredients:
- 1 purple cabbage head; cut into thin strips
- 4 prosciutto slices
- 1 red onion; thinly sliced
- 1 green apple; cored and chopped
- 1/2 cup pecans; toasted
- A handful watercress
- Black pepper to the taste
- 1/2 cup olive oil
- 1 garlic clove; minced
- 1/4 cup balsamic vinegar
- 1 tsp. honey
- 1/2 tsp. mustard
- A pinch of sea salt

Instructions:
1. Place prosciutto slices on a lined baking sheet, place in the oven at 350 °F and cook for 15 minutes.
2. Leave prosciutto to cool down and chop it.
3. In a salad bowl mix cabbage with prosciutto, onion, apple pieces, watercress and pecans and toss.
4. In another bowl; mix olive oil with honey, vinegar, garlic, mustard, a pinch of salt and black pepper and whisk well. Drizzle this over your salad and serve.

Nutrition Facts Per Serving: Calories: 110; Fat: 0.8g; Fiber: 1g; Carbs: 2g; Protein: 7g

Cuban Radish Salad

(Prep + Cook Time: 10 minutes | **Servings**: 4)

Ingredients:
- 6 radishes; sliced
- 1 romaine lettuce head; chopped
- 1 avocado; pitted, peeled and chopped
- 2 tomatoes; roughly chopped
- 1 red onion; chopped

For the salad dressing:
- 1/4 cup apple cider vinegar
- 1/2 cup olive oil
- 1/4 cup lime juice
- 3 garlic cloves; minced
- A pinch of sea salt
- Black pepper to the taste

Instructions:
1. In a salad bowl; mix radishes with lettuce leaves, avocado, onion and tomatoes and stir.
2. In another bowl; mix vinegar with oil, lime juice, garlic, a pinch of salt and black pepper and whisk well. Add this to salad, toss to coat and serve.

Nutrition Facts Per Serving: Calories: 100; Fat: 0.6g; Fiber: 1g; Carbs: 2g; Protein: 4g

Shrimp Cobb Salad

(Prep + Cook Time: 14 minutes | **Servings**: 4)

Ingredients:
- 1 lb. shrimp; peeled and deveined
- 4 bacon strips; cooked and chopped
- 1 tbsp. bacon fat
- 1 tsp. garlic powder
- A pinch of sea salt
- Black pepper to the taste
- 6 cups romaine lettuce leaves; chopped
- 4 eggs; hard-boiled, peeled and chopped
- 1-pint cherry tomatoes; halved
- 1 avocado; pitted, peeled and chopped

For the vinaigrette:
- 1 garlic clove, minced
- 2 tbsp. Paleo mayonnaise
- 2 tbsp. vinegar
- 3 tbsp. avocado oil

Instructions:
1. In a bowl mix garlic with mayo, vinegar and avocado oil, whisk well and leave aside for now.
2. Heat up a pan with the bacon fat over medium high heat, add shrimp, season with a pinch of salt, some black pepper and garlic powder, cook for 2 minutes, flip, cook for 2 minutes more and transfer them to a salad bowl.
3. Add tomatoes, avocado pieces, lettuce leaves, bacon and egg pieces and stir. Add the vinaigrette you've made earlier, toss to coat and serve.

Nutrition Facts Per Serving: Calories: 150; Fat: 1g; Fiber: 2g; Carbs: 6g; Protein: 10g

Avocado Salad

(Prep + Cook Time: 10 minutes | **Servings**: 2)

Ingredients:
- 1 avocado; pitted, peeled and chopped
- 1 tbsp. onion; chopped
- 5 oz. canned wild tuna; flaked
- Juice of 1 lemon
- Black pepper to the taste

Instructions:
1. In a salad bowl; mix avocado with onion, tuna, black pepper and lemon juice, toss well and serve.

Nutrition Facts Per Serving: Calories: 90; Fat: 0g; Fiber: 1g; Carbs: 0g; Protein: 12g

Watermelon Salad

(Prep + Cook Time: 1 hour 10 minutes | **Servings**: 4)

Ingredients:
- 8 cups mixed salad greens
- 4 cups watermelon; cubed
- 1/4 cup mayonnaise
- 1½ tbsp. honey
- 2 tsp. balsamic vinegar
- 1 tsp. poppy seeds
- A pinch of sea salt
- Black pepper to the taste

Instructions:
1. In a salad bowl; mix salad greens with watermelon cubes.
2. In another bowl; mix mayo with honey, vinegar and poppy seeds, whisk well and keep in the fridge for 1 hour. Drizzle this over salad, season with a pinch of salt and black pepper to the taste, toss to coat well and serve.

Nutrition Facts Per Serving: Calories: 120; Fat: 0.5g; Fiber: 1g; Carbs: 0g; Protein: 6g

Rich Salad

(**Prep + Cook Time**: 10 minutes | **Servings**: 1)

Ingredients:
- 1 chicken breast; cooked and sliced
- 1 medium lettuce head; chopped
- 1 sweet potato; boiled and cubed
- 1 tbsp. pumpkin seeds
- 6 black olives; pitted and chopped
- 1 tbsp. olive oil
- 1 tbsp. balsamic vinegar

Instructions:
1. In a salad bowl; mix chicken breast slices with lettuce, sweet potato, pumpkin seeds, olives, olive oil and balsamic vinegar, stir well and serve right away.

Nutrition Facts Per Serving: Calories: 130; Fat: 2g; Fiber: 1g; Carbs: 4g; Protein: 8g

Hearty Chicken Salad

(**Prep + Cook Time**: 1 hour 10 minutes | **Servings**: 6)

Ingredients:
- 1 rotisserie chicken; chopped
- 1 apple; cored and chopped
- 1/4 cup cranberries; dried
- 1/4 cup chives; chopped
- 1/4 cup red onion; chopped
- 1 celery stalk; chopped
- A pinch of sea salt
- Black pepper to the taste
- 2 cups mayonnaise
- 8 handfuls arugula
- 7 avocados; pitted, peeled and chopped

For the vinaigrette:
- 1 garlic clove, minced
- 1/2 cup olive oil
- 1 tsp. mustard
- 3 tbsp. lemon juice
- Black pepper to the taste

Instructions:
1. In a salad bowl; mix chicken meat with apple, cranberries, chives, onion, celery, arugula, avocados, mayo, a pinch of salt and black pepper to the taste and toss well.
2. In a small bowl; mix oil with garlic, mustard, black pepper and lemon juice and whisk well. Add this to salad, toss again well and leave aside at room temperature for 1 hour before serving.

Nutrition Facts Per Serving: Calories: 180; Fat: 3g; Fiber: 3g; Carbs: 6g; Protein: 20g

Autumn Salad

(**Prep + Cook Time**: 14 minutes | **Servings**: 4)

Ingredients:

For the salad dressing:
- 2 garlic cloves; minced
- 1/3 cup coconut milk
- 1/4 cup avocado oil
- 1 tbsp. parsley; chopped
- 1/3 cup cashew butter
- 1 tbsp. sesame seeds
- 1/2 cup green onion; chopped
- 2 tbsp. tamari sauce
- 2 tbsp. lemon juice
- 2 tbsp. vinegar
- A pinch of sea salt
- Black pepper to the taste

For the salad:
- 3 sweet potatoes; cut with a spiralizer
- 2 tbsp. water
- 1 tbsp. parsley; chopped

Instructions:
1. In your blender, mix cashew butter with 1 tbsp. parsley, green onion, sesame seeds, vinegar, tamari sauce, lemon juice, garlic, coconut milk, a pinch of salt and black pepper and pulse really well.
2. Add the oil gradually and blend again well.

3. Put sweet potato noodles in a bowl; add the water, place in your microwave and steam at High for 4 minutes.
4. Drain potato noodles, transfer to a bowl and add 1 tbsp. parsley. Add dressing, toss to coat and serve.

Nutrition Facts Per Serving: Calories: 300; Fat: 4g; Fiber: 4g; Carbs: 10g; Protein: 6g

Russian Salad

(Prep + Cook Time: 10 minutes | **Servings:** 4)

Ingredients:
- 1/2 cup walnuts; chopped
- 1/4 cup Paleo mayo anise
- 1½ lbs. beets; roasted, peeled and grated
- 1/2 cup raisins
- 2 garlic cloves; minced
- 1/4 cup parsley; chopped
- A pinch of sea salt
- Black pepper to the taste

Instructions:
1. In a salad bowl; mix grated beets with walnuts, raisins, garlic, parsley, salt and pepper and stir.
2. Add mayo, stir well and serve cold.

Nutrition Facts Per Serving: Calories: 150; Fat: 4g; Fiber: 3g; Carbs: 3g; Protein: 8g

Tomato Salad

(Prep + Cook Time: 10 minutes | **Servings:** 4)

Ingredients:
- 1 bunch kale; chopped
- 12 cherry tomatoes; halved
- 2 handful green beans
- 3 tbsp. Paleo mayonnaise
- 1 tsp. mustard

Instructions:
1. In a salad bowl; mix tomatoes with green beans and kale.
2. In a small bowl; mix mayo with mustard and whisk well. Add this to salad, toss to coat and serve.

Nutrition Facts Per Serving: Calories: 110; Fat: 2g; Fiber: 1g; Carbs: 3g; Protein: 5g

Tomato and Chicken Salad

(Prep + Cook Time: 10 minutes | **Servings:** 6)

Ingredients:
- 3 cups chicken; cooked and shredded
- 2 lbs. cherry tomatoes; halved
- 1/2 cup red onion; chopped
- 3 tbsp. oil
- 4 tbsp. balsamic vinegar
- A pinch of sea salt
- Black pepper to the taste
- 2 tbsp. basil; chopped
- 2 tbsp. chives; chopped
- 2 tbsp. parsley; chopped
- 1 tbsp. thyme; chopped

Instructions:
1. In a salad bowl; mix chicken with tomatoes, onion, basil, chives, parsley and thyme and stir.
2. In a small bowl; mix oil with vinegar, a pinch of salt and black pepper and whisk well. Add this to salad, toss to coat and serve.

Nutrition Facts Per Serving: Calories: 140; Fat: 3g; Fiber: 1g; Carbs: 2g; Protein: 16g

Radish and Eggs Salad

(Prep + Cook Time: 20 minutes | **Servings**: 2)

Ingredients:
- 8 radishes; sliced
- 2 eggs
- 1/2 cup green onions; chopped
- 1 tbsp. mayonnaise
- 1/2 tsp. mustard
- 1 tbsp. lemon juice
- A pinch of sea salt
- Black pepper to the taste
- A few lettuce leaves; chopped

Instructions:
1. Put water in a pot, add eggs, bring to a boil over medium high heat, cook for 10 minutes, transfer eggs to a bowl filled with ice water, leave them to cool down, peel and chop them.
2. In a salad bowl; mix lettuce leaves with chopped eggs, green onions and radishes. Add mustard, mayo, lemon juice, a pinch of salt and black pepper, toss to coat well and serve.

Nutrition Facts Per Serving: Calories: 110; Fat: 1g; Fiber: 2g; Carbs: 4g; Protein: 10g

Beetroot Salad

(Prep + Cook Time: 35 minutes | **Servings**: 2)

Ingredients:
- 2 garlic cloves; minced
- 4 chicken thighs; skin on
- 2 tsp. oregano; dried
- Juice of 1/2 lemon

For the pumpkin:
- 1/2 butternut squash; chopped
- 1½ tsp. fennel seeds

For the beetroot:
- 2 beetroots; cooked, peeled and cut into medium pieces
- 1/3 cup walnuts; chopped

For the salad dressing:
- 3 cups salad leaves; torn
- 1/2 tsp. maple syrup
- 2 tbsp. olive oil
- 1 tbsp. vinegar
- A pinch of sea salt
- Black pepper to the taste
- 2 tbsp. coconut oil
- 2 tbsp. olive oil

- 1 tbsp. olive oil

- 1 tbsp. vinegar
- 1/4 tsp. cinnamon powder
- 1 tbsp. maple syrup

- 1/2 tsp. mustard
- A pinch of sea salt
- Black pepper to the taste

Instructions:
1. In a bowl; mix chicken thighs with 2 garlic cloves, oregano juice from 1/2 lemon, 2 tbsp. oil, a pinch of salt and black pepper, stir; leave aside for 10 minutes and discard marinade.
2. Heat up a pan with the coconut oil over medium high heat, add chicken pieces, cook for 5 minutes on each side, transfer to a cutting board, leave aside to cool down, shred and put in a bowl.
3. In a bowl; mix butternut squash with fennel seeds, a pinch of salt, some black pepper and 1 tbsp. oil, toss well, spread on a lined baking sheet, place in the oven at 360 °F for 20 minutes.
4. Leave butternut squash pieces to cool down and add them to the bowl with the chicken.
5. In a bowl; mix beetroots with 1 tbsp. vinegar and black pepper to the taste, stir well and add to chicken salad as well.
6. Heat up a pan over medium high heat, add walnuts, maple syrup and cinnamon, stir; toast for a few minutes, take off heat, cool down and add to salad bowl.
7. In a small bowl; mix 2 tbsp. oil with 1 tbsp. vinegar, 1/2 tsp. maple syrup, mustard, a pinch of salt and some black pepper and whisk well. Add salad leaves to the salad bowl; add salad dressing, toss to coat well and serve.

Nutrition Facts Per Serving: Calories: 160; Fat: 3g; Fiber: 4g; Carbs: 5g; Protein: 20g

Cucumber and Tomato Salad

(Prep + Cook Time: 10 minutes | Servings: 4)

Ingredients:
- 1½ lbs. cucumber; sliced
- 1 cup mixed colored tomatoes; halved
- 2 tbsp. red vinegar
- 3 tbsp. olive oil
- 1 tsp. oregano; chopped
- 2 tbsp. mint; chopped
- 1/2 cup red onion; chopped
- 2 tbsp. parsley; chopped
- 2 tbsp. dill; chopped
- A pinch of sea salt
- Black pepper to the taste

Instructions:
1. In a bowl; mix cucumber with tomatoes, onion, mint, parsley, oregano, dill, salt and pepper and stir.
2. Add vinegar and oil, toss to coat and serve.

Nutrition Facts Per Serving: Calories: 90; Fat: 0g; Fiber: 1g; Carbs: 0g; Protein: 7g

Kale and Avocado Salad

(Prep + Cook Time: 10 minutes | Servings: 4)

Ingredients:
- 2 basil leaves; chopped
- 1 garlic clove; minced
- 1 avocado; pitted, peeled and chopped
- 1 bunch kale; chopped
- 1 cup grapes; seedless and halved
- 1/4 cup pumpkin seeds
- 1/3 cup red onion; chopped
- 2 tbsp. olive oil
- 1 tsp. maple syrup
- 3 tbsp. lemon juice

Instructions:
1. In a salad bowl; mix kale with avocado, grapes, pumpkin seeds and onion and stir;
2. In another bowl; mix oil with maple syrup, lemon juice, basil and garlic and whisk well. Add this to salad, toss to coat and serve.

Nutrition Facts Per Serving: Calories: 120; Fat: 1g; Fiber: 1g; Carbs: 2g; Protein: 11g

Grilled Shrimp Salad

(Prep + Cook Time: 1 hour 8 minutes | Servings: 4)

Ingredients:
- 4 bacon slices; cooked and crumbled
- 12 oz. shrimp; peeled and deveined
- 4 cups mixed salad greens
- 1 avocado; pitted, peeled and chopped
- 1/4 cup ghee; melted
- 1/2 tsp. dill; dried
- 1/4 tsp. smoked paprika
- A pinch of sea salt
- Black pepper to the taste
- A handful cherry tomatoes; halved
- 2 tbsp. scallions; chopped

Instructions:
1. In a bowl; mix ghee with a pinch of salt, black pepper, dill and paprika and stir well. Put shrimp in a bowl; add half of the ghee mix over them toss well and leave aside in the fridge for 1 hour.
2. Heat up a pan over medium high heat, add shrimp, cook for 3 minutes on each side and transfer to a bowl.
3. Add the rest of the ghee mix, bacon, mixed greens, avocado, tomatoes and scallions, toss everything well and serve.

Nutrition Facts Per Serving: Calories: 200; Fat: 3g; Fiber: 5g; Carbs: 7g; Protein: 15g

Chicken Salad and Raspberry Dressing

(Prep + Cook Time: 20 minutes | **Servings**: 4)

Ingredients:
For the salad dressing:
- 6 oz. raspberries
- 1 shallot; chopped
- 1 tbsp. raspberry vinegar
- 2/3 cup walnuts; chopped
- A pinch of sea salt
- Black pepper to the taste
- 1/4 cup olive oil

For the salad:
- 1 yellow bell pepper; chopped
- 2 chicken breast halves
- 8 oz. strawberries; halved
- 1 avocado; pitted, peeled and chopped
- 1/2 tsp. garlic powder
- 1 tbsp. olive oil
- 1/4 tsp. smoked paprika
- 1/4 tsp. turmeric
- Black pepper to the taste
- 1 tbsp. ghee
- 5 oz. baby arugula
- 1/4 red cabbage; shredded
- 1 cup blueberries

Instructions:
1. Put walnuts in your food processor, blend well and transfer to a bowl.
2. Add vinegar, raspberries, shallots, oil, a pinch of salt and black pepper, whisk well and leave aside for now.
3. Meanwhile; in a bowl, mix 1 tbsp. oil with garlic powder, black pepper, paprika and turmeric and whisk well.
4. Brush chicken breast halves with this mix, place them on your grill after you've greased it with the ghee and cook them over medium high heat for 4 minutes on each side.
5. Transfer chicken to a cutting board, leave them to cool down a bit, slice and transfer them to a salad bowl.
6. Add strawberries, avocado, cabbage, blueberries, bell pepper and arugula. Add salad dressing you've made at the beginning, toss to coat and serve.

Nutrition Facts Per Serving: Calories: 150; Fat: 3g; Fiber: 2g; Carbs: 5g; Protein: 18g

Figs and Cabbage Salad

(Prep + Cook Time: 16 minutes | **Servings**: 4)

Ingredients:
- 1 red cabbage head; shredded
- 2 figs; cut into quarters
- 2 tbsp. olive oil
- A pinch of sea salt
- Black pepper to the taste
- 1/4 cup balsamic vinegar
- 1/2 tsp. oregano; dried
- 1 yellow onion; chopped
- 1 tbsp. maple syrup
- A handful oregano; chopped

Instructions:
1. In a bowl mix cabbage with a pinch of salt and some black pepper, stir well and leave aside.
2. Heat up a pan with half of the oil over medium heat, add onion, stir and cook for 4 minutes.
3. Add dried oregano and vinegar, stir; cook for 5 minutes and take off heat. Add maple syrup, some black pepper and stir well.
4. In a salad bowl; mix squeezed cabbage with onions mix, figs and the rest of the oil, toss to coat and serve with fresh oregano on top.

Nutrition Facts Per Serving: Calories: 140; Fat: 2g; Fiber: 2g; Carbs: 4g; Protein: 9g

Vegetable Recipes

Tomato and Mushroom Skewers

(Prep + Cook Time: 20 minutes | **Servings:** 4)

Ingredients:
- 1 lb. mushroom caps
- 4 cups cherry tomatoes
- 1 tbsp. raw honey
- Black pepper to the taste
- 2 tbsp. Dijon mustard
- 4 tbsp. extra virgin olive oil
- 4 garlic cloves; minced
- 1/2 cup cilantro; minced
- 1/4 cup ghee
- 1/2 cup parsley; minced

Instructions:
1. In a bowl; mix mustard with olive oil, pepper and honey and whisk well.
2. Arrange mushrooms and tomatoes on skewers alternating pieces, brush them with the mustard mix, arrange on preheated grill over medium high heat and cook for 3 minutes on each side.
3. Heat up apan with the ghee over medium high heat, add garlic, stir and cook for 3 minutes.
4. Add cilantro, parsley, salt and pepper to the taste and cook for 2 minutes more. Divide skewers on plates, drizzle herb sauce on top and serve.

Nutrition Facts Per Serving: Calories: 138; Fat: 5g; Carbs: 15g; Fiber: 0g; Protein: 4g

Potato Bites

(Prep + Cook Time: 40 minutes | **Servings:** 4)

Ingredients:
- 2 sweet potatoes; thinly sliced
- 1 cup salsa
- 4 oz. bacon; already cooked and crumbled
- 1 tsp. chili powder
- 1/2 tsp. garlic powder
- 1/2 tsp. paprika
- 2 tbsp. extra virgin olive oil
- Black pepper to the taste
- Some cilantro; finely chopped

For the guacamole:
- 2 avocados; pitted, peeled and chopped
- 1 garlic clove; minced
- 1/4 cup red onions; chopped
- 1 tbsp. lime juice
- 1/2 cup tomatoes; finely chopped

Instructions:
1. In a bowl; mix avocados with lime juice, garlic, red onions and tomatoes, stir well, cover and keep in the fridge for now.
2. In a bowl; mix potato slices with the olive oil, chili powder, garlic powder, paprika and pepper and toss to coat.
3. Spread potatoes on a lined baking sheet, introduce in the oven at 450 °F and bake for 10 minutes on each side.
4. Take potato slices out of the oven, top each with guacamole, bacon, salsa and chopped cilantro. Divide between plates and serve.

Nutrition Facts Per Serving: Calories: 240; Fat: 6g; Carbs: 10g; Fiber: 3; Sugar: 0.4g; Protein: 17g

Stuffed Zucchinis

(Prep + Cook Time: 30 minutes | **Servings**: 4)

Ingredients:
- 2 tomatoes; chopped
- 1 eggplant; chopped
- 2 zucchinis; cut into halves lengthwise
- 1 yellow onion; chopped
- A pinch of sea salt
- Black pepper to the taste
- 1/2 bunch parsley; finely chopped
- 3 tbsp. extra virgin olive oil
- 2 garlic cloves; minced

Instructions:
1. Remove flesh from zucchini halves, season them with a pinch of sea salt and pepper, leave aside for 10 minutes and pat dry them,
2. Heat up a pan with 1 tbsp. oil over medium high heat, add onion, stir and cook for 4 minutes.
3. Add garlic, stir and cook 1 minute. Add the rest of the oil, eggplant and chopped zucchini flesh, stir and cook for 10 minutes.
4. Add tomatoes, parsley and pepper to the taste, stir and cook for 5 minutes more.
5. Fill zucchini halves with this mix, place on preheated grill over medium high heat, cook for 3 minutes, divide between plates and serve right away.

Nutrition Facts Per Serving: Calories: 130; Fat: 6g; Carbs: 9g; Fiber: 2; Sugar: 0g; Protein: 8g

Veggie Mix and Scallops

(Prep + Cook Time: 14 minutes | **Servings**: 4)

Ingredients:
- 2 mangos; peeled and chopped
- 1 cucumber; sliced
- 1 cup cauliflower rice; already cooked
- 1 tbsp. ginger; grated
- 2 tsp. lime juice
- 1/2 cup cilantro; chopped
- 2 tsp. olive oil
- 1½ lbs. sea scallops
- Black pepper to the taste

Instructions:
1. In a bowl; mix cucumber slices with mangos, ginger, lime juice, half of the oil, cilantro and black pepper to the taste and stir well.
2. Pat dry scallops and season them with some pepper.
3. Heat up a pan with the rest of the oil over medium high heat, add scallops and cook for 2 minutes on each side. Divide scallops on plates, add cauliflower rice and mango and cucumber salad on the side and serve.

Nutrition Facts Per Serving: Calories: 180; Fat: 3g; Fiber: 2g; Carbs: 4g; Protein: 14g

Broccoli and Cauliflower Fritters

(Prep + Cook Time: 20 minutes | **Servings**: 8)

Ingredients:
- 1 cup broccoli; chopped
- 1½ cups cauliflower; chopped
- A pinch of sea salt
- Black pepper to the taste
- 1 tbsp. coconut flour
- 2 eggs
- 1 tbsp. coconut oil for frying
- 2 tbsp. homemade mayonnaise
- 1 tbsp. extra virgin olive oil
- 1 tbsp. coriander; finely chopped
- 1/2 garlic clove; grated
- 1 tsp. lime juice

Instructions:
1. In a bowl; mix cauliflower with broccoli, eggs, coconut flour, a pinch of sea salt and pepper to the taste and stir very well.
2. Shape small patties and arrange them on a plate.

3. Heat up a pan with the coconut oil over medium high heat, add veggies fritters, cook for 4 minutes on each side, transfer them to paper towels, drain grease and arrange on a platter.
4. In a bowl; mix mayo with olive oil, coriander, garlic and lime juice and stir well. Serve you fritters with mayo mix.

Nutrition Facts Per Serving: Calories: 140; Fat: 3.8g; Carbs: 13g; Fiber: 3.3; Sugar: 8g; Protein: 7.3

Stuffed Mushrooms

(Prep + Cook Time: 20 minutes | **Servings:** 4)

Ingredients:
- 12 big mushrooms; stems removed
- A pinch of sea salt
- Black pepper to the taste
- 1 small tomato; diced
- 1/4 cup homemade paleo pesto
- 2 tbsp. extra virgin olive oil

Instructions:
1. Brush mushrooms with the olive oil and season them with a pinch of sea salt and pepper to the taste.
2. Heat up a pan over medium high heat, add mushrooms and cook them for 5 minutes on each side. Transfer them to a platter, fill each with pesto sauce, top with diced tomatoes and serve.

Nutrition Facts Per Serving: Calories: 80; Fat: 4g; Carbs: 5g; Fiber: 0g; Protein: 4g

Baked Yuka with Tomato Sauce

(Prep + Cook Time: 35 minutes | **Servings:** 3)

Ingredients:
- 1 yucca root; cut into strips
- 1/2 tsp. garlic powder
- 2 tbsp. coconut oil

For the sauce:
- 1 tomato; grated and skin discarded
- 1 garlic clove; grated
- 1 tbsp. vinegar
- Black pepper to the taste
- 1/2 tsp. smoked paprika
- 1/2 tsp. onion powder
- 2 tbsp. extra virgin olive oil
- A pinch of sea salt

Instructions:
1. Put yucca strips in a bowl; drizzle with coconut oil, sprinkle pepper, garlic powder, onion powder and paprika, toss to coat, spread on a lined baking sheet, introduce in the oven at 390 °F and bake for 25 minutes.
2. Meanwhile; in a bowl, mix tomato with olive oil, a pinch of sea salt, vinegar and garlic and stir very well.
3. Take yucca out of the oven, transfer to plates and serve with tomato sauce drizzled on top.

Nutrition Facts Per Serving: Calories: 230; Fat: 2.7g; Carbs: 51g; Fiber: 2.5g; Protein: 2g

Onion Rings

(Prep + Cook Time: 21 minutes | **Servings:** 40 pieces)

Ingredients:
- 2/3 cup cashew meal
- A pinch of sea salt
- Black pepper to the taste
- 1 big red onion; sliced and rings separated
- 1 tsp. garlic powder
- 1/2 tsp. sweet paprika
- 1 tsp. onion powder
- 3 eggs

Instructions:
1. In a bowl; mix eggs with a pinch of sea salt and pepper and whisk well.
2. In another bowl; mix cashew meal with pepper, garlic and onion powder and sweet paprika and stir well.
3. Dip each onion ring in eggs and then in cashew meal mix, spread them on a lined baking sheet, introduce in the oven at 425 °F and bake for 10 minutes.

4. Transfer onion rings to preheated broiler and broil for 1 minute. Leave onion rings to cool down, divide between bowls and serve as a snack.

Nutrition Facts Per Serving: Calories: 134; Fat: 3.6g; Carbs: 14g; Fiber: 1.5g; Protein: 4.5

Stuffed Eggplant

(**Prep + Cook Time**: 1 hour 10 minutes | **Servings**: 2)

Ingredients:
- 1 eggplant
- 2 tomatoes; finely chopped
- 3 thyme springs
- 1 garlic clove; minced
- 3 tbsp. extra virgin olive oil
- A pinch of sea salt
- Black pepper to the taste
- Lemon juice from 1/2 lemon

Instructions:
1. Place eggplant on a lined baking sheet, introduce in the oven at 400 °F and bake for 30 minutes.
2. Take eggplant out of the oven, leave aside to cool down, cut in half lengthways, drizzle each half with 1 tbsp. olive oil, introduce in the oven again at 350 °F and bake for 25 more minutes.
3. Take eggplant halves out of the oven, leave aside for 5 minutes, discard flesh and sprinkle halves with some of the lemon juice, a pinch of sea salt and pepper.
4. In a bowl; mix tomatoes with thyme, garlic and chopped eggplant flesh and stir.
5. Add lemon juice, pepper and 1 tbsp. olive oil and stir everything well. Scoop this into eggplant halves, divide on a plate and serve.

Nutrition Facts Per Serving: Calories: 180; Fat: 22g; Carbs: 8.5g; Fiber: 3.4; Sugar: 2g; Protein: 10g

Eggplant Jam

(**Prep + Cook Time**: 1 hour 10 minutes | **Servings**: 6)

Ingredients:
- 3 eggplants; sliced lengthwise
- A splash of hot sauce
- 1/4 cup water
- 1 tbsp. parsley; chopped
- 2 tbsp. lemon juice
- 2 tsp. sweet paprika
- 2 garlic cloves; minced
- A pinch of sea salt
- A pinch of cinnamon; ground
- 1tsp. cumin; ground

Instructions:
1. Sprinkle some salt on eggplant slices and leave them aside for 10 minutes.
2. Pat dry eggplant slices, brush them with half of the oil, place on a lined baking sheet, place in the oven at 375 degrees F, bake for 25 minutes flipping them halfway and leave them aside to cool down.
3. In a bowl; mix paprika with garlic, cinnamon, cumin, water and hot sauce and stir well.
4. Add baked eggplant pieces and mash them with a fork.
5. Heat up a pan with the rest of the oil over medium-low heat, add eggplant mix, stir and cook for 20 minutes. Add lemon juice and parsley, stir; take off heat, divide into small bowls and serve.

Nutrition Facts Per Serving: Calories: 150; Fat: 3g; Fiber: 2g; Carbs: 6g; Protein: 15g

Veggies and Fish Mix

(**Prep + Cook Time**: 42 minutes | **Servings**: 4)

Ingredients:
- 1 cup hot water
- 1 eggplant; chopped
- 3 cups cherry tomatoes; halved
- 1 tbsp. maple syrup
- 2 tbsp. olive oil
- 1 tsp. Paleo Tabasco sauce
- 1 lb. tuna; cubed
- 1 tsp. balsamic vinegar
- 1/2 cup basil; chopped
- Black pepper to the taste
- A pinch of sea salt

Instructions:
1. In a bowl; mix eggplant pieces with a pinch of salt and black pepper and stir.
2. Heat up a pan with 1 tbsp. oil over medium heat, add eggplant, cook for 6 minutes stirring often and transfer to a bowl.
3. Heat up the pan again with the rest of the oil over medium heat, add tomatoes, cover pan and cook for 6 minutes shaking the pan from time to time.
4. Return eggplant pieces to the pan, add maple syrup, vinegar and hot water, stir; cover and cook for 10 minutes.
5. Add tuna and Tabasco sauce, stir; cover pan again, reduce heat to medium-low and simmer for 10 minutes more. Sprinkle basil on top, divide veggies and tuna mix between plates and serve.

Nutrition Facts Per Serving: Calories: 120; Fat: 1g; Fiber: 2g; Carbs: 5g; Protein: 12g

Roasted Tomatoes

(**Prep + Cook Time**: 1 hour 10 minutes | **Servings**: 4)

Ingredients:
- 1 lb. cherry tomatoes; halved
- 1 big red onion; cut into wedges
- 2 red bell peppers; chopped
- 2 garlic cloves; minced
- 1 tsp. thyme; dried
- 1 tsp. oregano; dried
- 3 bay leaves
- 2 tbsp. olive oil
- 1 tbsp. balsamic vinegar
- A pinch of sea salt
- Black pepper to the taste

Instructions:
1. In a baking dish mix tomatoes with onions, garlic, a pinch of sea salt, black pepper, thyme, oregano, bay leaves, half of the oil and half of the vinegar, toss to coat, place in the oven at 350 °F and roast them for 1 hour.
2. Meanwhile; in your food processor, mix bell peppers with a pinch of sea salt, black pepper, the rest of the oil and the rest of the vinegar and blend very well.
3. Discard bay leaves, divide roasted tomatoes, garlic and onions on plates, drizzle the bell peppers sauce over them and serve.

Nutrition Facts Per Serving: Calories: 123; Fat: 1g; Fiber: 1g; Carbs: 2g; Protein: 10g

Cucumber Salsa

(**Prep + Cook Time**: 1 hour 10 minutes | **Servings**: 12)

Ingredients:
- 2 cucumbers; chopped
- 1/2 cup green bell pepper; chopped
- 2 tomatoes; chopped
- 1 jalapeno pepper; chopped
- 1 yellow onion; chopped
- 1 garlic clove; minced
- 2 tsp. cilantro; chopped
- 1 tsp. parsley; chopped
- 2 tbsp. lime juice
- 1/2 tsp. dill weed
- A pinch of sea salt
- Black pepper to the taste

Instructions:
1. In a bowl; mix cucumbers with jalapeno, tomatoes, green pepper, garlic, onion, a pinch of sea salt and pepper to the taste.
2. Add parsley, cilantro, dill and lime juice and stir well again. Keep in the fridge for 1 hour and serve.

Nutrition Facts Per Serving: Calories: 70; Fat: 0.2g; Carbs: 1g; Fiber: 2. protein 17

Veggies Dish with Tasty Sauce

(Prep + Cook Time: 35 minutes | **Servings**: 4)

Ingredients:
- 2 carrots; chopped
- 8 mushrooms; sliced
- 4 zucchinis; cut in thin noodles
- 2 cups spinach; torn
- 2 yellow squash; halved and sliced
- 1 tbsp. coconut oil
- 1 cup coconut milk
- Juice of 1 lemon
- A pinch of sea salt
- Black pepper to the taste

For the pesto:
- 1/2 cup extra virgin olive oil
- 2 cups basil
- 1/3 cup pine nuts
- 3 garlic clove; chopped
- A pinch of sea salt
- Black pepper to the taste

Instructions:
1. In your food processor, mix basil with nuts and garlic and pulse well.
2. Add oil, a pinch of salt and pepper, pulse well again, transfer to a bowl and leave aside.
3. Steam carrots, squash, zucchini and mushrooms in a bamboo steamer for 8 minutes, transfer them to a colander, season with a pinch of sea salt and pepper, leave aside for 10 minutes, pat dry them and put in a bowl.
4. Heat up a pan with the oil over medium high heat, add half of the coconut milk, salt and pepper and bring to a boil stirring all the time.
5. Add the pesto you've made, lemon juice and the rest of the coconut milk and stir again.
6. Add steamed veggies, stir and cook for 2 minutes. Add spinach, more salt and pepper if needed, stir; cook for 2 minutes more, transfer to bowls and serve.

Nutrition Facts Per Serving: Calories: 260; Fat: 12g; Carbs: 17g; Fiber: 13; Sugar: 5g; Protein: 18g

Surprise Dinner Dish

(Prep + Cook Time: 1 hour 45 minutes | **Servings**: 5)

Ingredients:
- 1 lb. sausage; casings removed
- 1 paleo coconut bread; cubed
- 2 tbsp. ghee; melted
- 3 celery stalks; chopped
- 1 fennel; chopped
- 4 garlic cloves; chopped
- 1 yellow onion; chopped
- 8 oz. mushrooms; chopped
- 1 pear; chopped
- 1 red bell pepper; chopped
- 1 tbsp. thyme; chopped
- 2 tbsp. parsley; chopped
- 1/2 cup white wine
- A pinch of sea salt
- Black pepper to the taste
- 1 tsp. oregano; dried
- 3 eggs; whisked
- 2 cups chicken stock

Instructions:
1. Spread paleo bread cubes on a lined baking sheet, introduce in the oven at 300 degrees f and bake for 20 minutes.
2. Toss bread cubes, introduce in the oven again, bake for 20 minutes more, take out of the oven and leave aside for now.
3. Heat up a pan over medium high heat, add sausage, break with a fork, brown for a few minutes, transfer to a bowl and leave aside for now as well.
4. Return pan to medium high heat, add 1 tbsp. ghee, melt and add garlic, fennel, onion and celery, stir and cook for 10 minutes.
5. Transfer veggies to the bowl along with the sausage and stir everything.
6. Return the pan to medium high heat again, melt the rest of the ghee and add red pepper, mushrooms and wine.
7. Stir, cook until wine evaporates, take off heat and add this to the bowl with the veggies and the sausage.

8. Add thyme, oregano, a pinch of sea salt, pepper, parsley, bread cubes and 1½ cups stock, stir everything and leave aside for 10 minutes.
9. Add the rest of the stock and stir everything again.
10. Pour the veggies mix in a greased baking dish, spread whisked eggs all over, introduce in the oven at 400 degrees F, cover with tin foil and bake for 30 minutes.
11. Remove foil and bake for 15 more minutes. Divide between plates and serve.

Nutrition Facts Per Serving: Calories: 220; Fat: 12g; Carbs: 5g; Fiber: 0.6g; Protein: 17.5

Watercress Soup

(**Prep + Cook Time**: 30 minutes | **Servings**: 4)

Ingredients:
- 8 oz. watercress
- 14 oz. veggie stock
- 12 oz. sweet potatoes; peeled and chopped
- 1 celery stick; chopped
- 1 onion; chopped
- 1 tbsp. lemon juice
- A pinch of nutmeg; ground
- 4 oz. canned coconut milk
- A pinch of sea salt
- Black pepper to the taste
- 1 tbsp. olive oil

Instructions:
1. Heat up a pot with the oil over medium heat, add onion and celery, stir and cook for 5 minutes.
2. Add sweet potato pieces and stock, stir; bring to a simmer, cover and cook on a low heat for 10 minutes.
3. Add watercress, stir; cover pot again and cook for 5 minutes.
4. Blend this with an immersion blender, add a pinch of nutmeg, lemon juice, salt, pepper and coconut milk, bring to a simmer again, divide into bowls and serve.

Nutrition Facts Per Serving: Calories: 159; Fat: 8g; Fiber: 3g; Carbs: 6g; Protein: 16g

Kohlrabi Dish

(**Prep + Cook Time**: 1 hour 10 minutes | **Servings**: 2)

Ingredients:
- 3 kohlrabi; peeled and thinly sliced
- A pinch of sea salt
- 1/3 cup parsley; chopped
- 2 tbsp. lard; melted
- Black pepper to the taste
- 4 tbsp. ghee

Instructions:
1. Arrange kohlrabi slices on the bottom of a baking dish.
2. Drizzle some of the lard over them, season with a pinch of salt and pepper and some of the parsley.
3. Add another layer of kohlrabi, drizzle more lard, season with pepper and parsley again and continue with kohlrabi slices again.
4. Finish with parsley.
5. Cover dish with tin foil, introduce in the oven at 350 °F and bake for 30 minutes.
6. Uncover dish, add ghee, introduce in the oven again and bake for 30 more minutes. Take the dish out of the oven, leave aside to cool down, slice, divide between plates and serve.

Nutrition Facts Per Serving: Calories: 207; Fat: 11g; Carbs: 18g; Fiber: 9.8; Sugar: 7g; Protein: 11.1

Avocado Spread

(Prep + Cook Time: 10 minutes | **Servings**: 4)

Ingredients:
- 2 avocados; pitted and peeled
- 4 bacon strips; cooked and crumbled
- 2 garlic cloves; minced
- 5 cherry tomatoes; halved
- 1 jalapeno pepper; chopped
- 1/2 red onion; chopped
- Juice of 1/2 lime
- A pinch of sea salt
- Black pepper to the taste

Instructions:
1. Put avocados in a bowl and mash them well.
2. Add garlic, jalapeno, onion, a pinch of salt, black pepper, lime juice and bacon and stir well. Top with cherry tomatoes halves and serve.

Nutrition Facts Per Serving: Calories: 140; Fat: 2g; Fiber: 2g; Carbs: 4g; Protein: 12g

Celery Casserole

(Prep + Cook Time: 30 minutes | **Servings**: 8)

Ingredients:
- 1 white onion; finely chopped
- 1 celery head; chopped
- 2½ tbsp. ghee
- 1½ tbsp. coconut flour
- 1/2 tsp. nutmeg
- A pinch of sea salt
- Black pepper to the taste
- 1½ cups coconut milk
- 2 tbsp. extra virgin olive oil
- 1/2 cup flax meal

Instructions:
1. Heat up a pan with 1 tbsp. olive oil over medium high heat, add celery, stir and cook for a few minutes until it browns a bit.
2. Add a pinch of sea salt and pepper, stir and transfer to a baking dish.
3. Heat up the same pan with the rest of the olive oil over medium heat, add onions, stir and cook for 4 minutes.
4. Add 1½ tbsp. ghee, stir well and cook for 1-2 minutes.
5. Add coconut flour, stir well for a few minutes and take off heat.
6. Add coconut milk, pepper to the taste and nutmeg and stir very well.
7. Return to medium heat and stir for 2 minutes more.
8. Add the rest of the ghee and flax meal, stir and pour everything over celery.
9. Toss to coat, introduce in the oven at 350 °F and bake for 15 minutes until it becomes golden. Take casserole out of the oven, leave aside to cool down, cut, divide between plates and serve.

Nutrition Facts Per Serving: Calories: 147; Fat: 9.2g; Carbs: 11.3g; Fiber: 1.5; Sugar: 2.1g; Protein: 3.1

Bell Peppers Stuffed with Tuna

(Prep + Cook Time: 20 minutes | **Servings**: 4)

Ingredients:
- 2 bell peppers; tops cut off, cut in halves and seeds removed
- 1 tbsp. capers; chopped
- 2 tbsp. tomato puree
- 4 oz. canned tuna; drained and flaked
- 1 scallion; chopped
- 1 tomato; chopped
- Black pepper to the taste

Instructions:
1. Place bell pepper halves on a lined baking sheet, place in preheated broiler over medium high heat, boil for 4 minutes and then leave them aside to cool down.
2. Meanwhile; in a bowl mix capers with tomato puree, tuna, tomato, black pepper and scallion and stir well.

3. Stuff bell peppers with this mix, place in preheated broiler again and cook for 5 minutes. Divide between plates and serve.

Nutrition Facts Per Serving: Calories: 140; Fat: 2g; Fiber: 4g; Carbs: 6g; Protein: 15g

Falafel

(**Prep + Cook Time**: 65 minutes | **Servings**: 4)

Ingredients:
- 2 cups cauliflower florets
- 1 cup yellow onion; chopped
- 1 zucchini; chopped
- 1/2 cup parsley; chopped
- 4 garlic cloves; minced
- 1/4 tsp. chili powder
- 1/2 cup cilantro; chopped
- 2 tsp. cumin
- A pinch of sea salt
- Black pepper to the taste
- 1/2 cup almond flour
- 1/2 tsp. turmeric
- Zest from 1 lemon
- 1 egg; whisked
- Coconut oil

Instructions:
1. In your food processor, mix cilantro, onion, parsley and garlic, blend well and transfer to a bowl.
2. In your food processor, also mix cauliflower with zucchini, blend very well and pour over onion mix.
3. Add chili powder, lemon zest, cumin, turmeric, egg, almond flour, a pinch of salt and pepper to the taste and stir well.
4. Spread some coconut oil on a lined baking sheet, arrange falafels, introduce in the oven at 375 °F and bake for 40 minutes, brushing them with some more coconut oil halfway.

Nutrition Facts Per Serving: Calories: 230; Fat: 14g; Carbs: 15g; Fiber: 2g; Protein: 22g

Eggplant Dish

(**Prep + Cook Time**: 50 minutes | **Servings**: 3)

Ingredients:
- 5 medium eggplants; sliced into rounds
- 2 garlic cloves; minced
- 1/2 cup olive oil
- 1 tsp. thyme; chopped
- 2 tbsp. balsamic vinegar
- 1 tsp. mustard
- Black pepper to the taste
- A pinch of sea salt
- 1 tsp. maple syrup

Instructions:
1. In a bowl; mix vinegar with thyme, mustard, garlic, oil, salt, pepper and maple syrup and whisk very well.
2. Arrange eggplant round on a lined baking sheet, place in the oven at 425 °F and roast for 40 minutes. Divide eggplants between plates and serve.

Nutrition Facts Per Serving: Calories: 120; Fat: 2g; Fiber: 2g; Carbs: 5g; Protein: 15g

Endive Bites

(**Prep + Cook Time**: 25 minutes | **Servings**: 4)

Ingredients:
- 4 slices bacon
- 16 endives leaves
- 1 cup cherry tomatoes; sliced
- A pinch of sea salt
- 2 tsp. white wine vinegar
- 1 tbsp. chives; chopped
- Black pepper to the taste
- 1 tbsp. extra virgin olive oil

Instructions:
1. Arrange bacon slices on a lined baking sheet, introduce in the oven at 400 °F and bake for 20 minutes.
2. Drain grease, transfer bacon to a cutting board, leave aside to cool down, crumble and put in a bowl.

3. In another bowl; mix tomatoes with chives, oil, a pinch of salt, pepper and vinegar and stir well. Divide this mix into endive leaves, sprinkle crumbled bacon on top of each, divide between plates and serve.

Nutrition Facts Per Serving: Calories: 120; Fat: 1g; Carbs: 10g; Fiber: 10; Sugar: 1g; Protein: 6g

Zucchini Noodles and Capers Sauce

(Prep + Cook Time: 10 minutes | **Servings**: 4)

Ingredients:
- 15 kalamata olives; pitted
- 8 oz. cherry tomatoes; halved
- 4 zucchinis; cut with a spiralizer
- 1 garlic clove
- 1 tbsp. capers; drained
- A pinch of sea salt
- Black pepper to the taste
- A pinch of red pepper flakes
- 2 tbsp. olive oil
- A handful basil; torn
- Juice of 1/2 lemon

Instructions:
1. In your food processor, mix capers with a pinch of sea salt, black pepper, pepper flakes and olives and blend well.
2. Transfer this to a bowl; add basil, oil and tomatoes, stir well and leave aside for 10 minutes. Divide zucchini noodles on plates, add tomatoes and capers sauce, toss to coat well and serve.

Nutrition Facts Per Serving: Calories: 100; Fat: 1g; Fiber: 2g; Carbs: 2g; Protein: 6g

Grilled Cherry Tomatoes

(Prep + Cook Time: 36 minutes | **Servings**: 4)

Ingredients:
- 1 romaine lettuce head; chopped
- A handful basil; chopped
- 1 cucumber; sliced
- 3 handfuls spinach; chopped
- 2 avocados; pitted, peeled and cubed
- 2 scallions; chopped
- 1/2 cup almonds; chopped
- 3 handfuls green beans; blanched and chopped

For the tomatoes skewers:
- 24 cherry tomatoes
- 3 garlic cloves; minced
- 3 tbsp. balsamic vinegar
- 2 tbsp. olive oil
- 1 tbsp. thyme; chopped
- A pinch of sea salt
- Black pepper to the taste

For the salad dressing:
- 2 tbsp. balsamic vinegar
- A pinch of sea salt
- Black pepper to the taste
- 4 tbsp. olive oil

Instructions:
1. In a salad bowl; mix lettuce with spinach, cucumber, basil, avocado pieces, scallions, almonds and green beans.
2. In a smaller bowl; mix 4 tbsp. oil with 2 tbsp. balsamic vinegar, a pinch of sea salt and black pepper and whisk well.
3. Add this to salad, toss to coat and leave aside for now.
4. In a bowl; mix 2 tbsp. oil with 3 tbsp. vinegar, 3 garlic cloves, thyme, a pinch of sea salt and black pepper and whisk well.
5. Add tomatoes, toss to coat and leave aside for 30 minutes.
6. Drain marinade, skewer 6 tomatoes on one skewer and repeat with the rest of the tomatoes.
7. Place skewers on preheated grill over medium high heat, grill for 3 minutes on each side and divide between plates. Serve with the salad you've made earlier on the side.

Nutrition Facts Per Serving: Calories: 140; Fat: 1g; Fiber: 1g; Carbs: 2g; Protein: 12g

Rutabaga Noodles and Cherry Tomatoes

(Prep + Cook Time: 35 minutes | **Servings:** 4)

Ingredients:
For the sauce:
- 1 garlic clove; minced
- 3/4 cup cashews; soaked for a couple of hours and drained
- 2 tbsp. Nutritional yeast
- 1/2 cup veggie stock
- 1 tbsp. shallot; chopped
- A pinch of sea salt
- Black pepper to the taste
- 2 tsp. lemon juice

For the pasta:
- 1 cup cherry tomatoes; halved
- 5 tsp. olive oil
- 1/4 tsp. garlic powder
- 2 rutabagas, peeled and cut into thin noodles

Instructions:
1. Place tomatoes and rutabaga noodles on a lined baking sheet, drizzle the oil over them, season with a pinch of sea salt, black pepper and garlic powder, toss to coat, place in the oven at 400 °F and bake for 20 minutes.
2. Meanwhile; in a food processor, mix garlic with shallots, cashews, veggie stock, Nutritional yeast, lemon juice, a pinch of sea salt and black pepper to the taste and blend well.
3. Divide rutabaga pasta between plates, top with tomatoes and drizzle the sauce over them.

Nutrition Facts Per Serving: Calories: 230; Fat: 2g; Fiber: 5g; Carbs: 10g; Protein: 8g

Stuffed Baby Peppers

(Prep + Cook Time: 10 minutes | **Servings:** 4)

Ingredients:
- 12 baby bell peppers; cut into halves lengthwise and seeds removed
- 1/4 tsp. red pepper flakes; crushed
- 1 lb. shrimp; cooked, peeled and deveined
- 6 tbsp. jarred Paleo pesto
- A pinch of sea salt
- Black pepper to the taste
- 1 tbsp. lemon juice
- 1 tbsp. olive oil
- A handful parsley; chopped

Instructions:
1. In a bowl; mix shrimp with pepper flakes, Paleo pesto, a pinch of salt, black pepper, lemon juice, oil and parsley and whisk very well.
2. Divide this into bell pepper halves, arrange on plates and serve.

Nutrition Facts Per Serving: Calories: 130; Fat: 2g; Fiber: 1g; Carbs: 3g; Protein: 15g

Garlic Sauce

(Prep + Cook Time: 20 minutes | **Servings:** 4)

Ingredients:
- 2 garlic cloves; minced
- 3 eggplants; cut into halves and thinly sliced
- 1 red chili pepper; chopped
- 1 green onion stalk; chopped
- 1 tbsp. ginger; grated
- 2 tbsp. avocado oil
- 1 tbsp. coconut aminos
- 1 tbsp. balsamic vinegar

Instructions:
1. Heat up a pan with half of the oil over medium high heat, add eggplant slices, cook for 2 minutes, flip, cook for 3 minutes more and transfer to a plate.
2. Heat up the pan with the rest of the oil over medium heat, add chili pepper, garlic, green onions and ginger, stir and cook for 1 minute.

3. Return eggplant slices to the pan, stir and cook for 1 minute. Add coconut aminos and vinegar, stir; divide between plates and serve.

Nutrition Facts Per Serving: Calories: 130; Fat: 2g; Fiber: 4g; Carbs: 7g; Protein: 9g

Paleo Pancakes

(Prep + Cook Time: 25 minutes | Servings: 4)

Ingredients:
- 1/2 cup almond flour
- 1/2 cup tapioca flour
- 1 small red onion; chopped
- 1 Serrano chili pepper; minced
- 1 small piece of ginger; grated
- A handful cilantro; chopped
- Coconut oil for frying
- A pinch of sea salt
- Black pepper to the taste
- 1 cup coconut milk
- 1/2 tsp. chili powder
- 1/4 tsp. turmeric

Instructions:
1. In a bowl; mix almond and tapioca flour with milk, chili powder, a pinch of sea salt, pepper and turmeric and stir well.
2. Add onion, Serrano pepper, cilantro and ginger and stir very well.
3. Heat up a pan with the oil over medium high heat, pour 1/4 cup pancakes mix, spread, cook for 4 minutes on each side and transfer to a plate. Repeat with the rest of the batter and serve pancakes with green chutney.

Nutrition Facts Per Serving: Calories: 198; Fat 6.2g; Carbs: 30g; Fiber: 5.9; Sugar: 4g; Protein: 8.5

Sweet Potatoes and Cabbage Bake

(Prep + Cook Time: 1 hour 20 minutes | Servings: 4)

Ingredients:
- 8 sweet potatoes; cut into thin matchsticks
- 1 carrot; sliced
- 2½ cups green cabbage; shredded
- 4 oz. pancetta; chopped
- 3 tomatoes; sliced
- 2 garlic cloves; minced
- A pinch of sea salt
- Black pepper to the taste
- 1 tsp. thyme; dried

Instructions:
1. In a baking dish, mix cabbage with potatoes, garlic and carrot.
2. Add thyme, a pinch of sea salt and pepper and pancetta and toss to coat.
3. Spread tomato slices over veggie mix, cover dish with tin foil, introduce in the oven at 350 °F and bake for 35 minutes.
4. Discard tin foil and bake veggies for 30 more minutes. Take the dish out of the oven, leave aside to cool down, divide between plates and serve.

Nutrition Facts Per Serving: Calories: 190; Fat: 0.5g; Carbs: 43g; Fiber: 7g; Protein: 5.9

Mexican Stuffed Peppers

(Prep + Cook Time: 30 minutes | Servings: 4)

Ingredients:
- 4 bell peppers; tops cut off and seeds removed
- 1/2 cup tomato juice
- 2 tbsp. jarred jalapenos; chopped
- 4 chicken breasts
- 1 cup tomatoes; chopped
- 1/4 cup yellow onion; chopped
- 1/4 cup green peppers; chopped
- 2 cups Paleo salsa
- A pinch of sea salt
- 2 tsp. onion powder
- 1/2 tsp. red pepper; crushed
- 1 tsp. chili powder
- 1/2 tsp. garlic powder
- 1/4 tsp. oregano
- 1 tsp. cumin; ground

Instructions:
1. In your slow cooker, mix chicken breasts with tomato juice, jalapenos, tomatoes, onion, green peppers, a pinch of salt, onion powder, red pepper, chili powder, garlic powder, oregano and cumin, stir well, cover and cook on Low for 6 hours.
2. Shred meat using 2 forks and stir everything well.
3. Stuff bell peppers with this mix, place them into a baking dish, pour salsa over them, place in the oven at 350 °F and bake for 20 minutes. Divide stuffed peppers on plates and serve.

Nutrition Facts Per Serving: Calories: 240; Fat: 4g; Fiber: 3g; Carbs: 7g; Protein: 20g

Artichokes and Tomatoes Dip

(Prep + Cook Time: 40 minutes | **Servings:** 4)

Ingredients:
- 2 artichokes; cut in halves and trimmed
- Juice from 3 lemons
- 4 sun-dried tomatoes; chopped
- A bunch of parsley; chopped
- A bunch of basil; chopped
- 1 garlic clove; minced
- 4 tbsp. olive oil
- Black pepper to the taste

Instructions:
1. In a bowl; mix artichokes with lemon juice from 1 lemon, some black pepper and toss to coat.
2. Transfer to a pot, add water to cover, bring to a boil over medium high heat, cook for 30 minutes and drain.
3. In your food processor, mix the rest of the lemon juice with tomatoes, parsley, basil, garlic, black pepper and olive oil and blend really well.
4. Divide artichokes between plates and top each with the tomatoes dip.

Nutrition Facts Per Serving: Calories: 140; Fat: 1g; Fiber: 1g; Carbs: 3g; Protein: 9g

Artichokes with Horseradish Sauce

(Prep + Cook Time: 55 minutes | **Servings:** 2)

Ingredients:
- 3 cups artichoke hearts
- 1 tbsp. horseradish; prepared
- 2 tbsp. mayonnaise
- 1 tsp. lemon juice
- 1 tbsp. lemon juice
- A pinch of sea salt
- Black pepper to the taste

Instructions:
1. In a bowl; mix horseradish with mayo, a pinch of sea salt, black pepper and 1 tsp. lemon juice, whisk well and leave aside for now.
2. Arrange artichoke hearts on a lined baking sheet, drizzle 2 tbsp. olive oil over them, 1 tbsp. lemon juice and sprinkle a pinch of salt and some black pepper.
3. Toss to coat well, place in the oven at 425 °F and roast them for 45 minutes. Divide artichoke hearts between plates and serve with the horseradish sauce on top.

Nutrition Facts Per Serving: Calories: 300; Fat: 3g; Fiber: 12g; Carbs: 16g; Protein: 10g

Zucchini Noodles with Tomatoes and Spinach

(Prep + Cook Time: 30 minutes | **Servings:** 6)

Ingredients:
- 3 zucchinis; cut with a spiralizer
- 16 oz. mushrooms; sliced
- 1/4 cup sun dried tomatoes; chopped
- 1/2 cup cherry tomatoes; halved
- 2 cups marinara sauce
- 2 cups spinach; chopped
- 2 tbsp. olive oil
- 1 tsp. garlic; minced
- A pinch of sea salt
- Black pepper to the taste
- A pinch of cayenne pepper
- A handful basil; chopped

Instructions:
1. Put zucchini noodles in a bowl; season them with a pinch of salt and black pepper and leave them aside for 10 minutes.
2. Heat up a pan with the oil over medium high heat, add garlic, stir and cook for 1 minute.
3. Add mushrooms, stir and cook for 4 minutes.
4. Add sun dried tomatoes, stir and cook for 4 minutes more.
5. Add cherry tomatoes, spinach, cayenne, marinara and zucchini noodles, stir and cook for 6 minutes more. Sprinkle basil on top, toss gently, divide between plates and serve.

Nutrition Facts Per Serving: Calories: 120; Fat: 1g; Fiber: 1g; Carbs: 2g; Protein: 9g

Eggplant Hash

(Prep + Cook Time: 40 minutes | **Servings**: 4)

Ingredients:
- 1/2 lb. cherry tomatoes; halved
- 1 eggplant; roughly chopped
- 1/2 cup olive oil
- 1 tsp. Tabasco sauce
- 1/4 cup basil; chopped
- 1/4 cup mint; chopped
- A pinch of sea salt
- Black pepper to the taste

Instructions:
1. Put eggplant pieces in a bowl; add a pinch of salt, toss to coat, leave aside for 20 minutes and drain using paper towels.
2. Heat up a pan with half of the oil over medium high heat, add eggplant, cook for 3 minutes, flip, cook them for 3 minutes more and transfer to a bowl.
3. Heat up the same pan with the rest of the oil over medium high heat, add tomatoes and cook them for 8 minutes stirring from time to time.
4. Return eggplant pieces to the pan and also add a pinch of salt, black pepper, basil, mint and Tabasco sauce. Stir, cook for 2 minutes more, divide between plates and serve.

Nutrition Facts Per Serving: Calories: 120; Fat: 1g; Fiber: 4g; Carbs: 8g; Protein: 15g

Stuffed Peppers

(Prep + Cook Time: 50 minutes | **Servings**: 4)

Ingredients:
- 1/4 cup ghee; melted
- 6 colored bell peppers
- 1 garlic head; cloves peeled and chopped
- 10 anchovy fillets
- 15 walnuts

Instructions:
1. Place bell peppers on a lined baking sheet, place in preheated broiler, cook for 20 minutes and leave them to cool down.
2. Heat up a pan with the ghee over low heat, add garlic, stir and cook for 10 minutes.
3. Grind walnuts in a coffee grinder and add this powder to the pan.
4. Also add anchovy and stir well.
5. Peel burnt skin off peppers, discard tops, cut in halves and remove skins. Divide pepper halves on plates, divide anchovy mix on them and serve.

Nutrition Facts Per Serving: Calories: 140; Fat: 3g; Fiber: 3g; Carbs: 6g; Protein: 14g

Spinach and Mushroom Dish

(Prep + Cook Time: 25 minutes | **Servings:** 2)

Ingredients:
- 6 mushrooms; chopped
- A handful cherry tomatoes; cut in halves
- 3 handfuls spinach; torn
- 1 tsp. ghee
- 2 tbsp. extra virgin olive oil
- 1 small red onion; sliced
- 1/2 tsp. lemon rind; diced
- 1 garlic clove; minced
- A pinch of sea salt
- Black pepper to the taste
- A pinch of nutmeg
- A drizzle of lemon juice

Instructions:
1. Heat up a pan with the ghee over medium high heat, add mushrooms, stir; cook for 4 minutes and transfer them to a plate.
2. Heat up the same pan with the olive oil over medium high heat, add onion, stir and cook for 3 minutes.
3. Add tomatoes, a pinch of sea salt, pepper, lemon rind, nutmeg and garlic, stir and cook for 3 minutes more.
4. Add spinach, stir and cook for 2-3 minutes. Add lemon juice at the end, stir gently, transfer to plates and serve with mushrooms on top.

Nutrition Facts Per Serving: Calories: 120; Fat: 4.5g; Carbs: 7g; Fiber: 2.5g; Protein: 3.4

Cherry Mix

(Prep + Cook Time: 34 minutes | **Servings:** 4)

Ingredients:
- 3 cups cherry tomatoes; halved
- 1/4 tsp. cumin; ground
- 1 tbsp. sherry vinegar
- 1 tsp. coconut sugar
- 1 red onion; chopped
- 2 cucumbers; sliced
- 1/4 cup olive oil
- A pinch of sea salt
- Black pepper to the taste

Instructions:
1. Put cherry tomatoes in a bowl; season with coconut sugar, a pinch of salt and black pepper and leave aside for 30 minutes.
2. Drain tomatoes and pour juices into a pan.
3. Heat this up over medium heat, add cumin and vinegar and bring to a simmer.
4. Cook for 4 minutes, take off heat and mix with olive oil. Add tomatoes, onion and cucumber to this mix, toss well, divide between plates and serve.

Nutrition Facts Per Serving: Calories: 120; Fat: 1g; Fiber: 2g; Carbs: 2g; Protein: 7g

Stuffed Poblanos

(Prep + Cook Time: 50 minutes | **Servings:** 4)

Ingredients:
- 1 white onion; chopped
- 8 oz. mushrooms; chopped
- 10 poblano peppers; one side of them sliced and reserved
- 1 tbsp. olive oil
- Cooking spray
- 2 tsp. garlic; minced
- A pinch of sea salt
- Black pepper to the taste
- 1/2 cup cilantro; chopped

Instructions:
1. Place poblano boats in a baking dish which you've sprayed with some cooking spray.
2. Heat up a pan with the oil over medium high heat, add chopped poblano pieces, onion and mushrooms, stir and cook for 5 minutes.
3. Add garlic, cilantro, salt and black pepper, stir and cook for 2 minutes.

4. Divide this into poblano boats, introduce them in the oven at 375 °F and bake for 30 minutes. Divide between plates and serve.

Nutrition Facts Per Serving: Calories: 150; Fat: 3g; Fiber: 2g; Carbs: 4g; Protein: 10g

Tomato Quiche

(**Prep + Cook Time**: 30 minutes | **Servings**: 2)

Ingredients:
- 1 bunch basil; chopped
- 4 eggs
- 1 garlic clove; minced
- A pinch of sea salt
- Black pepper to the taste
- 1/2 cup cherry tomatoes; halved
- 1/4 cup almond cheese

Instructions:
1. In a bowl; mix eggs with a pinch of sea salt, black pepper, almond cheese and basil and whisk well.
2. Pour this into a baking dish, arrange tomatoes on top, place in the oven at 350 °F and bake for 20 minutes. Leave quiche to cool down, slice and serve.

Nutrition Facts Per Serving: Calories: 140; Fat: 1g; Fiber: 1g; Carbs: 2g; Protein: 10g

Liver Stuffed Peppers

(**Prep + Cook Time**: 25 minutes | **Servings**: 4)

Ingredients:
- 1/2 lb. chicken livers; chopped
- 4 bacon slices; chopped
- 1 white onion; chopped
- 4 garlic cloves; chopped
- 4 bell peppers; tops cut off and seeds removed
- A pinch of sea salt
- Black pepper to the taste
- 1/2 tsp. lemon zest; grated
- 1/4 tsp. thyme; chopped
- 1/4 tsp. dill; chopped
- A drizzle of olive oil
- A handful parsley; chopped

Instructions:
1. Heat up a pan over medium heat, add bacon, stir and cook for 2 minutes.
2. Add onion and garlic, stir and cook for 2 minutes.
3. Add livers, a pinch of salt and black pepper, stir; cook for 5 minutes and take off heat.
4. Transfer this to your food processor, blend very well, transfer to a bowl and aside for 10 minutes.
5. Add thyme, oil, parsley, lemon zest and dill, stir well and Stuff each bell pepper with this mix. Serve right away.

Nutrition Facts Per Serving: Calories: 150; Fat: 3g; Fiber: 2g; Carbs: 5g; Protein: 12g

Stuffed Portobello Mushrooms

(**Prep + Cook Time**: 30 minutes | **Servings**: 4)

Ingredients:
- 10 basil leaves
- 1 cup baby spinach
- 3 garlic cloves; chopped
- 1 cup almonds; roughly chopped
- 1 tbsp. parsley
- 2 tbsp. Nutritional yeast
- 1/4 cup olive oil
- 8 cherry tomatoes; halved
- A pinch of sea salt
- Black pepper to the taste
- 4 Portobello mushrooms; stem removed and chopped

Instructions:
1. In your food processor, mix basil with spinach, garlic, almonds, parsley, Nutritional yeast, oil, a pinch of salt, black pepper to the taste and mushroom stems and blend well.
2. Stuff each mushroom with this mix, place them on a lined baking sheet, place in the oven at 400 °F and bake for 20 minutes. Divide between plates and serve right away.

Nutrition Facts Per Serving: Calories: 145; Fat: 3g; Fiber: 2g; Carbs: 6g; Protein: 17g

Zucchini Noodles and Pesto

(Prep + Cook Time: 20 minutes | **Servings:** 4)

Ingredients:
- 6 zucchinis; trimmed and cut with a spiralizer
- 1 cup basil
- 1 avocado; pitted and peeled
- A pinch of sea salt
- Black pepper to the taste
- 3 garlic cloves; chopped
- 1/4 cup olive oil
- 2 tbsp. olive oil
- 1 lb. shrimp; peeled and deveined
- 1/4 cup pistachios
- 2 tbsp. lemon juice
- 2 tsp. old bay seasoning

Instructions:
1. In a bowl; mix zucchini noodles with a pinch of sea salt and some black pepper, leave aside for 10 minutes and squeeze well.
2. In your food processor, mix pistachios with black pepper, basil, avocado, lemon juice and a pinch of salt and blend well.
3. Add 1/4 cup oil, blend again and leave aside for now.
4. Heat up a pan with 1 tbsp. oil over medium high heat, add garlic, stir and cook for 1 minute.
5. Add shrimp and old bay seasoning, stir; cook for 4 minutes and transfer to a bowl.
6. Heat up the same pan with the rest of the oil over medium high heat, add zucchini noodles, stir and cook for 3 minutes.
7. Divide on plates, add pesto on top and toss to coat well. top with shrimp and serve.

Nutrition Facts Per Serving: Calories: 140; Fat: 1g; Fiber: 1g; Carbs: 5g; Protein: 14g

Spaghetti Squash and Tomatoes

(Prep + Cook Time: 60 minutes | **Servings:** 4)

Ingredients:
- 1/4 cup pine nuts
- 2 cups basil; chopped
- 1 spaghetti squash; halved lengthwise and seedless
- Black pepper to the taste
- A pinch of sea salt
- 1 tsp. garlic; minced
- 1½ tbsp. olive oil
- 1 cup mixed cherry tomatoes; halved
- 1/2 cup olive oil
- 2 garlic cloves; minced

Instructions:
1. Place spaghetti squash halves on a lined baking sheet, place in the oven at 375 °F and bake for 40 minutes.
2. Leave squash to cool down and make your spaghetti out of the flesh.
3. In your food processor, mix pine nuts with a pinch of salt, basil and 2 garlic cloves and blend well.
4. Add 1/2 cup olive oil, blend again well and transfer to a bowl.
5. Heat up a pan with 1½ tbsp. oil over medium high heat, add tomatoes, a pinch of salt, some black pepper and 1 tsp. garlic, stir and cook for 2 minutes. Divide spaghetti squash on plates, add tomatoes and the basil pesto on top.

Nutrition Facts Per Serving: Calories: 150; Fat: 1g; Fiber: 2g; Carbs: 4g; Protein: 12g

Daikon Rolls

(Prep + Cook Time: 15 minutes | **Servings**: 4)

Ingredients:
- 1/2 cup pumpkin seeds
- 2 green onions; chopped
- 1/2 bunch cilantro; roughly chopped
- 2 tbsp. avocado oil
- 1 tbsp. lime juice
- 2 tsp. water
- A pinch of sea salt
- Black pepper to the taste
- 2 daikon radishes; sliced lengthwise into long strips
- 1 small cucumber; cut into matchsticks
- 1/2 avocado; pitted, peeled and sliced
- Handful microgreens

Instructions:
1. In your food processor, mix pumpkin seeds with a pinch of sea salt, pepper, cilantro and green onions and blend very well.
2. Add avocado oil gradually and lime juice and blend very well again. Add water and blend some more.
3. Spread this on each daikon slice, add cucumber matchsticks, avocado slices and micro greens, roll them, seal edges, divide between plates and serve.

Nutrition Facts Per Serving: Calories: 140; Fat: 0g; Carbs: 23g; Fiber: 0g; Protein: 0

Glazed Carrots

(Prep + Cook Time: 25 minutes | **Servings**: 4)

Ingredients:
- 1 lb. carrots; sliced
- 1 tbsp. coconut oil
- 1 tbsp. ghee
- 1/2 cup pineapple juice
- 1 tsp. ginger; grated
- 1/2 tbsp. maple syrup
- 1/2 tsp. nutmeg
- 1 tbsp. parsley; chopped

Instructions:
1. Heat up a pan with the ghee and the oil over medium high heat, add ginger, stir and cook for 2 minutes.
2. Add carrots, stir and cook for 5 minutes.
3. Add pineapple juice, maple syrup and nutmeg, stir and cook for 5 minutes more. Add parsley, stir; cook for 3 minutes, divide between plates and serve.

Nutrition Facts Per Serving: Calories: 100; Fat: 0.5g; Fiber: 1g; Carbs: 3g; Protein: 7g

Cauliflower Pizza

(Prep + Cook Time: 40 minutes | **Servings**: 6)

Ingredients:
- 1½ cups mashed cauliflower
- A pinch of sea salt
- Black pepper to the taste
- 1/2 cup almond meal
- 1½ tbsp. flax seed; ground
- 2/3 cup water
- 1/2 tsp. oregano; dried
- 1/2 tsp. garlic powder
- Pizza sauce for serving
- Spinach leaves; chopped and already cooked for serving
- Mushrooms; sliced and cooked for serving

Instructions:
1. In a bowl; mix flax seed with water and stir well.
2. In a bowl; mix cauliflower with almond meal, flax seed mix, a pinch of sea salt, pepper, oregano and garlic powder, stir well, shape small pizza crusts, spread them on a lined baking sheet and bake them in the oven at 420 °F and bake for 15 minutes.
3. Take pizzas out of the oven, spread pizza sauce, spinach and mushrooms on them, introduce in the oven again and bake 10 more minutes. Divide between plates and serve.

Nutrition Facts Per Serving: Calories: 150; Fat: 8g; Carbs: 20g; Fiber: 1g; Protein: 9g

Cucumber Wraps

(Prep + Cook Time: 40 minutes | **Servings**: 4)

Ingredients:
For the mayo:
- 1 cup macadamia nuts
- 1 tbsp. coconut aminos
- 3 tbsp. lemon juice
- 1 tbsp. agave
- 1 tsp. caraway seeds
- 1/3 cup dill; chopped
- A pinch of sea salt
- Some water

For the filling:
- 1 cup alfalfa sprouts
- 1 red bell pepper; cut into thin strips
- 2 carrots; cut into thin matchsticks
- 1 cucumber; cut into thin matchsticks
- 1 cup pea shoots
- 4 Paleo coconut wrappers

Instructions:
1. Put macadamia nuts in a bowl; add water to cover, leave aside for 30 minutes and drain well.
2. In your food processor, mix nuts with coconut aminos, lemon juice, agave, caraway seeds, a pinch of salt and dill and blend very well.
3. Add some water and blend again until you obtain a smooth mayo.
4. Divide alfalfa sprouts, bell pepper, carrot, cucumber and pea shoots on each coconut wrappers, spread dill mayo over them, wrap, cut each in half and serve.

Nutrition Facts Per Serving: Calories: 140; Fat: 3g; Fiber: 3g; Carbs: 5g; Protein: 12g

Garlic Tomatoes

(Prep + Cook Time: 60 minutes | **Servings**: 4)

Ingredients:
- 1 lb. mixed cherry tomatoes
- 4 garlic cloves; crushed
- 3 thyme springs; chopped
- A pinch of sea salt
- Black pepper to the taste
- 1/4 cup olive oil

Instructions:
1. In a baking dish, mix tomatoes with a pinch of sea salt, black pepper, olive oil and thyme, toss to coat, place in the oven at 325 °F and bake for 50 minutes. Divide tomatoes and pan juices between plates and serve.

Nutrition Facts Per Serving: Calories: 100; Fat: 0g; Fiber: 1g; Carbs: 1g; Protein: 6g

Grilled Artichokes

(Prep + Cook Time: 35 minutes | **Servings**: 4)

Ingredients:
- 2 artichokes; trimmed and halved
- Juice of 1 lemon
- 1 tbsp. lemon zest grated
- 1 rosemary spring; chopped
- 2 tbsp. olive oil
- A pinch of sea salt
- Black pepper to the taste

Instructions:
1. Put water in a pot, add a pinch of salt and lemon juice, bring to a boil over medium high heat, add artichokes, boil for 15 minutes, drain and leave them to cool down.
2. Drizzle olive oil over them, season with black pepper to the taste, sprinkle lemon zest and rosemary, stir well and place them on your preheated grill.
3. Grill artichokes over medium high heat for 5 minutes on each side, divide them between plates and serve.

Nutrition Facts Per Serving: Calories: 120; Fat: 1g; Fiber: 2g; Carbs: 6g; Protein: 7g

Pork Stuffed Bell Peppers

(Prep + Cook Time: 36 minutes | **Servings**: 4)

Ingredients:
- 1 lb. pork; ground
- 1 tsp. Cajun spice
- 1 tbsp. olive oil
- 1 tbsp. tomato paste
- 6 garlic cloves; minced
- 1 yellow onion; chopped
- 4 big bell peppers; tops cut off and seeds removed
- A pinch of sea salt
- Black pepper to the taste

Instructions:
1. Heat up a pan with the oil over medium high heat, add garlic and onion, stir and cook for 4 minutes.
2. Add meat, stir and cook for 10 minutes more.
3. Add a pinch of salt, black pepper, tomato paste and Cajun seasoning, stir and cook for 3 minutes more.
4. Stuff bell peppers with this mix, place them on preheated grill over medium high heat, grill for 3 minutes on each side, divide between plates and serve.

Nutrition Facts Per Serving: Calories: 140; Fat: 3g; Fiber: 2g; Carbs: 3g; Protein: 10g

Carrots and Lime

(Prep + Cook Time: 40 minutes | **Servings**: 6)

Ingredients:
- 1¼ lbs. baby carrots
- 3 tbsp. ghee; melted
- 8 garlic cloves; minced
- A pinch of sea salt
- Black pepper to the taste
- Zest of 2 limes; grated
- 1/2 tsp. chili powder

Instructions:
1. In a bowl; mix baby carrots with ghee, garlic, a pinch of salt, black pepper to the taste and chili powder and stir well.
2. Spread carrots on a lined baking sheet, place in the oven at 400 °F and roast for 15 minutes.
3. Take carrots out of the oven, shake baking sheet, place in the oven again and roast for 15 minutes more. Divide between plates and serve with lime on top.

Nutrition Facts Per Serving: Calories: 100; Fat: 1g; Fiber: 1g; Carbs: 1g; Protein: 7g

Eggplant Casserole

(Prep + Cook Time: 60 minutes | **Servings**: 4)

Ingredients:
- 1 lb. beef; ground
- 2 eggplants; sliced
- 3 tbsp. olive oil
- 1 garlic clove; minced
- 3/4 cup tomato sauce
- 1/2 bunch basil; chopped
- A pinch of sea salt
- Black pepper to the taste

Instructions:
1. Heat up a pan with 1 tbsp. oil over medium high heat, add eggplant slices, cook for 5 minutes on each side, transfer them to paper towels, drain grease and leave them aside.
2. Heat up another pan with the rest of the oil over medium high heat, add garlic, stir and cook for 1 minute.
3. Add beef, stir and cook for 5 minutes more.
4. Add tomato sauce, stir and cook for 5 minutes more.
5. Add a pinch of sea salt and black pepper, stir; take off heat and mix with basil.
6. Place one layer of eggplant slices into a baking dish, add one layer of beef mix and repeat with the rest of the eggplant slices and beef.
7. Place in the oven at 350 °F and bake for 30 minutes. Leave eggplant casserole to cool down, slice and serve.

Nutrition Facts Per Serving: Calories: 342; Fat: 23g; Fiber: 7g; Carbs: 10g; Protein: 23g

Warm Watercress Mix

(Prep + Cook Time: 20 minutes | **Servings:** 4)

Ingredients:
- 1 lb. watercress; chopped
- 1/4 cup olive oil
- 1 garlic clove; cut in halves
- 1 bacon slice; cooked and crumbled
- 1/4 cup hazelnuts; chopped
- Black pepper to the taste
- 1/4 cup pine nuts

Instructions:
1. Heat up a pan with the oil over medium heat, add garlic clove halves, cook for 2 minutes and discard.
2. Heat up the pan with the garlic oil again over medium heat, add hazelnuts and pine nuts, stir and cook for 6 minutes.
3. Add bacon, black pepper to the taste and watercress, stir; cook for 2 minutes, divide between plates and serve right away.

Nutrition Facts Per Serving: Calories: 100; Fat: 1g; Fiber: 2g; Carbs: 2g; Protein: 6g

Artichokes Dish

(Prep + Cook Time: 60 minutes | **Servings:** 4)

Ingredients:
- 16 mushrooms; sliced
- 1/3 cup tamari sauce
- 1/3 cup olive oil
- 4 tbsp. balsamic vinegar
- 4 garlic cloves; minced
- 1 tbsp. lemon juice
- 1 tsp. oregano; dried
- 1 tsp. rosemary; dried
- 1/2 tbsp. thyme; dried
- A pinch of sea salt
- Black pepper to the taste
- 1 sweet onion; chopped
- 1 jar artichoke hearts
- 4 cups spinach
- 1 tbsp. coconut oil
- 1 tsp. garlic; minced
- 1 cauliflower head; florets separated
- 1/2 cup veggie stock
- 1 tsp. garlic powder
- A pinch of nutmeg; ground

Instructions:
1. In a bowl; mix vinegar with tamari sauce, lemon juice, 4 garlic cloves, olive oil, oregano, rosemary, thyme, a pinch of salt, black pepper and mushrooms, toss to coat well and leave aside for 30 minutes.
2. Transfer these to a lined baking sheet and bake them in the oven at 350 °F for 30 minutes.
3. In your food processor, mix cauliflower with a pinch of sea salt and black pepper and pulse until you obtain your rice.
4. Heat up a pan over medium high heat, add cauliflower rice, toast for 2 minutes, add nutmeg, garlic powder, black pepper and stock, stir and cook until stock evaporated.
5. Heat up a pan with the coconut oil over medium heat, add onion, artichokes, 1 tsp. garlic and spinach, stir and cook for a few minutes. Divide cauliflower rice on plates, top with artichokes and mushrooms and serve.

Nutrition Facts Per Serving: Calories: 200; Fat: 3g; Fiber: 2g; Carbs: 7g; Protein: 18g

Cucumber Noodles and Shrimp

(Prep + Cook Time: 25 minutes | **Servings:** 4)

Ingredients:
- 1 lb. shrimp; peeled and deveined
- 1 tbsp. Paleo tamari sauce
- 3 tbsp. coconut aminos
- 1 tbsp. sriracha
- 1 tbsp. balsamic vinegar
- 1/2 cup warm water
- 1 tbsp. honey
- 3 tbsp. lemongrass; chopped
- 1 tbsp. ginger; dried
- 1 tbsp. olive oil

For the cucumber noodles:

- 2 cucumbers; cut with a spiralizer
- 1 carrot; cut into thin matchsticks
- 1/4 cup balsamic vinegar
- 1/4 cup ghee; melted
- 1/4 cup peanuts; roasted
- 2 tbsp. sriracha sauce
- 1 tbsp. coconut aminos
- 1 tbsp. ginger; grated
- A handful mint; chopped

Instructions:
1. In a bowl; mix 3 tbsp. coconut aminos with 1 tbsp. vinegar, 1 tbsp. tamari, 1 tbsp. sriracha, warm water, honey, lemongrass, 1 tbsp. ginger, 1 tbsp. olive oil and whisk well.
2. Add shrimp, toss to coat and leave aside for 20 minutes.
3. Heat up your grill over medium high heat, add shrimp, cook them for 3 minutes on each side and transfer to a bowl.
4. In a bowl; mix cucumber noodles with carrot, ghee, 1/4 cup vinegar, 2 tbsp. Sriracha, 1 tbsp. coconut aminos, 1 tbsp. ginger, peanuts and mint and stir well. Divide cucumber noodles on plates, top with shrimp and serve.

Nutrition Facts Per Serving: Calories: 140; Fat: 1g; Fiber: 2g; Carbs: 3g; Protein: 8g

Baked Eggplant

(**Prep + Cook Time**: 40 minutes | **Servings**: 3)

Ingredients:
- 2 eggplants; sliced
- A pinch of sea salt
- Black pepper to the taste
- 1 cup almonds; ground
- 1 tsp. garlic; minced
- 2 tsp. olive oil

Instructions:
1. Grease a baking dish with some of the oil and arrange eggplant slices on it.
2. Season them with a pinch of salt and some black pepper and leave them aside for 10 minutes.
3. In your food processor, mix almonds with the rest of the oil, garlic, a pinch of salt and black pepper and blend well.
4. Spread this over eggplant slices, place in the oven at 425 °F and bake for 30 minutes. Divide between plates and serve.

Nutrition Facts Per Serving: Calories: 140; Fat: 1g; Fiber: 1g; Carbs: 3g; Protein: 15g

Purple Carrots

(**Prep + Cook Time**: 1 hour 10 minutes | **Servings**: 2)

Ingredients:
- 6 purple carrots; peeled
- A drizzle of olive oil
- 2 tbsp. sesame seeds paste
- 6 tbsp. water
- 3 tbsp. lemon juice
- 1 garlic clove; minced
- A pinch of sea salt
- Black pepper to the taste
- White and sesame seeds

Instructions:
1. Arrange purple carrots on a lined baking sheet, sprinkle a pinch of salt, black pepper and a drizzle of oil, place in the oven at 350 °F and bake for 1 hour.
2. Meanwhile; in your food processor, mix sesame seeds paste with water, lemon juice, garlic, a pinch of sea salt and black pepper and pulse really well.
3. Spread this over carrots, toss gently, divide between plates and sprinkle sesame seeds on top.

Nutrition Facts Per Serving: Calories: 100; Fat: 1g; Fiber: 1g; Carbs: 5g; Protein: 10g

Stuffed with Beef

(Prep + Cook Time: 1 hour 5 minutes | **Servings**: 2)

Ingredients:
- 1 lb. beef; ground
- 1 tsp. coriander; ground
- 1 onion; chopped
- 3 garlic cloves; minced
- 2 tbsp. coconut oil
- 1 tbsp. ginger; grated
- 1/2 tsp. cumin
- 1/2 tsp. turmeric
- 1 tbsp. hot curry powder
- A pinch of sea salt
- 1 egg
- 4 bell peppers; cut in halves and seeds removed
- 1/3 cup raisins
- 1/3 cup walnuts; chopped

Instructions:
1. Heat up a pan with the oil over medium high heat, add onion, stir and cook for 4 minutes.
2. Add garlic, stir and cook for 1 minute.
3. Add beef, stir and cook for 10 minutes.
4. Add coriander, ginger, cumin, curry powder, a pinch of salt and turmeric and stir well.
5. Add walnuts and raisins, stir take off heat and mix with egg.
6. Divide this mix into pepper halves, place them on a lined baking sheet, place in the oven at 350 °F and bake for 40 minutes. Divide between plates and serve.

Nutrition Facts Per Serving: Calories: 240; Fat: 4g; Fiber: 3g; Carbs: 7g; Protein: 12g

Carrot Hash

(Prep + Cook Time: 55 minutes | **Servings**: 4)

Ingredients:
- 3/4 lb. beef; ground
- 1 yellow onion; chopped
- 1 tbsp. olive oil
- 6 bacon slices; chopped
- 3 cups carrots; chopped
- A pinch of sea salt
- Black pepper to the taste
- 2 scallions; chopped

Instructions:
1. Place carrots on a lined baking sheet, drizzle the oil, season with a pinch of salt and some black pepper, toss to coat, place in the oven at 425 °F and bake for 25 minutes.
2. Meanwhile; heat up a pan over medium high heat, add bacon and fry for a couple of minutes.
3. Add onion and beef and some black pepper, stir and cook for 7-8 minutes more.
4. Take carrots out of the oven, add them to the beef and bacon mix, stir and cook for 10 minutes. Sprinkle scallions on top, divide between plates and serve.

Nutrition Facts Per Serving: Calories: 160; Fat: 2g; Fiber: 1g; Carbs: 2g; Protein: 12g

Snacks & Appetizers Recipes

Stuffed Mushrooms

(Prep + Cook Time: 30 minutes | **Servings**: 8)

Ingredients:
- 1 lb. cremini mushrooms caps
- 3 tbsp. olive oil
- A pinch of cayenne pepper

For the dip:
- 1 cup coconut cream
- 1/2 cup mayonnaise
- 2 tbsp. coconut oil
- 1 yellow onion; finely chopped
- A pinch of smoked paprika
- Onion dip

- 1/4 tsp. white pepper
- 1/4 tsp. garlic powder
- 2 tbsp. green onions chopped

Instructions:
1. Heat up a pan with 2 tbsp. coconut oil over medium heat, add onion, garlic powder and white pepper, stir; cook for 10 minutes, take off heat and leave aside to cool down.
2. In a bowl; mix mayo with coconut cream, green onions and caramelized onions, stir well and keep in the fridge for now.
3. Season mushroom caps with a pinch of cayenne pepper and paprika and drizzle the olive oil over them.
4. Rub them, place on preheated grill over medium high heat and cook them for 5 minutes on each side. Arrange them on a platter, fill each with some of the onion dip and serve them cold!

Nutrition Facts Per Serving: Calories: 150; Fat: 3g; Fiber: 2g; Carbs: 4g; Protein: 6g

Avocado Boats

(Prep + Cook Time: 10 minutes | **Servings**: 2)

Ingredients:
- 5 oz. canned tuna; drained and flaked
- Juice of 1 lemon
- 1 avocado; pitted and cut in halves
- Black pepper to the taste
- 1 tbsp. yellow onion; chopped
- A pinch of sea salt

Instructions:
1. Scoop most of the avocado flesh and put it in a bowl.
2. Add lemon juice, onion, black pepper to the taste, a pinch of salt and tuna and stir everything very well. Fill avocado cups with this mix and serve them.

Nutrition Facts Per Serving: Calories: 100; Fat: 2g; Fiber: 1g; Carbs: 3g; Protein: 5g

Pepperoni Bites

(Prep + Cook Time: 15 minutes | **Servings**: 24 pieces)

Ingredients:
- 1/3 cup tomatoes; chopped
- 1/2 cup bell peppers; mixed and chopped
- 24 pepperoni sliced
- 1/2 cup paleo marinara sauce
- 4 oz. almond cheese; cubed
- 2 tbsp. basil; chopped
- Black pepper to the taste

Instructions:
1. Divide pepperoni slices into a muffin tray. Divide tomato and bell pepper pieces into pepperoni cups.
2. Also divide Paleo marinara sauce, basil and almond cheese cubes.
3. Sprinkle black pepper at the end, introduce cups in the oven at 400 °F and bake for 10 minutes.
4. Leave your pepperoni cups to cool down a bit, transfer them to a platter and serve.

Nutrition Facts Per Serving: Calories: 120; Fat: 2g; Fiber: 1g; Carbs: 3g; Protein: 5g

Egg Cups

(Prep + Cook Time: 25 minutes | **Servings**: 12)

Ingredients:
- 12 eggs
- A drizzle of avocado oil
- 8 asparagus spears; chopped
- A pinch of sea salt
- Black pepper to the taste
- 12 bacon strips; cooked

Instructions:
1. Divide bacon strips into 12 muffin cups.
2. Crack an egg in each, add asparagus pieces on top, season with a pinch of sea salt and black pepper, place in the oven at 400 °F and bake for 15 minutes. Leave egg cups to cool down, transfer them to a platter and serve.

Nutrition Facts Per Serving: Calories: 200; Fat: 13g; Fiber: 1g; Carbs: 1g; Protein: 10g

Roasted Eggplant Spread

(Prep + Cook Time: 1 hour 10 minutes | **Servings**: 4)

Ingredients:
- 1 eggplant; cut into halves lengthwise
- 2 tbsp. lemon juice
- 2 tbsp. olive oil
- 1 garlic head; peeled
- Black pepper to the taste
- A pinch of sea salt

Instructions:
1. Place eggplant halves and the garlic head on a lined baking sheet, drizzle some of the oil over them, place in the oven at 350 °F and bake for 1 hour.
2. Leave eggplant and garlic to cool down, peel eggplant halves and put everything in your food processor.
3. Add a pinch of salt, black pepper, lemon juice and the rest of the oil and pulse really well. Transfer eggplant spread to a bowl and serve right away.

Nutrition Facts Per Serving: Calories: 100; Fat: 2g; Fiber: 1g; Carbs: 1g; Protein: 2g

Cauliflower Popcorn

(Prep + Cook Time: 35 minutes | **Servings**: 1)

Ingredients:
- 1 small cauliflower head; chopped
- 1/2 tsp. chives; dried
- 1/2 tsp. onion powder
- A pinch of sea salt
- A drizzle of avocado oil

Instructions:
1. In a bowl; mix cauliflower popcorn with a pinch of salt and the oil.
2. Toss to coat and spread them on a lined baking sheet.
3. Place in the oven at 450 °F and bake for 15 minutes.
4. Take baking sheet out of the oven, flip popcorn and then bake for 15 minutes more. Transfer popcorn to a bowl; add chives and onion powder, stir and serve them.

Nutrition Facts Per Serving: Calories: 80; Fat: 1g; Fiber: 0g; Carbs: 0g; Protein: 2g

Cabbage Chips

(Prep + Cook Time: 2 hours 10 minutes | **Servings**: 8)

Ingredients:
- 1/2 red cabbage head; leaves separated and halved
- 1/2 green cabbage head; leaves separated and halved
- A drizzle of olive oil
- Black pepper to the taste
- A pinch of sea salt

Instructions:
1. Spread cabbage leaves on a lined baking sheet, place in the oven at 200 °F and bake for 2 hours.

2. Take cabbage chips out of the oven, drizzle oil over them, sprinkle salt and black pepper, rub well, transfer to a bowl and serve as a Paleo snack.

Nutrition Facts Per Serving: Calories: 80; Fat: 1g; Fiber: 0g; Carbs: 1g; Protein: 2g

Appetizer Salad

(Prep + Cook Time: 10 minutes | **Servings**: 4)

Ingredients:
- 4 oz. prosciutto; cut into very thin strips
- 1 big romaine lettuce head; chopped
- 1/2 cup artichoke hearts; chopped
- 4 oz. pepperoni; cubed
- 1/2 cup pickled hot peppers; chopped
- 1/2 cup black olives; pitted and chopped
- A drizzle of Italian dressing

For the dressing:
- 3/4 cup avocado oil
- 1/4 cup red wine vinegar
- 1 tbsp. parsley; chopped
- 1 garlic clove; minced
- 1 tsp. oregano; dried
- Black pepper to the taste
- A pinch of sea salt

Instructions:
1. In a bowl; mix parsley with garlic, oregano, a pinch of salt, black pepper, oil and vinegar and whisk well.
2. In a salad bowl; mix prosciutto with romaine lettuce, artichoke hearts, pepperoni, hot peppers and olives. Add salad dressing, toss to coat and serve as a Paleo appetizer.

Nutrition Facts Per Serving: Calories: 100; Fat: 1g; Fiber: 2g; Carbs: 2g; Protein: 4g

Sun Dried Tomatoes Spread

(Prep + Cook Time: 55 minutes | **Servings**: 6)

Ingredients:
- 1 cauliflower head; florets separated
- 1/2 cup sun-dried tomatoes; chopped
- 10 garlic cloves
- 4 tbsp. tahini
- 4 tbsp. lemon juice
- 5 tbsp. olive oil
- 1 tsp. basil; dried
- Black pepper to the taste
- 1 tsp. cumin; ground
- A pinch of sea salt

Instructions:
1. Put cauliflower florets and garlic cloves on a lined baking sheet, drizzle 1 tbsp. oil over them, toss to coat, place in the oven at 400 °F and bake for 45 minutes flipping once.
2. Leave cauliflower and garlic to cool down and transfer to your blender.
3. Add sun-dried tomatoes, 4 tbsp. oil, black pepper, 1/2 tsp. cumin, tahini paste, a pinch of salt and lemon juice and blend until you obtain a paste.
4. Transfer to a bowl; sprinkle the rest of the cumin and dried basil on top and serve.

Nutrition Facts Per Serving: Calories: 90; Fat: 2g; Fiber: 2g; Carbs: 3g; Protein: 1g

Hummus

(Prep + Cook Time: 50 minutes | **Servings**: 4)

Ingredients:
- 1 cauliflower head; florets separated
- 1 small eggplant; chopped
- 1 small red bell pepper; chopped
- 4 tbsp. sesame seeds paste
- 5 tbsp. olive oil
- 4 tbsp. lemon juice
- 1 tsp. garlic powder
- Black pepper to the taste
- 1/2 tsp. cumin
- A pinch of paprika for serving
- A pinch of sea salt

Instructions:
1. Arrange eggplant, cauliflower and bell pepper pieces on a lined baking sheet.

2. Drizzle 1 tbsp. over them, toss to coat and bake in the oven at 400 °F for 40 minutes.
3. Leave veggies to cool down and transfer them to your blender.
4. Add sesame seeds paste, salt, pepper, 4 tbsp. oil, garlic powder, cumin and lemon juice and blend until you obtain a paste.
5. Transfer to a bowl; sprinkle paprika on top and serve as a Paleo snack.

Nutrition Facts Per Serving: Calories: 90; Fat: 1g; Fiber: 1g; Carbs: 3g; Protein: 6g

Mixed Snack

(**Prep + Cook Time**: 1 hour 35 minutes | **Servings**: 6)

Ingredients:
- 1 cup raw cashews; halved
- 21/4 cup walnuts; chopped
- 1/3 cup stevia
- 1 cup coconut flakes; unsweetened
- 5 tbsp. coconut oil
- 1 tsp. vanilla extract
- 2 cups banana slices; dried
- 3/4 cup dark chocolate chips

Instructions:
1. In your crock pot, mix cashews with walnuts, stevia, oil, vanilla extract and coconut flakes, cover and cook on High for 1 hour.
2. Turn crock pot to Low and cook for 30 minutes. Spread all these on a lined baking sheet and leave them aside to cool down.
3. Mix them with chocolate chips and banana slices, transfer to a bowl and serve as a snack.

Nutrition Facts Per Serving: Calories: 222; Fat: 12g; Fiber: 3g; Carbs: 10g; Protein: 6g

Baked Zucchini Chips

(**Prep + Cook Time**: 22 minutes | **Servings**: 4)

Ingredients:
- 1 zucchini; thinly sliced
- A pinch of sea salt
- Black pepper to the taste
- 1 tsp. thyme; dried
- 1 egg
- 1 tsp. garlic powder
- 1 cup almond flour

Instructions:
1. In a bowl; whisk the egg with a pinch of salt.
2. Put flour in another bowl and mix it with thyme, black pepper and garlic powder.
3. Dredge zucchini slices in the egg mix and then in flour.
4. Arrange chips on a lined baking sheet, place in the oven at 450 °F and bake for 6 minutes.
5. Flip chips, cook them for 6 minutes more and transfer to a bowl. Serve your zucchini chips cold.

Nutrition Facts Per Serving: Calories: 110; Fat: 4g; Fiber: 3g; Carbs: 6g; Protein: 6g

Stuffed Eggs

(**Prep + Cook Time**: 10 minutes | **Servings**: 8)

Ingredients:
- 4 eggs; hard-boiled, peeled and cut in halves
- 1 avocado; pitted, peeled and chopped
- A pinch of sea salt
- Black pepper to the taste
- 1 tsp. cilantro; chopped
- A pinch of garlic powder

Instructions:
1. Place egg halves on a platter and scoop egg yolks.
2. In a bowl; mix egg yolks with avocado, cilantro, a pinch of sea salt, black pepper to the taste and garlic powder.
3. Mash everything well and then stuff egg whites with this mix. Serve them as a Paleo appetizer.

Nutrition Facts Per Serving: Calories: 60; Fat: 4g; Fiber: 1g; Carbs: 1g; Protein: 3g

Coconut Bars

(**Prep + Cook Time**: 30 minutes | **Servings**: 10)

Ingredients:
- 1 cup coconut flakes; unsweetened
- 2 cups cashews
- 1¼ cups figs; dried
- 1 tsp. vanilla extract
- A pinch of sea salt
- 1/3 cup dark chocolate chips
- 1 tbsp. protein powder
- 1 tbsp. cocoa powder

Instructions:
1. In your food processor, mix figs with vanilla, cashews, a pinch of saltg; Protein: powder, cocoa powder and coconut and blend them well.
2. Transfer this into a baking dish and press well. Put chocolate chips in a heatproof bowl; place in your microwave for 1 minute until it melts.
3. Pour this over coconut mix, spread well, place in your freezer for 20 minutes, cut into bars and serve as a Paleo snack.

Nutrition Facts Per Serving: Calories: 234; Fat: 12g; Fiber: 3g; Carbs: 6g; Protein: 6g

Paleo Hummus

(**Prep + Cook Time**: 10 minutes | **Servings**: 6)

Ingredients:
- 1/2 cup cashews; soaked for 2 hours and drained
- 1 garlic clove; minced
- 1 tbsp. olive oil
- 2 tbsp. lemon juice
- 1/2 cup pumpkin puree
- 2 tbsp. sesame paste
- 1/4 tsp. cumin; ground
- A pinch of cayenne pepper
- A pinch of sea salt
- 1/2 tsp. pumpkin spice

Instructions:
1. In your food processor, mix soaked cashews with lemon juice, pumpkin puree, sesame paste, garlic, cumin, pepper, sea salt and pumpkin spice and blend really well.
2. Add oil gradually and blend again well. Transfer to a bowl and serve as a Paleo snack.

Nutrition Facts Per Serving: Calories: 60; Fat: 1g; Fiber: 2g; Carbs: 6g; Protein: 1g

Party Meatballs

(**Prep + Cook Time**: 50 minutes | **Servings**: 20)

Ingredients:
- 1 lb. turkey meat; ground
- 1 tbsp. coconut oil
- 1 yellow onion; chopped
- 1 egg
- 1 cup almond flour
- 3 tbsp. hot sauce
- 1 tsp. Italian seasoning
- A pinch of sea salt
- Black pepper to the taste
- 2 tbsp. parsley; chopped
- Paleo marinara sauce for serving

Instructions:
1. In a bowl; mix turkey meat with half of the flour, a pinch of salt, black pepper, Italian seasoning, parsley, onion, egg and hot sauce and stir well.
2. Put the rest of the flour in another bowl. Shape 20 turkey meatballs and dip each one in flour.
3. Heat up a pan with the oil over medium high heat, add meatballs, cook them for 4 minutes on each side, transfer to paper towels, drain grease and place all of them on a platter.
4. Serve them with some Paleo marinara sauce on the side.

Nutrition Facts Per Serving: Calories: 70; Fat: 3g; Fiber: 0.6g; Carbs: 2g; Protein: 6g

Chicken Appetizer

(Prep + Cook Time: 30 minutes | **Servings**: 2)

Ingredients:
- 3 chicken breasts; skinless, boneless and cut into small strips
- 1 cup coconut flour
- 3 tbsp. curry powder
- 2 tsp. turmeric; ground
- 1 tbsp. cumin powder
- 1 tbsp. garlic powder
- Black pepper to the taste

Instructions:
1. In a bowl; mix curry powder with flour, turmeric, cumin, garlic powder and black pepper and stir well.
2. Add chicken strips, toss well to coat and arrange them on a lined baking sheet.
3. Place in the oven at 350 °F and bake for 20 minutes. Transfer chicken strips to a bowl and serve them cold.

Nutrition Facts Per Serving: Calories: 100; Fat: 2g; Fiber: 3g; Carbs: 4g; Protein: 2g

Delicious Crackers

(Prep + Cook Time: 3 hours 10 minutes | **Servings**: 40)

Ingredients:
- 1/2 cup chia seeds
- 1 cup flaxseed; ground
- 1/2 cup pumpkin seeds
- 1/3 cup sesame seeds
- 1¼ cups water
- 1/2 tsp. garlic powder
- 1 tsp. thyme; dried
- 1 tsp. basil; dried
- A pinch of sea salt

Instructions:
1. Put pumpkin seeds in your food processor, pulse really well and transfer them to a bowl.
2. Add flaxseed, sesame seeds, chia, salt, water, garlic powder, thyme and basil and stir well until they combine.
3. Spread this on a lined baking sheet, press well, cuts into 40 pieces, place in the oven at 200 °F and bake for 3 hours. Leave your crackers to cool down before serving them as a snack.

Nutrition Facts Per Serving: Calories: 60; Fat: 1g; Fiber: 2g; Carbs: 2g; Protein: 3g

Beef Jerky

(Prep + Cook Time: 12 hours 10 minutes | **Servings**: 6)

Ingredients:
- 2½ lbs. beef; thinly sliced
- 1/2 cup coconut aminos
- 2 tbsp. gluten free liquid smoke
- 1/4 cup coconut sugar
- 1/4 cup apple cider vinegar
- A pinch of sea salt
- Small ginger pieces; thinly sliced

Instructions:
1. In a bowl; mix vinegar with coconut sugar, aminos, liquid smoke, ginger and a pinch of salt and stir well.
2. Add meat slices, toss to coat well, cover and keep in the fridge for 6 hours.
3. Transfer meat slices to your preheated dehydrator at 165 °F and dehydrate them for 6 hours. Transfer beef jerky to a bowl and serve as a snack.

Nutrition Facts Per Serving: Calories: 140; Fat: 2g; Fiber: 3g; Carbs: 7g; Protein: 7g

Watermelon Wraps

(Prep + Cook Time: 10 minutes | **Servings**: 20)

Ingredients:
- 4 watermelon slices
- 1 avocado; peeled, pitted and chopped
- 1/2 cup cucumber; chopped
- 1/4 cup red onion; chopped
- 1 tsp. coconut aminos
- 1 tsp. lime juice

Instructions:
1. Cut 20 circles of watermelon using a cookie cutter.
2. In a bowl; mix onion with avocado, aminos, cucumber and lime juice and stir well. Divide this into watermelon circles, place them on a platter and serve right away.

Nutrition Facts Per Serving: Calories: 80; Fat: 1g; Fiber: 1g; Carbs: 2g; Protein: 2g

Chicken Skewers

(Prep + Cook Time: 3 hours 15 minutes | **Servings**: 4)

Ingredients:
- 4 chicken breasts; cubed
- 3/4 cup lemon garlic powder
- 2 tbsp. parsley
- Black pepper to the taste

Instructions:
1. In a bowl; mix chicken with lemon garlic, black pepper and parsley, stir well, cover and keep in the fridge for 3 hours.
2. Arrange chicken pieces on skewers, place them all on preheated grill and cook for 15 minutes, flipping once. Arrange skewers on a platter and serve.

Nutrition Facts Per Serving: Calories: 150; Fat: 3g; Fiber: 2g; Carbs: 4g; Protein: 8g

Chicken Strips

(Prep + Cook Time: 30 minutes | **Servings**: 4)

Ingredients:
- 1 lb. chicken tenders
- 1 egg; whisked
- A pinch of sea salt
- 1/3 cup coconut; unsweetened and shredded
- 1/4 cup coconut flour

Instructions:
1. In a bowl; mix coconut with coconut flour and a pinch of sea salt and stir.
2. Put whisked egg in another bowl.
3. Dip chicken pieces in egg, then in coconut mixture and arrange them all on a lined baking sheet.
4. Place in the oven at 350 °F and bake for 25 minutes flipping pieces halfway. Transfer chicken strips to a bowl and serve them with a Paleo dip on the side.

Nutrition Facts Per Serving: Calories: 400; Fat: 23g; Fiber: 5g; Carbs: 8g; Protein: 12g

Zucchini Rolls

(Prep + Cook Time: 15 minutes | **Servings**: 4)

Ingredients:
- 3 zucchinis; thinly sliced lengthwise
- 14 bacon slices
- 1/2 cup sun-dried tomatoes; drained and chopped
- 4 tbsp. raspberry vinegar
- 1/2 cup basil; chopped
- A pinch of sea salt
- Black pepper to the taste

Instructions:
1. Place zucchini slices in a bowl; sprinkle a pinch of sea salt and vinegar over them and leave aside for 10 minutes.
2. Drain well and season with black pepper to the taste.

3. Divide bacon slices, chopped sun dried tomatoes and basil over zucchini ones, roll each and secure with a toothpick and arrange them on a lined baking sheet. Place in the oven at 400 °F for 5 minutes, then arrange them on a platter and serve as an appetizer.

Nutrition Facts Per Serving: Calories: 243; Fat: 12g; Fiber: 3g; Carbs: 5g; Protein: 14g

Guacamole

(Prep + Cook Time: 10 minutes | **Servings**: 4)

Ingredients:
- 3 green onions; chopped
- 3 avocados; pitted, peeled and roughly chopped
- A pinch of pink salt
- 1 tsp. garlic powder
- 4 radishes; chopped
- Juice from 1 lime

Instructions:
1. In your food processor mix onions with avocados, garlic powder, salt and lime juice and pulse a few times.
2. Transfer to a bowl; add radishes, stir and serve cold.

Nutrition Facts Per Serving: Calories: 60; Fat: 4g; Fiber: 0g; Carbs: 3g; Protein: 1g

Butternut Squash Bites

(Prep + Cook Time: 50 minutes | **Servings**: 4)

Ingredients:
- 2 lbs. butternut squash; cut into medium cubes
- 15 bacon slices; cut in halves
- 1 tsp. chili powder
- 1 tsp. garlic powder
- 1 tsp. sweet paprika
- Black pepper to the taste

Instructions:
1. In a bowl; mix butternut squash cubes with chili powder, black pepper, garlic powder and paprika and toss to coat.
2. Wrap squash pieces in bacon slices, place them all on a lined baking sheet, place in the oven at 350 °F and bake for 20 minutes.
3. Take baking sheet out of the oven, flip pieces and bake them for 20 minutes more. Arrange squash bites on a platter and serve.

Nutrition Facts Per Serving: Calories: 132; Fat: 2g; Fiber: 2g; Carbs: 4g; Protein: 6g

Mushroom and Broccoli Appetizer

(Prep + Cook Time: 30 minutes | **Servings**: 4)

Ingredients:
- 10 mushroom caps
- 1/2 tsp. dry mango powder
- 1/2 tsp. chili powder
- 1 cup broccoli florets
- 1 tsp. garam masala
- 1 tsp. ginger and garlic paste
- 1/2 tsp. turmeric powder
- A drizzle of olive oil
- A pinch of sea salt
- Black pepper to the taste

Instructions:
1. In a bowl; mix mango powder with chili powder, garam masala, ginger paste, turmeric, salt, pepper and oil and stir very well.
2. Add mushroom caps and broccoli florets, toss to coat well and keep in the fridge for 20 minutes.
3. Arrange these on skewers, place them on preheated grill over medium high heat, cook for 5 minutes on each side and transfer to a platter. Serve them with a tasty Paleo mayo on the side.

Nutrition Facts Per Serving: Calories: 120; Fat: 2g; Fiber: 1g; Carbs: 2g; Protein: 5g

Mushroom Boats

(Prep + Cook Time: 40 minutes | **Servings**: 4)

Ingredients:
- 1 lb. Mexican chorizo; chopped
- 1 lb. big white mushroom caps; stems separated and chopped
- 3 tbsp. coconut oil
- 1 yellow onion; chopped
- A pinch of black pepper

Instructions:
1. Heat up a pan with 2 tbsp. oil over medium heat, add mushrooms stems, stir and cook them for 3 minutes.
2. Add the rest of the oil, onion and a pinch of black pepper, stir and cook for 7 minutes.
3. Transfer this mix to a bowl; add chorizo and stir well.
4. Stuff mushrooms with this mix, place them on a lined baking sheet and bake in the oven at 400 °F for 20 minutes. Arrange mushrooms on a platter and serve them.

Nutrition Facts Per Serving: Calories: 245; Fat: 23g; Fiber: 2g; Carbs: 4g; Protein: 13g

Nuts Snack

(Prep + Cook Time: 26 minutes | **Servings**: 4)

Ingredients:
- 1 egg white
- 16 oz. mixed raw nuts
- Black pepper to the taste
- A pinch of sea salt
- 1 tsp. sage; dried
- 1/2 tsp. smoked paprika
- 1 tbsp. rosemary; chopped
- 1 tbsp. garlic powder

Instructions:
1. In a bowl; whisk egg white with a pinch of sea salt.
2. Put nuts in another bowl and add egg white to them.
3. Add black pepper, sage, paprika, rosemary and garlic powder and stir everything really well.
4. Spread this on a lined baking sheet, place in the oven at 300 °F and roast for 8 minutes.
5. Flip nuts and bake them for 8 minutes more. Leave nuts to cool down, divide into bowls and serve as a snack.

Nutrition Facts Per Serving: Calories: 100; Fat: 3g; Fiber: 1g; Carbs: 5g; Protein: 6g

Carrot Balls

(Prep + Cook Time: 25 minutes | **Servings**: 14)

Ingredients:
- 1 cup baby carrots; grated
- 3/4 cup pecans
- 1 egg white; whisked well
- 1/2 tsp. cinnamon powder
- 1 tbsp. honey
- 2 tbsp. coconut flour
- 2 tbsp. flaxseed; ground

Instructions:
1. In a bowl; mix baby carrots with egg white, cinnamon, pecans, honey, flaxseed and coconut flour and stir well.
2. Shape 14 balls from this mix, place them on a lined baking sheet, place in the oven at 350 °F and bake for 15 minutes. Leave carrot balls to cool down before transferring them to a bowl and serving them.

Nutrition Facts Per Serving: Calories: 120; Fat: 2g; Fiber: 2g; Carbs: 4g; Protein: 5g

Cucumber Rolls

(Prep + Cook Time: 10 minutes | **Servings**: 3)

Ingredients:
- 1 cucumber; very thinly sliced
- 6 ham slices
- 1 jalapeno; chopped
- 3 tsp. Paleo mayonnaise
- 1 tsp. dill; chopped
- 6 green onions; chopped

Instructions:
1. Arrange ham slices on a working surface.
2. In a bowl; mix mayo with jalapeno, green onions and dill and stir well.
3. Spread some of this mix over 1 ham slice, add a cucumber slice at the end, roll cucumber around ham and secure with a toothpick. Repeat with the remaining ingredients and serve your cucumber rolls right away.

Nutrition Facts Per Serving: Calories: 70; Fat: 1g; Fiber: 2g; Carbs: 2g; Protein: 5g

Cauliflower Mini Hot Dogs

(Prep + Cook Time: 35 minutes | **Servings**: 6)

Ingredients:
- 12 small sausages
- 2 eggs; whisked
- 1 cup cauliflower riced
- 1½ tbsp. coconut oil
- 1/2 tsp. baking soda
- 1 tsp. apple cider vinegar
- 1/4 cup coconut flour
- 1 tsp. red pepper sauce
- A pinch of sea salt
- 1/4 tsp. smoked paprika
- 1/2 tsp. mustard powder
- A pinch of chili powder
- 2 tsp. jalapenos; chopped

Instructions:
1. In a bowl; mix riced cauliflower with coconut flour, eggs, oil, red pepper sauce, mustard, salt, chili powder, paprika and jalapenos.
2. In a bowl; mix baking soda with vinegar and stir well.
3. Add this to cauliflower mix and stir well.
4. Place 12 spoonfuls of this mix on a lined baking sheet, press 1 sausage in the center and top with other 12 spoonfuls of cauliflower mix.
5. Shape place in the oven at 400 °F and bake for 25 minutes. Arrange on a platter and serve them.

Nutrition Facts Per Serving: Calories: 140; Fat: 6g; Fiber: 2g; Carbs: 4g; Protein: 8g

Fried Peppers

(Prep + Cook Time: 23 minutes | **Servings**: 4)

Ingredients:
- 10 shishito peppers
- 1 garlic clove; minced
- Juice of 1/2 lemon
- 2 tsp. olive oil
- A pinch of sea salt
- Black pepper to the taste

Instructions:
1. Heat up a pan with the oil over medium high heat, add peppers, lemon juice, garlic, a pinch of salt and black pepper, stir and cook for 10 minutes.
2. Drain excess grease on paper towels, arrange on a small platter and serve.

Nutrition Facts Per Serving: Calories: 60; Fat: 1g; Fiber: 1g; Carbs: 1g; Protein: 2g

Apricot Bites

(**Prep + Cook Time**: 2 hours 40 minutes | **Servings**: 4)

Ingredients:
- 10 apricots; dried
- 10 bacon strips; cut in halves
- 10 oz. canned chestnuts
- 2 tsp. lemongrass; chopped
- 4 tbsp. garlic; minced
- 1/2 cup coconut aminos

Instructions:
1. Wrap a chestnut and an apricot in bacon and secure with a toothpick.
2. Repeat this with the rest of the chestnuts, apricots and bacon pieces.
3. Heat up a pan over medium heat, add garlic, stir and sauté it for 20 minutes.
4. Transfer garlic to a bowl when it's cold, add lemongrass and coconut aminos.
5. Add apricot bites, cover and leave them aside for 2 hours.
6. Spread apricot bites on a lined baking sheet, place in the oven at 350 °F and bake for 20 minutes. Arrange them on a platter and serve as an appetizer.

Nutrition Facts Per Serving: Calories: 130; Fat: 2g; Fiber: 2g; Carbs: 3g; Protein: 8g

Chicken Bites

(**Prep + Cook Time**: 55 minutes | **Servings**: 13)

Ingredients:
- 2 lbs. chicken breasts; cut into medium pieces
- 1 adobo chili pepper; chopped
- 1/5 cup paleo bbq sauce
- 13 pastrami slices

Instructions:
1. Put bbq sauce in a small pot and heat up over medium high heat.
2. Add chili, stir and bring to a boil.
3. Wrap chicken pieces in pastrami slices, secure them with a toothpick and place them in a baking dish.
4. Spoon the bbq sauce over them, place in the oven at 375 °F and bake for 45 minutes. Leave chicken bites to cool down, arrange them on a platter and serve.

Nutrition Facts Per Serving: Calories: 170; Fat: 3g; Fiber: 2g; Carbs: 4g; Protein: 10g

Wrapped Olives

(**Prep + Cook Time**: 45 minutes | **Servings**: 36)

Ingredients:
- 36 almond stuffed green olives
- A pinch of black pepper
- 12 bacon slices; each cut in 3 pieces

Instructions:
1. Wrap each olive with a bacon piece, secure them with a toothpick, sprinkle some black pepper all over, place them on a lined baking sheet, place in the oven at 400 °F and bake for 35 minutes.
2. Leave this tasty Paleo appetizer to cool down before arranging on a platter and serving.

Nutrition Facts Per Serving: Calories: 20; Fat: 2g; Fiber: 0g; Carbs: 0g; Protein: 0.4

Kale Chips And Yummy Dip

(Prep + Cook Time: 30 minutes | **Servings**: 6)

Ingredients:
- 1 bunch kale; leaves separated
- 1 tbsp. avocado oil
- A pinch of sea salt
- Black pepper to the taste

For the aioli dip:
- 3 rosemary springs; chopped
- 1/2 cup avocado oil
- 1/2 cup olive oil
- 3 garlic cloves; minced
- 1/2 tsp. mustard powder
- 1 egg yolk
- 2 tbsp. lemon juice

Instructions:
1. Pat dry kale leaves, arrange them on a lined baking sheet, drizzle 1 tbsp. avocado oil, sprinkle a pinch of sea salt and black pepper to the taste, place in the oven at 275 °F and bake for 20 minutes.
2. Meanwhile; in your food processor, mix egg yolk with mustard powder, lemon juice and garlic and blend well.
3. Add olive oil and avocado oil gradually and blend until you obtain a smooth paste.
4. Add rosemary, blend again well and transfer your dip to a bowl.
5. Take kale chips out of the oven, leave them to cool down and arrange them on a platter. Serve with aioli dip on the side.

Nutrition Facts Per Serving: Calories: 100; Fat: 2g; Fiber: 1g; Carbs: 1g; Protein: 6g

Rosemary Crackers

(Prep + Cook Time: 24 minutes | **Servings**: 40)

Ingredients:
- 1/4 cup coconut flour
- 1 cup almond flour
- 1/2 cup sesame seeds; toasted and ground
- 2 tbsp. tapioca flour
- A pinch of sea salt
- Black pepper to the taste
- 1 tsp. onion powder
- 1 tsp. rosemary; chopped
- 1/2 tsp. thyme; chopped
- 2 eggs
- 3 tbsp. olive oil

Instructions:
1. In a bowl; mix sesame seeds with coconut flour, almond flour, tapioca flour, salt, pepper, rosemary, thyme and onion powder and stir well.
2. In another bowl; whisk eggs with the oil and stir well. Add this to flour mix and knead until you obtain a dough.
3. Shape a disk out of this dough, flatten well and cut 40 crackers out of it.
4. Arrange them all on a lined baking sheet, place in the oven at 375 °F and bake for 14 minutes.
5. Leave your crackers to cool down and serve them as a tasty Paleo snack.

Nutrition Facts Per Serving: Calories: 50; Fat: 3g; Fiber: 1g; Carbs: 2g; Protein: 2g

Scallops Bites

(**Prep + Cook Time**: 26 minutes | **Servings**: 4)

Ingredients:
- 20 sea scallops
- 4 bacon slices
- 1/2 cup baby spinach leaves
- 1/4 cup red onion; chopped

For the sauce:
- 2 shallots; chopped
- 4 tbsp. balsamic vinegar
- 1/2 tsp. curry powder
- 1/2 tsp. red pepper; ground
- A pinch of sea salt
- 1 tbsp. coconut oil
- 1/4 tsp. honey
- 1 tbsp. bacon fat

Instructions:
1. Heat up a pan with 1 tbsp. oil over medium high heat, add bacon, stir; cook until it browns, transfer to paper towels, drain grease, cut into medium pieces and leave aside.
2. In a bowl; mix red pepper with curry powder and a pinch of sea salt and stir.
3. Add scallops and rub them well.
4. Heat up the same pan where you cooked the bacon over medium high heat, add scallops and cook them for 3 minutes on each side.
5. Heat up the same pan with 1 tbsp. bacon fat over medium high heat, add shallots, stir and cook them for 2 minutes.
6. Add honey and vinegar, stir; cook until everything thickens and take off heat.
7. Arrange bacon pieces on a platter.
8. Add spinach leaves and onion pieces.
9. Top with scallops, stick a toothpick in the middle of each and drizzle the sauce you've made on top. Enjoy this great Paleo appetizer!

Nutrition Facts Per Serving: Calories: 200; Fat: 3g; Fiber: 3g; Carbs: 6g; Protein: 10g

Oyster Spread

(**Prep + Cook Time**: 10 minutes | **Servings**: 4)

Ingredients:
- 4 oz. canned smoked oysters
- 2 tsp. coconut cream
- 1 tbsp. red onion; chopped
- 2 pinches cayenne pepper

Instructions:
1. Drain oysters and put them into a bowl.
2. Mash using a fork, add coconut cream, onion and cayenne, stir well, divide on Paleo crackers and serve as an appetizer!

Nutrition Facts Per Serving: Calories: 120; Fat: 2g; Fiber: 2g; Carbs: 5g; Protein: 10g

Dessert Recipes

Cherry Sorbet

(Prep + Cook Time: 2 hours and 20 minutes | **Servings**: 7)

Ingredients:
- 1/2 cup dark cocoa powder
- 3/4 cup Paleo red cherry jam
- 1/4 cup maple syrup
- 2 cups water

For the compote:
- 1 lb. cherries; pitted and cut in halves
- 2 tbsp. stevia

Instructions:
1. In a pan, mix cherry jam with cocoa and maple syrup, stir; bring to a boil, gradually add the water, stir again, remove from heat, leave aside to cool down completely.
2. Whisk this sorbet again, pour in a casserole and keep in the freezer for 1 hour.
3. For the compote, mix in a bowl; stevia with cherries, toss to coat and leave aside for 1 hour. When the time has passed, serve this compote with the sorbet.

Nutrition Facts Per Serving: Calories: 197; Fat: 1g; Fiber: 4g; Carbs: 9g; Protein: 2

Pumpkin Custard

(Prep + Cook Time: 1hour 10 minutes | **Servings**: 6)

Ingredients:
- 1½ cups pumpkin puree
- 2/3 cup maple syrup
- 1 cup coconut milk
- 2 tbsp. chia seeds ground and mixed with 5 tbsp. water
- 1 tbsp. baking powder
- 2 tsp. pumpkin pie spice
- A pinch of salt
- 1 tsp. cinnamon
- 1/2 tsp. vanilla
- Pumpkin seeds for serving

Instructions:
1. In a bowl; mix pumpkin puree with coconut milk, maple syrup, chia seeds mixed with water, baking powder, pumpkin pie spice, a pinch of salt, cinnamon and vanilla and stir well using your kitchen mixer.
2. Pour this into small ramekins, arrange them on a baking tray filled half way with hot water, place in the oven at 325 °F and bake for 1 hour.
3. Take custards out of the oven, leave them to cool down and serve with pumpkin seeds on top.

Nutrition Facts Per Serving: Calories: 151; Fat: 2g; Fiber: 2g; Carbs: 6g; Protein: 6g

Pumpkin Pudding

(Prep + Cook Time: 18 minutes | **Servings**: 4)

Ingredients:
- 1¾ cup almond milk
- 1/2 cup pumpkin puree
- 2 tbsp. tapioca starch
- 1/4 cup raw honey
- 1 tbsp. water
- 1 egg
- 1 tsp. vanilla extract
- 1/4 tsp. nutmeg; ground
- 1/2 tsp. cinnamon; ground
- 1/8 tsp. allspice; ground
- 1/4 tsp. ginger; ground

Instructions:
1. In a bowl; mix tapioca starch with water and stir well.
2. Put almond milk in a pot and mix with honey and egg.
3. Stir, bring to a boil and stir in the tapioca starch mix. Cook for 2 minutes and take off heat.
4. In a bowl; mix pumpkin puree with vanilla extract, nutmeg, cinnamon, allspice and ginger and stir well.
5. Pour this into almond milk mix, stir and place over medium high heat.

6. Cook for 4 minutes, transfer to dessert bowls and serve after you've chilled in the freezer for 2 hours.

Nutrition Facts Per Serving: Calories: 246; Fat: 5.3g; Carbs: 43g; Fiber: 0.5; Sugar: 5g; Protein: 6g

Chocolate Parfait

(**Prep + Cook Time**: 2 hours| **Servings**: 4)

Ingredients:
- 1 cup almond milk
- 2 tbsp. cocoa powder
- 1 tbsp. chia seeds
- A pinch of salt
- 1/2 tsp. vanilla extract

Instructions:
1. In a bowl; mix cocoa powder, almond milk, vanilla extract and chia seeds and stir well until they blend.
2. Transfer to a dessert glass, place in the fridge for 2 hours and then serve.

Nutrition Facts Per Serving: Calories: 130; Fat: 5g; Fiber: 2g; Carbs: 7g; Protein: 16g

Avocado Pudding

(**Prep + Cook Time**: 3 hours | **Servings**: 4)

Ingredients:
- 1 cup almond milk
- 2 avocados; peeled and pitted
- 3/4 cup maple syrup
- 3/4 cup cocoa powder
- 1 tsp. vanilla extract
- 1/4 tsp. cinnamon
- Walnuts chopped for serving

Instructions:
1. Put avocados in your kitchen blender and pulse well. Add cocoa powder, almond milk, maple syrup, cinnamon and vanilla extract and pulse well again.
2. Pour into serving bowls, top with walnuts and keep in the fridge for 2-3 hours before you serve it.

Nutrition Facts Per Serving: Calories: 231; Fat: 8g; Fiber: 5g; Carbs: 7g; Protein: 2.9

Raspberry Popsicles

(**Prep + Cook Time**: 2 hours 15 minutes | **Servings**: 4)

Ingredients:
- 1½ cups raspberries
- 2 cups water

Instructions:
1. Put raspberries and water in a pan, heat up over medium heat, bring to a boil and simmer for 15 minutes.
2. Take off heat, pour the mix into an ice cube tray, add a popsicle stick in each, introduce in the freezer and chill for 2 hours.

Nutrition Facts Per Serving: Calories: 58; Fat: 0.4g; Carbs: 0g; Fiber: 2. protein 1.4

Poached Rhubarb

(**Prep + Cook Time**: 15 minutes | **Servings**: 3)

Ingredients:
- 1½ cup maple syrup
- 4½ cups rhubarbs cut into medium pieces.
- Juice of 1 lemon
- Some thin lemon zest strips
- 1 vanilla bean
- 1½ cups water

Instructions:
1. Put the water in a pan.
2. Add maple syrup, vanilla bean, lemon juice and lemon zest.
3. Stir, bring to a boil and add rhubarb. Reduce heat, simmer for 5 minutes, take off heat and transfer rhubarb to a bowl.
4. Allow liquid to cool down, discard vanilla bean and serve.

Nutrition Facts Per Serving: Calories: 108; Fat: 1g; Fiber: 0g; Carbs: 0g; Protein: 1g

Passion Fruit Pudding

(Prep + Cook Time: 65 minutes | **Servings**: 6)

Ingredients:
- 1 cup Paleo passion fruit curd
- 4 passion fruits; pulp and seeds
- 3½ oz. maple syrup
- 3 eggs
- 2 oz. ghee; melted
- 3½ oz. almond milk
- 1/2 cup almond flour
- 1/2 tsp. baking powder

Instructions:
1. Put half of the passion fruit curd in a bowl and leave aside.
2. In another bowl; mix the rest of the curd with passion fruit seeds and pulp and stir.
3. Divide this into 6 teacups.
4. In a bowl; whisk eggs with maple syrup, ghee, the reserved curd, baking powder, milk and flour and stir well.
5. Divide this into the 6 cups as well, put them in an oven pan, fill the pan halfway with water, place in the oven at 200 °F and bake for 50 minutes. Take puddings out of the oven, leave aside to cool down and serve!

Nutrition Facts Per Serving: Calories: 430; Fat: 22g; Fiber: 3g; Carbs: 7g; Protein: 8g

Pomegranate Fudge

(Prep + Cook Time: 2 hours 5 minutes | **Servings**: 6)

Ingredients:
- 1/2 cup coconut milk
- 1 tsp. vanilla extract
- 1½ cups dark chocolate; chopped
- 1/2 cup almonds; chopped
- 1/2 cup pomegranate seeds

Instructions:
1. Put milk in a pan and heat up over medium low heat.
2. Add chocolate and stir for 5 minutes.
3. Take off heat, add vanilla extract, half of the pomegranate seeds and half the of the nuts and stir.
4. Pour this into a lined baking pan, spread, sprinkle a pinch of salt, the rest of the pomegranate arils and nuts, cover and keep in the fridge for a few hours. Cut, arrange on a platter and serve.

Nutrition Facts Per Serving: Calories: 68; Fat: 0.9g; Fiber: 4g; Carbs: 6g; Protein: 0.2

Summer Carrot Cake

(Prep + Cook Time: 3 hour 15 minutes | **Servings**: 6)

Ingredients:
For the cashew frosting:
- 2 cups cashews; soaked
- 2 tbsp. lemon juice
- 2 tbsp. coconut oil; melted
- 1/3 cup maple syrup
- Water

For the cake:
- 1 cup pineapple; dried and chopped
- 2 carrots; chopped
- 1½ cups coconut flour
- 1 cup dates; pitted
- 1/2 cup dry coconut
- 1/2 tsp. cinnamon

Instructions:
1. In your blender, mix cashews with lemon juice, coconut oil, maple syrup and some apple, pulse very well, transfer to a bowl and leave aside for now.
2. Put carrots in your food processor and pulse them a few times.
3. Add flour, dates, pineapple, coconut and cinnamon and pulse very well again.
4. Pour half of this mix into a springform pan and spread evenly.
5. Add 1/3 of the frosting and also spread.

6. Add the rest of the cake mix and the rest of the frosting.
7. Place in the freezer and keep until it's hard enough. Cut and serve.

Nutrition Facts Per Serving: Calories: 140; Fat: 3.7g; Fiber: 4g; Carbs: 8g; Protein: 4.3

Green Apple Smoothie

(Prep + Cook Time: 10 minutes | **Servings**: 3)

Ingredients:
- 1 big green apple; cored and cut into medium cubes
- 1 cup baby spinach
- 1 tbsp. pure maple syrup
- A pinch of cardamom
- 1/2 tsp. cinnamon
- 1/2 tsp. vanilla extract

Instructions:
1. Put apple cubes in your food processor.
2. Add spinach, maple syrup, vanilla extract, cardamom and cinnamon and blend until you obtain a smooth cream. Pour into 2 glasses and serve right away!

Nutrition Facts Per Serving: Calories: 145; Fat: 0.8g; Fiber: 3g; Carbs: 8g; Protein: 4g

Cupcakes

(Prep + Cook Time: 1 hour 10 minutes | **Servings**: 6)

Ingredients:
- 16 oz. mulberries; dried
- 16 oz. dates; pitted and chopped
- 3 oz. almond butter
- 3 oz. raw beet juice powder
- 3 oz. spirulina powder
- 8 oz. coconut water
- 1 tsp. cinnamon; ground
- 1½ cups raw cashews

Instructions:
1. In your food processor, mix mulberries with dates, cinnamon and butter and blend very well.
2. Scoop this mix into a cupcake pan and leave aside.
3. Clean your food processor, mix spirulina powder with half of the cashews and half of the coconut water, blend well, transfer to a bowl and leave aside.
4. Clean your blender again, add beet powder with the rest of the cashews and the coconut water and pulse well.
5. Decorate half of the cupcakes with the beets frosting and the other half with the spirulina powder one. Keep cupcakes in the fridge for 1 hour and serve them.

Nutrition Facts Per Serving: Calories: 340; Fat: 11g; Fiber: 2g; Carbs: 7g; Carbs: 9g; Protein: 15g

Hazelnut Balls

(Prep + Cook Time: 30 minutes | **Servings**: 4)

Ingredients:
- 10 hazelnuts; roasted
- 1 cup hazelnuts; roasted and chopped
- 1 tsp. vanilla extract
- 2 tbsp. raw cocoa powder
- 1/4 cup maple syrup

Instructions:
1. Put 1/2 cup chopped hazelnuts in your food processor and blend well. Add vanilla extract, cocoa powder and maple syrup and blend again well.
2. Roll the 10 hazelnuts in cocoa powder mix, dip them in the rest of the chopped hazelnuts and arrange balls on a lined baking sheet.
3. Introduce in the freezer for 20 minutes and then serve them.

Nutrition Facts Per Serving: Calories: 47; Fat: 2g; Carbs: 11g; Fiber: 0.1; Sugar: 7g; Protein: 2g

Strawberry Cobbler

(**Prep + Cook Time**: 50 minutes | **Servings**: 8)

Ingredients:
- 3/4 cup maple syrup
- 6 cups strawberries; halved
- 1/8 tsp. baking powder
- 1 tbsp. lemon juice
- 1/2 cup coconut flour
- 1/8 tsp. baking soda
- 1/2 cup water
- 3½ tbsp. coconut oil
- A drizzle of avocado oil

Instructions:
1. Grease a baking dish with a drizzle of avocado oil and leave aside.
2. In a bowl; mix strawberries with maple syrup, sprinkle some flour and add lemon juice.
3. Stir very well and pour into baking dish.
4. In another bowl; mix flour with baking powder and soda and stir well.
5. Add coconut and mix until the whole thing crumbles in your hands.
6. Add 1/2 cup water and spread over strawberries.
7. Place in the oven at 375 °F and bake for 30 minutes. Take cobbler out of the oven, leave aside for 10 minutes and then serve.

Nutrition Facts Per Serving: Calories: 275; Fat: 9g; Fiber: 4g; Carbs: 9g; Protein: 4

Caramel Ice Cream

(**Prep + Cook Time**: 16 minutes | **Servings**: 6)

Ingredients:
For the caramel sauce:
- 3/4 cup stevia
- 1/2 cup coconut milk

For the ice cream:
- 12 oz. firm almond cheese
- 1 can coconut milk
- 2 tbsp. maple syrup
- 1 tsp. vanilla extract
- 100 drops liquid stevia
- 2 tsp. guar guar

Instructions:
1. In a pan, heat up over medium high heat 1/2 cup coconut milk, 3/4 cup stevia and maple syrup.
2. Stir well, bring to a boil, reduce heat to low and simmer for 3-4 minutes.
3. Take off heat, add vanilla extract, stir and leave in the fridge to cool down completely.
4. In your food processor, mix canned coconut milk, almond cheese, a pinch of salt and the caramel and pulse well.
5. Add guar guar and blend again well.
6. Take mix from the fridge and transfer to an ice cream maker. When the ice cream is done, transfer to bowls and serve with caramel on top.

Nutrition Facts Per Serving: Calories: 161; Fat: 7, fiber 1g; Carbs: 10g; Protein: 3.2

Fruit Jelly

(**Prep + Cook Time**: 10 minutes | **Servings**: 2)

Ingredients:
- 1 lbs. grapefruit jelly
- 1/2 lb. coconut cream
- A handful fresh berries for serving
- A handful nuts; roughly chopped for serving

Instructions:
1. In your food processor, combine grapefruit jelly with coconut cream and blend very well. Add berries and nuts, toss gently, transfer to dessert cups and serve right away!

Nutrition Facts Per Serving: Calories: 70; Fat: 29g; Carbs: 4.4g; Fiber: 1g; Protein: 3.5; Sugar: 1

Stuffed Apples

(Prep + Cook Time: 50 minutes | **Servings**: 4)

Ingredients:
- 4 apples; peeled
- 1 cup fresh blueberries
- 2 tsp. lemon juice
- 1/2 cup apple juice
- 1/2 tsp. cinnamon; ground
- 4 tbsp. almond meal
- 4 tbsp. coconut flakes

Instructions:
1. Scoop the inside of each apple, brush them with lemon juice and place in a baking dish.
2. Fill apples with blueberries and sprinkle cinnamon on top.
3. Spread the rest of the blueberries in the baking dish, pour apple juice, sprinkle almond meal and coconut flakes on each apple, introduce everything in the oven at 375 °F and bake for 40 minutes.
4. Take apples out of the oven, leave them to cool down, divide between plates and serve.

Nutrition Facts Per Serving: Calories: 169; Fat: 1.4g; Carbs: 38g; Fiber: 4.7; Sugar: 31g; Protein: 3.8

Carrot Cupcakes

(Prep + Cook Time: 1 hour 10 minutes | **Servings**: 6)

Ingredients:
- 1 cup almonds
- 2 cups carrot pulp
- 1 cup dates; chopped
- 1/2 tsp. ginger; grated
- 1 tsp. cinnamon powder
- A pinch of nutmeg
- 3/4 cup raisins

For the frosting:
- 1 cup cashews; soaked for 1 hour and drained
- A splash of water
- 1 tsp. lemon juice
- 6 dates; pitted, soaked for 1 hour and drained

Instructions:
1. In your food processor, mix 1 cup walnuts with 1 cup dates, carrot pulp, 1 tsp. cinnamon, ginger, a pinch of nutmeg and the raisins and blend very well.
2. Divide this between cupcakes tins and push it well.
3. Clean your food processor, add 1 cup cashews, 6 dates, a splash of water and the lemon juice and blend these as well. Divide the frosting on the cupcakes, introduce them in the fridge and keep there for 1 hour.

Nutrition Facts Per Serving: Calories: 150; Fat: 5g; Fiber: 2g; Carbs: 7g; Protein: 1.4

Intense Cheesecake

(Prep + Cook Time: 6 hours 10 minutes | **Servings**: 4)

Ingredients:

For the white layer:
- 1½ cups cashews; soaked overnight
- 6 tbsp. lemon juice
- 6 tbsp. maple syrup
- 1 tsp. vanilla extract
- 5 tbsp. coconut oil

For the yellow layer:
- 1/2 tsp. cinnamon
- 1½ tsp. turmeric
- 1 cup mango chopped

For the orange layer:
- 1½ carrots; chopped
- 1 cup dried apricots
- 1 tbsp. lemon juice
- 2 tbsp. coconut oil; melted
- 1 tbsp. maple syrup
- 1 tsp. cinnamon
- A pinch of turmeric

Instructions:
1. In your blender, mix 1½ cups cashews with 6 tbsp. lemon juice, 6 tbsp. maple syrup, 5 tbsp. coconut oil and 1 tsp. vanilla extract, blend very well, transfer to a bowl and leave aside.
2. Clean your food processor and add 1 cup mango.
3. Mix with turmeric and cinnamon, blend well, transfer to a bowl and also leave aside.
4. Clean your food processor again and add apricots.
5. Mix with carrots, 2 tbsp. coconut oil, 1 tbsp. lemon juice, 1 tbsp. maple syrup, 1 tsp. cinnamon and a pinch of turmeric, blend well and transfer to a third bowl.
6. Pour orange layer into a springform pan and spread evenly on the bottom.
7. Pour the yellow layer on top and also spread well. End with the white layer, spread, keep cheese cake in the freezer for 6 hours, cut and serve it.

Nutrition Facts Per Serving: Calories: 170; Fat: 6g; Fiber: 4g; Carbs: 6g; Protein: 12g

Hazelnut Pancakes

(Prep + Cook Time: 35 minutes | **Servings:** 4)

Ingredients:
- 1/4 cup coconut milk
- 1 banana; peeled and mashed
- 4 eggs
- 1 tsp. vanilla extract
- 1½ cups hazelnut meal
- 2 tbsp. coconut flour
- 1/2 tsp. baking soda
- Ghee for cooking

For the sauce:
- 2 blood oranges; peeled and sliced
- 2 tbsp. coconut oil
- 1 tbsp. lemon juice
- Juice from 1 blood orange
- 2 tsp. honey
- 1 vanilla bean

Instructions:
1. Heat up a pan with the coconut oil over medium heat, add orange juice, lemon juice, honey and vanilla bean, bring to a boil and simmer for 15 minutes stirring from time to time.
2. In a bowl; mix eggs with vanilla extract and coconut milk and stir. Add mashed banana, coconut flour, baking soda and hazelnut meal and stir very well.
3. Heat up a pan with the ghee over medium heat, spoon 1/4 cup pancake mix, spread a bit, cook for 3 minutes on one side, flip, cook for 1 more minute and transfer to a plate.
4. Repeat this with the rest of the batter and serve pancakes with orange slices on the side and with the orange sauce on top.

Nutrition Facts Per Serving: Calories: 90; Fat: 4.2g; Carbs: 10g; Fiber: 0.5; Sugar: 2.7g; Protein: 2.4

Tomato Cake

(Prep + Cook Time: 40 minutes | **Servings:** 4)

Ingredients:
- 3/4 cup maple syrup
- 1 cup tomatoes chopped
- 1/2 cup extra virgin olive oil
- 1½ cups coconut flour
- 1 tsp. cinnamon
- 1 tsp. baking powder
- 1 tsp. baking soda
- 2 tbsp. apple cider vinegar

Instructions:
1. In a bowl; mix flour with baking powder, baking soda, cinnamon and maple syrup and stir well.
2. In another bowl; mix tomatoes with olive oil and vinegar and stir well.
3. Combine the 2 mixtures, stir well and pour everything into a greased round pan.
4. Introduce cake in the oven at 375 °F and bake for 30 minutes. Take cake out of the oven, leave aside to cool down, transfer to a platter, cut and serve it.

Nutrition Facts Per Serving: Calories: 153; Fat: 3.2g; Carbs: 28g; Fiber: 0.8; Sugar: 11.5g; Protein: 2.7

Dessert Smoothie Bowl

(Prep + Cook Time: 6 minutes | **Servings**: 4)

Ingredients:
- 1/2 cup coconut water
- 1½ cup avocado; chopped
- 2 tbsp. green tea powder
- 2 tsp. lime zest
- 1 tbsp. honey
- Melted coconut butter for serving
- 1 mango thinly sliced for serving

Instructions:
1. In your blender, mix water with avocado, green tea powder and lime zest and pulse well.
2. Add honey and pulse again well. Transfer to a bowl; top with coconut butter spread all over and with sliced mango and serve.

Nutrition Facts Per Serving: Calories: 337; Fat: 7g; Fiber: 8g; Carbs: 10g; Protein: 10.4

Pumpkin Cookies

(Prep + Cook Time: 30 minutes | **Servings**: 4)

Ingredients:
- 1/4 cup apple sauce
- 1½ cup pumpkin puree
- 1 tsp. vanilla extract
- 1/4 cup coconut milk
- 1 cup almond milk
- 1/2 tsp. pumpkin pie spice
- 1/2 cup coconut flour

Instructions:
1. In a bowl; mix applesauce with pumpkin puree, vanilla extract and coconut milk and stir very well. Add almond meal, pumpkin pie spice and coconut flour and stir well again.
2. Drop spoonfuls of batter on a lined baking sheet, flatten with a fork, introduce in the oven at 350 °F and bake for 25 minutes.
3. Take cookies out of the oven, leave aside to cool down, transfer to a platter and serve.

Nutrition Facts Per Serving: Calories: 140; Fat: 18g; Carbs: 22g; Fiber: 1.1g; Protein: 10g

Summer Sorbet

(Prep + Cook Time: 2 hours | **Servings**: 4)

Ingredients:
- 1 cup dates; pitted and chopped
- 3 cups plums; chopped
- 2½ cups water
- 1 tsp. lemon juice

Instructions:
1. Put dates and plums in your food processor t and blend well. Add water gradually and pulse a few more times.
2. Add lemon juice, pulse for a few more seconds, transfer to a bowl and keep in the freezer for 2 hours.
3. Scoop into dessert cups and serve right away!

Nutrition Facts Per Serving: Calories: 85; Fat: 0g; Carbs: 23g; Fiber: 0; Sugar: 1g; Protein: 1g

Summer Energy Bars

(**Prep + Cook Time**: 30 minutes | **Servings**: 6)

Ingredients:
- 1/4 cup cocoa nibs
- 1/4 cup hemp seeds
- 1/4 cup goji berries
- 1/4 cup coconut; shredded
- 8 dates; pitted and soaked
- 1 cup almonds; soaked for at least 3 hours
- 2 tbsp. cocoa powder

Instructions:
1. Put almonds in your food processor and blend them well.
2. Add hemp seeds, cocoa nibs, cocoa powder, goji, coconut and blend very well.
3. Add dates gradually and blend some more.
4. Transfer mix to a parchment paper, spread and press it. Cut in equal pieces and serve after you've kept them in the fridge for 30 minutes.

Nutrition Facts Per Serving: Calories: 140; Fat: 6g; Fiber: 3g; Carbs: 7g; Protein: 19g

Coconut Macaroons

(**Prep + Cook Time**: 50 minutes | **Servings**: 4)

Ingredients:
- 1 egg white
- 3 cups coconut flakes
- 2/3 cup almond milk
- 1/2 tsp. vanilla extract
- 1 tsp. lemon juice
- 1 tsp. lemon zest

For the lemon curd:
- 1/2 cup raw honey
- 2 egg yolks
- 2 eggs
- 5 tbsp. ghee; softened
- 1 tsp. lemon zest; grated
- 2/3 cup lemon juice

Instructions:
1. In a bowl; mix honey with ghee and stir with a mixer for 3 minutes.
2. Add 2 egg yolks and 2 eggs and mix again well. Add 2/3 cup lemon juice and mix 1 minute more.
3. Transfer this to a pot, heat up over medium-low heat and cook for 15 minutes stirring often.
4. Add 1 tsp. lemon zest, stir; take off heat, transfer to a bowl and keep in the fridge for now.
5. In a bowl; mix coconut flakes with almond milk, 1 egg white, vanilla extract, 1 tsp. lemon juice, 1 tsp. lemon zest and stir well.
6. Shape small cookies, arrange them on a lined baking sheet, introduce in the oven at 325 °F and bake 20 minutes.
7. Take cookies out of the oven, leave aside for 5 minutes and arrange them on a platter.
8. Fill each macaroon with the lemon curd you've made and serve.

Nutrition Facts Per Serving: Calories: 100; Fat: 4g; Carbs: 11g; Fiber: 2; Sugar: 9g; Protein: 1g

Cherry Jam

(**Prep + Cook Time**: 50 minutes | **Servings**: 4)

Ingredients:
- 6 cups cherries; pitted and roughly chopped
- 1 cup raw honey
- 1 tbsp. lemon juice

Instructions:
1. Put cherries in a pan, add honey and leave aside for 10 minutes.
2. Place pan over medium heat, bring to a simmer and mix with lemon juice.
3. Cook for 30 minutes, stirring all the time, take off heat and serve in small dessert bowls. Keep the rest in the fridge.

Nutrition Facts Per Serving: Calories: 50; Fat: 0g; Carbs: 12g; Fiber: 0; Sugar: 13g; Protein: 0

Chia Seeds Pudding

(Prep + Cook Time: 1 hour 10 minutes | **Servings**: 4)

Ingredients:
- 1 cup almond milk
- 1/2 cup pumpkin puree
- 2 tbsp. maple syrup
- 1/2 cup coconut milk
- 1/2 tsp. cinnamon powder
- 1/2 tsp. vanilla extract
- 1/4 tsp. ginger; grated
- 1/4 cup chia seeds

Instructions:
1. In a bowl; mix almond milk with coconut milk, pumpkin puree, cinnamon, maple syrup, vanilla and ginger and stir well.
2. Add chia seeds, stir and leave aside for 20 minutes. Divide into 4 glasses, cover and keep in the fridge for 1 hour.

Nutrition Facts Per Serving: Calories: 135; Fat: 7g; Fiber: 7g; Carbs: 10g; Protein: 6.5

Muffins

(Prep + Cook Time: 40 minutes | **Servings**: 8)

Ingredients:
- 1 cup almond butter
- 1 egg; whisked
- 3 bananas; chopped
- 1/2 cup cocoa powder
- 2 tbsp. raw honey
- 2 tsp. vanilla extract

Instructions:
1. In a bowl; mix almond butter with bananas, cocoa powder, egg, vanilla extract and honey and stir very well.
2. Pour this into a muffin tray, introduce in the oven at 375 °F and bake for 30 minutes. Leave muffins to cool down for 5 minutes, removed from muffin tray and serve.

Nutrition Facts Per Serving: Calories: 171; Fat: 19g; Carbs: 24g; Fiber: 1g; Protein: 10g

Spring Cheesecake

(Prep + Cook Time: 2 hours 10 minutes | **Servings**: 4)

Ingredients:
For the crust:
- 1/2 cup pecans
- 1/2 cup macadamia nuts
- 1/2 cup dates
- 1/2 cup walnuts

For the filling:
- 1 cup date paste
- 3 cups cashews; soaked for 3 hours
- 1/2 cup almond milk
- 2 cups strawberries
- 3/4 cup coconut oil
- 1/4 cup lime juice
- Sliced limes for serving
- Sliced strawberries for serving

Instructions:
1. Put nuts, walnuts, dates and pecans in your food processor and blend well.
2. Put 3 spoons of crust mix each part of a muffin tin, press well and leave aside for now.
3. Put cashews, strawberries, date paste, lime juice, almond milk and coconut oil in your food processor and blend very well.
4. Put 3 spoons of filling mix on top of crust mix, place in the freezer and keep for 2 hours. Transfer cheesecakes on a platter, top with strawberries and limes and serve.

Nutrition Facts Per Serving: Calories: 140; Fat: 2g; Fiber: 1g; Carbs: 8g; Protein: 2g

Mango Granita

(**Prep + Cook Time**: 6 hours 10 minutes | **Servings**: 6)

Ingredients:
- 4 cups mango; peeled and cubed
- 2 tbsp. lime juice
- 6 tbsp. maple syrup
- A pinch of salt
- A pinch of ground red pepper

Instructions:
1. Put mango, lime juice, maple syrup, salt and red pepper in a pan, bring to a boil, stir; reduce heat to low and simmer for 10 minutes.
2. Remove from heat, leave aside for 10 minutes, pour into your food processor, pulse a few times, strain into a bowl; discard solids, pour into a baking dish, place in the freezer and keep there for 6 hours scraping every hour. Scrape with a fork after 6 hours and serve!

Nutrition Facts Per Serving: Calories: 127; Fat: 0.3g; Fiber: 2g; Carbs: 5g; Protein: 0.7

Fruits Mix and Vinaigrette

(**Prep + Cook Time**: 20 minutes | **Servings**: 4)

Ingredients:
- 1 lb. strawberries; halved
- 1½ cups blueberries
- 1/4 cup basil leaves; torn
- 2 tbsp. lemon juice
- 1½ tbsp. maple syrup
- 1½ tbsp. champagne vinegar
- 1 tbsp. olive oil

Instructions:
1. In a pot, mix lemon juice with maple syrup and vinegar, bring to a boil at a medium high temperature, simmer for 15 minutes, add oil, stir and leave aside for 2 minutes.
2. In a bowl; mix blueberries with strawberries and lemon vinaigrette, toss to coat, sprinkle basil on top and serve!

Nutrition Facts Per Serving: Calories: 163; Fat: 4g; Fiber: 4g; Carbs: 10g; Protein: 2.1

Fruit Cream

(**Prep + Cook Time**: 6 hours 10 minutes | **Servings**: 6)

Ingredients:
- 1 cup apples; chopped
- 1 cup pineapple; chopped
- 1 cup chickoo; chopped
- 1 cup melon; chopped
- 1 cup papaya; chopped
- 1/2 tsp. vanilla powder
- 3/4 cup cashews
- Stevia to the taste
- Some cold water

Instructions:
1. Put cashews in a bowl; add some water on top, leave aside for 6 hours, drain them and put them in your food processor.
2. Blend them well and add cold water to cover them.
3. Also add stevia and vanilla, blend some more and keep in the fridge for now.
4. In a bowl; arrange a layer of mixed apples with pineapples, melon, papaya and chickoo.
5. Add a layer of cold cashew paste, another layer of fruits, another one of cashew paste and to with a layer of fruits. Serve right away!

Nutrition Facts Per Serving: Calories: 140; Fat: 1g; Fiber: 1g; Carbs: 3g; Protein: 2g

Almond and Fig Dessert

(Prep + Cook Time: 15 minutes | **Servings**: 4)

Ingredients:
- 12 figs cut in halves
- 1/4 cup maple syrup
- 1 cup almonds; toasted and chopped
- 2 tbsp. coconut butter

Instructions:
1. Heat up a pot with the butter over medium high heat and stir until it melts.
2. Add maple syrup and figs, stir well and cook for about 5 minutes.
3. Add almonds, stir gently and take off heat. Transfer to dessert bowls and serve right away!

Nutrition Facts Per Serving: Calories: 220; Fat: 6g; Fiber: 8g; Carbs: 9g; Protein: 12g

Chocolate Butter Cups

(Prep + Cook Time: 40 minutes | **Servings**: 4)

Ingredients:
- 1/2 cup soft coconut butter
- 1 cup dark chocolate; chopped
- 5 tbsp. almond flour
- 1 tsp. matcha powder+ some more for the topping
- 3 tbsp. maple syrup
- 1 tsp. coconut oil
- Cocoa nibs

Instructions:
1. In a bowl; mix coconut butter with almond flour, maple syrup and matcha powder, stir; cover and keep in the fridge for 10 minutes.
2. Put dark chocolate in a bowl; place it over another bowl filled with boiling water, stir until it melts and mix with coconut oil.
3. Spoon 2 tsp. of this melted mix in a muffin liner.
4. Repeat this with 7 other muffin liners.
5. Take 1 tbsp. matcha mix and shape a ball, place in a muffin liner, press to flatten it and repeat this with the rest of the muffin liners.
6. Top each with 1 tbsp. melted chocolate and spread evenly.
7. Sprinkle some matcha powder all over muffins.
8. Add cocoa nibs on top of each, introduce them in the freezer and keep there until they are solid. Take them out of the freezer, leave at room temperature for a few minutes and serve.

Nutrition Facts Per Serving: Calories: 230; Fat: 2g; Fiber: 1g; Carbs: 9g; Protein: 3g

Berry and Cashew Cake

(Prep + Cook Time: 5 hours 10 minutes | **Servings**: 6)

Ingredients:
For the crust:
- 1/2 cup dates; pitted
- 1 tbsp. water
- 1/2 tsp. vanilla
- 1/2 cup almonds

For the cake:
- 2½ cups cashews; soaked for 8 hours
- 1 cup blueberries
- 3/4 cup maple syrup
- 1 tbsp. coconut oil

Instructions:
1. In your food processor, mix dates with water, vanilla and almonds and pulse well.
2. Transfer dough to a working surface and flatten it. Arrange into a lined round pan and leave aside for now.
3. In your blender, mix maple syrup with coconut oil, cashews and blueberries and blend well.
4. Spread evenly on the crust, introduce cake in the freezer for 5 hours, leave at room temperature for 15 minutes, then cut and serve it.

Nutrition Facts Per Serving: Calories: 230; Fat: 0.5g; Fiber: 5g; Carbs: 12g; Protein: 4g

Almond Bars

(Prep + Cook Time: 37 minutes | **Servings**: 9)

Ingredients:
- 1/2 cup coconut butter
- 3/4 cup melted coconut oil
- 1/2 cup cocoa powder
- 1/2 cup maple syrup
- 1/4 cup dark chocolate; chopped
- 1/2 cup raspberries
- 1/4 cup almonds; roasted and chopped

Instructions:
1. Heat up a pan over medium heat, add coconut oil, coconut butter, maple syrup and cocoa powder and stir well until everything blends.
2. Add chocolate pieces, almonds and raspberries and stir again. Pour this mix into a lined baking tray, introduce in the freezer for 20 minutes, slice, arrange on plates and serve.

Nutrition Facts Per Serving: Calories: 120; Fat: 3.5g; Carbs: 5g; Fiber: 0g; Protein: 1g

Summer Lemon Fudge

(Prep + Cook Time: 30 minutes | **Servings**: 4)

Ingredients:
- 1/3 cup natural cashew butter
- 1½ tbsp. coconut oil
- 2 tbsp. coconut butter
- 5 tbsp. lemon juice
- 1/2 tsp. lemon zest
- A pinch of salt
- 1 tbsp. maple syrup

Instructions:
1. In a bowl; mix cashew butter with coconut one, coconut oil, lemon juice, lemon zest, a pinch of salt and maple syrup and stir until you obtain a creamy mix.
2. Line a muffin tray with some parchment paper, scoop 1 tbsp. of lemon fudge mix in each of the 10 pieces, place in the freezer and keep the for a few hours. Take out of the fridge 20 minutes before you serve them.

Nutrition Facts Per Serving: Calories: 72; Fat: 4g; Fiber: 0g; Carbs: 8g; Protein: 1g

Grapefruit Granita

(Prep + Cook Time: 4 hours 20 minutes | **Servings**: 6)

Ingredients:
- 64 oz. red grapefruit juice
- 1 cup water
- 1 cup maple syrup
- 1/2 cup mint; chopped
- Mint leaves for serving

Instructions:
1. Put 1 cup water in a pan, bring to a boil, add maple syrup, stir and take off heat. Add mint, cover and leave aside for 5 minutes.
2. Strain into a plastic container, discard mint, add grapefruit juice, cover, place in the freezer for 4 hours.
3. Take out of the freezer 15 minutes before you scrape with a fork and serve with mint leaves on top.

Nutrition Facts Per Serving: 120; Fat: 0.3g; Carbs: 2g; Fiber: 0.2g; Protein: 1g

Spring Ice Cream

(**Prep + Cook Time**: 2hours 3 minutes | **Servings**: 8)

Ingredients:
- 2 cans coconut milk
- 1/3 cup pure maple syrup
- 1/3 cup coconut nectar
- 1 tbsp. arrowroot powder
- 1/4 tsp. vanilla beans
- 1 tbsp. water

Instructions:
1. Fill 1/3 of a bowl with ice cubes, place another bowl on top and leave aside for now.
2. Pour coconut milk in a pot, reserve 2 tablespoons, put them in a bowl; mix with arrowroot starch and stir well.
3. Add arrowroot mix of coconut milk to the pot and stir.
4. Also add vanilla beans, maple syrup and coconut nectar, stir well, place on stove and heat up over medium heat.
5. Stir well, bring to a boil, boil for 2 minutes, take off heat and pour into the bowl you've placed over the ice.
6. Add water, stir well and leave aside for 1 hour and 30 minutes.
7. Pour this into your ice cream machine and turn on. Pour into a container, place in the freezer and leave it there for 20 minutes. Serve right away!

Nutrition Facts Per Serving: Calories: 136; Fat: 4g; Fiber: 2g; Carbs: 7g; Protein: 2g

Made in the USA
Middletown, DE
13 January 2020